# Multimodal Imaging Atlas of Cardiac Masses

# Multimodal Imaging Atlas of Cardiac Masses

Edited by

## Azin Alizadehasl

Professor of Cardiology, Echocardiologist, Cardio-Oncologist, Cardio-Oncology Research Center, Rajaie Cardiovascular Medical and Research Center, Iran University of Medical Sciences, Tehran, Iran

## Majid Maleki

Professor of Cardiology, Interventional CardioOncologist, EchoCardiologist, Cardio-Oncology Research Center, Rajaie Cardiovascular Medical and Research Center, Iran University of Medical Sciences, Tehran, Iran

ELSEVIER

Elsevier
Radarweg 29, PO Box 211, 1000 AE Amsterdam, Netherlands
The Boulevard, Langford Lane, Kidlington, Oxford OX5 1GB, United Kingdom
50 Hampshire Street, 5th Floor, Cambridge, MA 02139, United States

**Notices**
Knowledge and best practice in this field are constantly changing. As new research and experience broaden our understanding, changes in research methods, professional practices, or medical treatment may become necessary.

Practitioners and researchers must always rely on their own experience and knowledge in evaluating and using any information, methods, compounds, or experiments described herein. In using such information or methods they should be mindful of their own safety and the safety of others, including parties for whom they have a professional responsibility.

ISBN: 978-0-323-84906-7

For information on all Elsevier publications visit our website at https://www.elsevier.com/books-and-journals

*Publisher:* Dolores Meloni
*Acquisitions Editor:* Robin R. Carter
*Editorial Project Manager:* Sam W. Young
*Production Project Manager:* Kiruthika Govindaraju
*Cover Designer:* Miles Hitchen

Typeset by STRAIVE, India

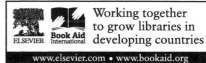

*This work is dedicated to our parents and patients with love and deep gratitude for their priceless support, encouragement, and patience.*

# Contents

# Contributors

**Amir Abdi**
School of Medicine, Islamic Azad University Tehran Medical Branch, Tehran, Iran

**Saifollah Abdi**
Cardiovascular Intervention Research Center, Rajaie Cardiovascular Medical and Research Center, Iran University of Medical Sciences, Tehran, Iran

**Azin Alizadehasl**
Cardio-Oncology Research Center, Rajaie Cardiovascular Medical and Research Center, Iran University of Medical Sciences, Tehran, Iran

**Rasoul Azarfarin**
Cardio-Oncology Research Center, Rajaie Cardiovascular Medical and Research Center, Iran University of Medical Sciences, Tehran, Iran

**Ana Barac**
Clinical Physiology Laboratory, NHLBI, National Institutes of Health, Bethesda, MD; Cardio-Oncology Program, MedStar Washington Hospital Center, Washington, DC; Georgetown University, Washington, DC, United States

**Mohamad Bashir**
Vascular and Endovascular Surgery, Health Education and Improvement Wales, Nantgarw, Wales, United Kingdom

**Charles Benton**
NHLBI, National Institutes of Health, Bethesda, MD, United States

**Mohammad Biglari**
Hematology-Oncology and Stem Cell Transplantation Research Center, Tehran University of Medical Sciences, Tehran, Iran

**Muath Bishawi**
Division of Cardiothoracic Surgery, Department of Surgery, Duke University Medical Center, Durham, NC, United States

**L. Maximillian Buja**
Department of Pathology and Laboratory Medicine, McGovern Medical School, The University of Texas Health Science Center at Houston (UTHealth); Cardiovascular Pathology, Texas Heart Institute, Houston, TX, United States

**Daniela Cardinale**
Cardioncology Unit, European Institute of Oncology, Istituto di Ricovero e Cura a Carattere Scientifico, Milan, Italy

**Marcus Carlsson**
NHLBI, National Institutes of Health; Clinical Physiology Laboratory, NHLBI, National Institutes of Health, Bethesda, MD; Lund University, Lund, Sweden; Georgetown University, Washington, DC, United States

**Vincenzo Caruso**
Cardioncology Unit, European Institute of Oncology, Istituto di Ricovero e Cura a Carattere Scientifico, Milan, Italy

**Edward P. Chen**
Division of Cardiothoracic Surgery, Department of Surgery, Duke University Medical Center, Durham, NC, United States

**Carlo Maria Cipolla**
Cardiology Department, European Institute of Oncology, Istituto di Ricovero e Cura a Carattere Scientifico, Milan, Italy

**Mahdi Daliri**
Heart Valve Disease Research Center, Rajaie Cardiovascular Medical and Research Center, Iran University of Medical Sciences, Tehran, Iran

**John A. Elefteriades**
Aortic Institute at Yale-New Haven Hospital, Yale University School of Medicine, New Haven, CT, United States

**Ata Firouzi**
Cardiovascular Intervention Research Center, Rajaie Cardiovascular Medical and Research Center, Iran University of Medical Sciences, Tehran, Iran

**Alireza Alizadeh Ghavidel**
Heart Valve Disease Research Center, Rajaie Cardiovascular Medical and Research Center, Iran University of Medical Sciences, Tehran, Iran

**Neha Gupta**
Cleveland Clinic Foundation, Cleveland, OH, United States

**Mahshid Hesami**
Surgical and Clinical Pathology, Rajaie Cardiovascular Medical and Research Center, Iran University of Medical Sciences, Tehran, Iran

**Saeid Hosseini**
Rajaie Cardiovascular Medical and Research Center, Tehran, Iran

**Ehsan Khalilipur**
Cardiovascular Intervention Research Center, Rajaie Cardiovascular Medical and Research Center, Iran University of Medical Sciences, Tehran, Iran

**Shirin Habibi Khorasani**
Cardio-Oncology Research Center, Rajaie Cardiovascular Medical and Research Center, Iran University of Medical Sciences, Tehran, Iran

**Hadi Malek**
Rajaie Cardiovascular Medical and Research Center, Iran University of Medical Sciences, Tehran, Iran

**Majid Maleki**
Cardio-Oncology Research Center, Rajaie Cardiovascular Medical and Research Center, Iran University of Medical Sciences, Tehran, Iran

**Amirhossein Mirhosseini**
Hematology-Oncology and Stem Cell Transplantation Research Center, Tehran University of Medical Sciences, Tehran, Iran

**Idhrees Mohammed**
Institute of Cardiac and Aortic Disorders, SRM Institutes for Medical Science, Vadapalani, Chennai, India

**Seyyed Asadollah Mousavi**
Hematology-Oncology and Stem Cell Transplantation Research Center, Tehran University of Medical Sciences, Tehran, Iran

**Kambiz Mozaffari**
Surgical and Clinical Pathology, Rajaie Cardiovascular Medical and Research Center, Iran University of Medical Sciences, Tehran, Iran

**Afsheen Nasir**
Yale University School of Medicine, New Haven, CT, United States

**Feridoun Noohi**
Cardio-Oncology Research Center, Rajaie Cardiovascular Medical and Research Center, Iran University of Medical Sciences, Tehran, Iran

**Joaquin Alfonso Palanca**
Barts and The London School of Medicine and Dentistry, Queen Mary University of London, London, United Kingdom

**Sahar Parkhideh**
RIOHCT, TUMS, Tehran, Iran

**Niloufar Akbari Parsa**
Echocardiography Department, Guilan University of Medical Sciences, Rasht, Iran

**Hamidreza Pouraliakbar**
Department of Radiology, CardioOncology Research Center, Iran University of Medical Sciences, Rajaie Cardiovascular Medical and Research Center, Tehran, Iran

**Kiara Rezaei-Kalantari**
Department of Radiology, CardioOncology Research Center, Iran University of Medical Sciences, Rajaie Cardiovascular Medical and Research Center, Tehran, Iran

**Shahrad Shadman**
NHLBI, National Institutes of Health, Bethesda, MD, United States

**Sheikh Mohammed Shariful Islam**
Institute for Physical Activity and Nutrition, School of Exercise and Nutrition Sciences, Deakin University, Melbourne, VIC, Australia

**Sidhant Singh**
Barts and The London School of Medicine and Dentistry, Queen Mary University of London, London, United Kingdom

**Avisa Tabib**
Heart Valve Disease Research Center, Rajaie Cardiovascular Medical and Research Center, Iran University of Medical Sciences, Tehran, Iran

**Sven Z.C.P. Tan**
Barts and The London School of Medicine and Dentistry, Queen Mary University of London, London, United Kingdom

**Nahid Yaghoobi**
Rajaie Cardiovascular Medical and Research Center, Iran University of Medical Sciences, Tehran, Iran

**Mohammad A. Zafar**
Aortic Institute at Yale-New Haven Hospital, Yale University School of Medicine, New Haven, CT, United States

# Preface

Why the reader should read this book. We believe the best answer is: this is the book about cardio-oncology we wanted when we were starting out.

What distinguishes this book from the others available is a strong emphasis on the practical points in multimodal imaging aspects of cardio-oncology sciences.

The intended audience is both those who are new to the field of cardio-oncology and those who are experienced in this area. This book is not intended to be an encyclopedia of the field, but has focused on many routine and daily issues that cardio-oncologists face in their routine practice. Because of this, many rare and complex problems are either mentioned only briefly or not at all, and the very complex topic of this field is touched on only lightly. In spite of this, this book can stand on its own as one of the first books to offer a practical guide.

Different chapters of this book on multimodality imaging in cardio-oncology offer many tips and tricks regarding the topics of the respective chapters. For each of the mentioned and presenting problems, there are lists of what the most likely potential diagnosis and findings are, as well as what findings would constitute sufficient negative evidence for cardio-oncology diseases being an explanation of the clinical problem.

Most of the image modalities were collected by the authors to make this book as practical as possible in the real world.

We believe this book will be very useful and it is recommended for any expert who works in the internal medicine branches of cardiology, oncology, hematology, and cardio-oncology. It is also recommended to all medical students, interns, residents, and fellows of the abovementioned fields to assist in becoming familiar with this very important and common world health problem.

**Azin Alizadehasl**
**Majid Maleki**

# Acknowledgments

Any book has a number of contributors both direct and indirect, and this book is no exception.

Most of the images used in this book were collected by the authors at the centers in which they work, and on their behalf by excellent sonographers, technicians, or their colleagues. We owe a great debt to all the authors, who gave their time and expertise and provided the images in order to make this book as rich as could be.

Expert secretarial help was provided by Sara Tayebi and Arefeh Ghorbani; also, our families have given their support to this effort, and understood the importance of the time spent on completing this book.

We owe a great debt to Elsevier, with special, sincere thanks and great appreciation to Robin Carter, Sam Young, and Kiruthika Govindaraju for their great help, support, and recommendations.

# History and physical examination of different cardiac masses

**Seyyed Asadollah Mousavi and Amirhossein Mirhosseini**

*Hematology-Oncology and Stem Cell Transplantation Research Center, Tehran University of Medical Sciences, Tehran, Iran*

## Key points

- Primary cardiac tumors (PCTs) are extremely rare that may be symptomatic or found incidentally.
- The signs and symptoms of cardiac tumors generally are determined by the location of the tumor in the heart and not by its histopathology.
- Cardiac myxoma is the most common benign heart tumor.
- The tumor plop sound is one of the classic and characteristic auscultation findings of cardiac myxoma. The other physical examination findings in cardiac tumors include prominent A wave with elevation of JVP; loud S1, S3, S4; and diastolic rumble.
- Malignant tumors are extremely rare and represent only 5% to 6% of PCTs. The most common are sarcomas.
- Cardiac metastases are 20–40 times more common than PCTs.
- Melanomas have the greatest propensity for cardiac involvement, and also carcinomas of the thorax, including breast, lung, and esophageal, are the most common carcinomas that metastasize to the heart.

Primary cardiac tumors (PCTs) are very rare [1]. As an example, in one series of over 12,000 autopsies, only seven were identified with an incidence of less than 0.1% [2]. Cardiac tumors may be symptomatic or found incidentally. In symptomatic patients, a mass can virtually always be detected by echocardiography, magnetic resonance imaging, and/or computed tomography. Because symptoms may mimic other cardiac conditions, the clinical challenge is to consider the possibility of a cardiac tumor so that the appropriate diagnostic test(s) can be conducted.

Multimodal Imaging Atlas of Cardiac Masses. https://doi.org/10.1016/B978-0-323-84906-7.00008-X

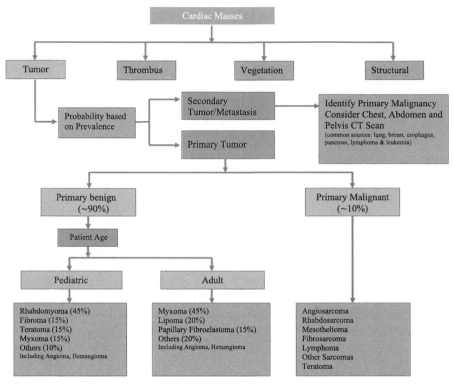

**FIG. 1.1**

Primary benign and malignant cardiac masses.

## Clinical manifestations

The signs and symptoms of cardiac tumors generally are determined by the location of the tumor in the heart and not by its histopathology [3].

### Mechanisms of symptom production

Cardiac tumors may cause symptoms through different mechanisms:

- Embolization which is usually systemic but can be pulmonic. Aortic valve and left atrial tumors were associated with greatest risk of embolization [4].
- Obstruction of the circulation through the heart or heart valves, producing symptoms of heart failure. Interference with the heart valves, causing regurgitation.

- Direct invasion of the myocardium, resulting in impaired left ventricular function, arrhythmias, heart block, or pericardial effusion with or without tamponade.
- Invasion of the adjacent lung may cause pulmonary symptoms and may mimic bronchogenic carcinoma. Constitutional or systemic symptoms.
- Left atrial tumors may release tumor fragments or thrombi into the systemic circulation and lead to neurological complications.

## *Physical examination of cardiac tumors*

**Table 1.2** Physical examination findings of cardiac tumors.

|  | Findings | Comments |
|---|---|---|
| Neck | Prominent A wave with elevation of JVP | |
| Heart | Loud S1 | Prolapsing of atrial tumor into the mitral valve orifice results in delay in closure of mitral valve producing |
| | Delay in P2 | Intensity of which depends on the absence or presence of pulmonary hypertension |
| | Tumor plop | Trial tumor striking against the endocardial wall may produce an early diastolic sound |
| | S3 and S4 | In some cases S3 and S4 may also be present |
| Murmur | Diastolic atrial rumble | Obstruction of mitral valve by the atrial tumor |
| | Systolic murmur at cardiac apex | Damaging of the mitral valves leading to mitral regurgitation |
| | Diastolic rumble | Obstruction of the tricuspid valve and a holosystolic murmur due to tricuspid regurgitation in right atrial tumors |

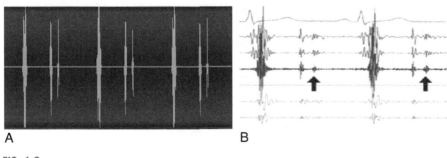

A                                             B

**FIG. 1.3**

(A) Single second heart sound followed by a tumor plop. (B) Phonocardiogram showing tumor plop sound recognized as a high pitched sound after second heart sound (*arrow*).

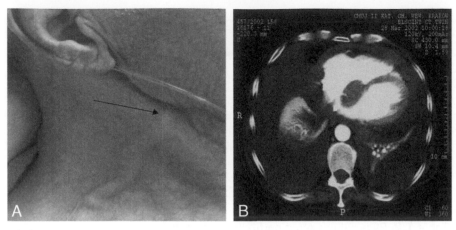

**FIG. 1.4**

(A) A 72-year-old man with primary cardiac lymphoma (diffuse large B-cell) with marked jugular venous distention. External jugular vein marked by an *arrow* (B). CT scan of the chest at the level of the heart. A tumor within the right atrium adhering to the interatrial septum. A pericardial effusion is visible.

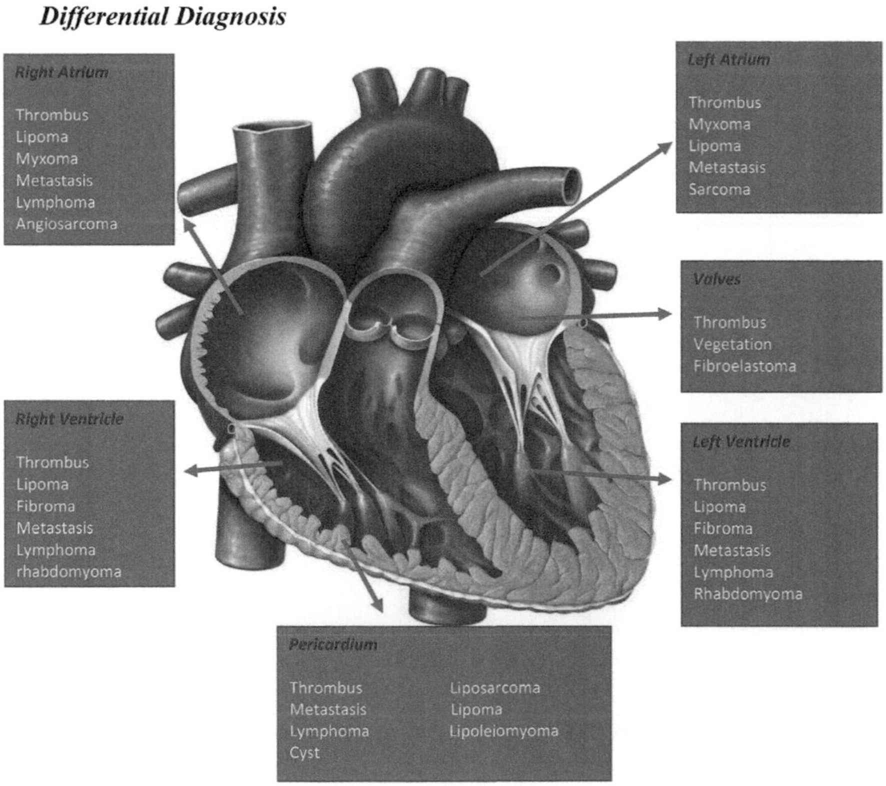

## *Differential Diagnosis*

**Right Atrium**

Thrombus
Lipoma
Myxoma
Metastasis
Lymphoma
Angiosarcoma

**Left Atrium**

Thrombus
Myxoma
Lipoma
Metastasis
Sarcoma

**Valves**

Thrombus
Vegetation
Fibroelastoma

**Right Ventricle**

Thrombus
Lipoma
Fibroma
Metastasis
Lymphoma
rhabdomyoma

**Left Ventricle**

Thrombus
Lipoma
Fibroma
Metastasis
Lymphoma
Rhabdomyoma

**Pericardium**

Thrombus          Liposarcoma
Metastasis        Lipoma
Lymphoma          Lipoleiomyoma
Cyst

**FIG. 1.5**

Differential diagnosis of cardiac masses according to the site of mass.

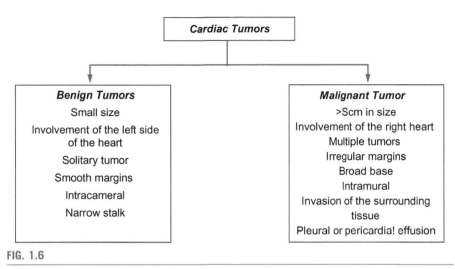

**FIG. 1.6**

Benign and malignant cardiac tumor characteristics.

## Histology of benign cardiac tumors

**Table 1.7** Histology of benign cardiac tumors.

| Tumors | Histopathology | References |
|---|---|---|
| Myxoma | Spindle or stellate cells, pseudovascular structure, myxoid matrix, hemorrhage, dystrophic calcification can be present | [5,6] |
| Lipoma | Mature adipocytes, occasionally with entrapped myocytes at the periphery | [7,8] |
| Fibroma | Fibroblasts and collagen bundles, some elastic fibers, calcification is a common finding | [5] |
| Rhabdomyoma | Spider cell (vacuolated enlarged cardiac myocyte with clear cytoplasm due to abundant glycogen) | [5,8] |
| Papillary fibroelastoma | Endocardium-coated fronds with an avascular collagenous core containing mucopolysaccharide and elastin | [7,9,10] |

Most PCTs are benign and include myxomas, rhabdomyomas, papillary fibroelastomas, fibromas, hemangiomas, lipomas, and leiomyomas. Myxoma is the most common pathological subtype [11]. Nonmyxoma subtypes, which mostly occur in children and adolescents, are less reported [11,12]. Benign tumors have favorable prognosis with a 30-day mortality of only 1% [11]. They are generally more common in older women [11,12], and according to their size and location, benign PCTs manifest with a wide array of symptoms. However, 13.3%–27.7% of cases occur in asymptomatic individuals and are detected incidentally [11].

*Myxoma*

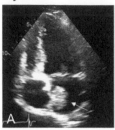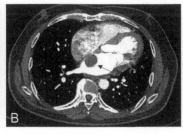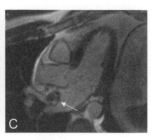

**FIG. 1.8**

Left atrial myxoma in a 64-year-old man who presented with embolic events. (A) Large mobile mass (*white arrow*) seen on transthoracic echocardiography attached to the interatrial septum. (B) Low-attenuated, well-circumscribed mass with a smooth surface (*black arrow*) seen on cardiac computed tomography (CT). (C) Heterogeneous uptake in left atrial mass (*white arrow*) on late gadolinium imaging on cardiac magnetic resonance (CMR).

Cardiac myxomas are the most common PCT [12] and be derived from mesenchymal cell precursors [13]. They form intracavitary masses, which are most commonly found in the left atrium attached by a stalk to the fossa ovalis and also may be seen in the right atrium in children [13,14]. Myxomas are morphologically divided into two groups: polypoid and papillary. The former, when large, may present with obstructive symptoms with a "tumor plop" being occasionally heard on auscultation. In contrast, papillary myxoma causes embolic events. In both variants, constitutional symptoms like fatigue, fever, and weight loss have also been reported. Calcification is seen in approximately 14% of patients and is more commonly associated in right-sided lesions [15].

**Table 1.9** Myxoma signs and symptoms.

| Symptoms | Incidence (%) |
|---|---|
| Dvsonea on exertion | >75 |
| Paroxysmal dyspnea | −25 |
| Fever | −50 |
| Weight loss | −25 |
| Severe dizziness/syncope | −20 |
| Sudden death | −15 |
| Hemoptysis | −15 |

*Lipoma*

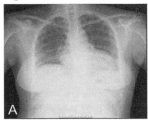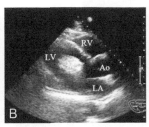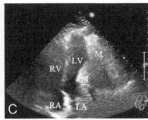

**FIG. 1.10**

Multimodality images demonstrating left ventricular infiltrating lipoma. (A) The X-ray indicated an enlarged heart. (B) The mass in the left ventricle (LV) by echocardiography in parasternal long-axis view. (C) The masses at the intracardiac and extracardiac site of LV in apex four-chamber view. Ao indicates aorta; LA, left atrial; M, mass; RA, right atrial; and RV, right ventricle.

Lipoma is the second most common primary benign cardiac neoplasm (8%–12%) and commonly occurs in middle-aged and older adults [16]. Approximately 50% of lipomas originate from the subendocardial layer, and the other arises from the subepicardial or myocardial layers [16]. They are typically asymptomatic but may cause arrhythmias or valvular dysfunction and ischemic chest pain due to compression of the coronary arteries [17].

*Papillary Fibroelastoma*

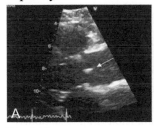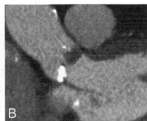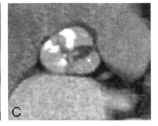

**FIG. 1.11**

Papillary fibroelastoma in a 78-year-old woman presenting with embolic events. (A) Long-axis, zoomed-in view of a small independent mobile structure (*white arrow*) attached to the aortic valve. (B and C) Hypodense mass (*white arrows*) between the right and left leaflets with frondlike papillary appearance on cardiac CT.

Papillary fibroelastomas are rare and often found on the valves. They are best visualized on echocardiography and can present with embolic complications. Surgical excision is reserved for large left-sided tumors. Papillary fibroelastoma is rare and constitutes 11.5% of all PCTs [18]. They are found on the valvular endocardium of the aortic and mitral valves followed by the tricuspid valve and the endocardium, which consists of 75% of all valvular tumors [19].

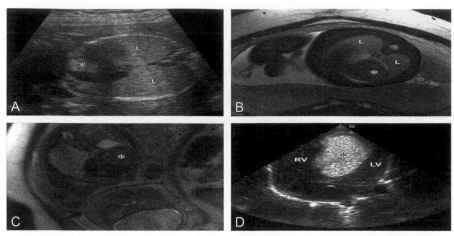

**FIG. 1.12**

Rhabdomyoma. (A) Transverse US image obtained in a fetus at 22 weeks of gestation shows a hyperechoic mass (*) in the interventricular septum. $L$ = lung. (B and C) Axial half-Fourier acquisition single-shot turbo spin-echo (HASTE) (Siemens Healthcare, Erlangen, Germany) (B) and coronal true fast imaging with steady-state precession (FISP) (C) fetal MR images obtained at 34 weeks of gestation in the same patient as in a show a large mass (*) arising from the interventricular septum, consistent with a rhabdomyoma. $L$ = lung. (D) Oblique postnatal echocardiogram shows a large echogenic rhabdomyoma (*) in the ventricular septum that fills almost the entire right ventricle ($RV$) and a portion of the left ventricle ($LV$).

Rhabdomyoma is the most common pediatric PCT and typically presents during the first year of life [20]. These tumors usually are multiple in 90% of patients and often involve the atria and ventricles with equal distribution on the right and left side of the heart [8]. Association with tuberous sclerosis is well established [21]. Rhabdomyomas can lead to arrhythmia and present with palpitations and syncopal symptoms. Cavity protrusion that results in flow obstruction may result in heart failure symptoms [22]. Rhabdomyomas usually spontaneously regress; therefore, serial echocardiography is recommended as a follow-up.

*Fibroma*

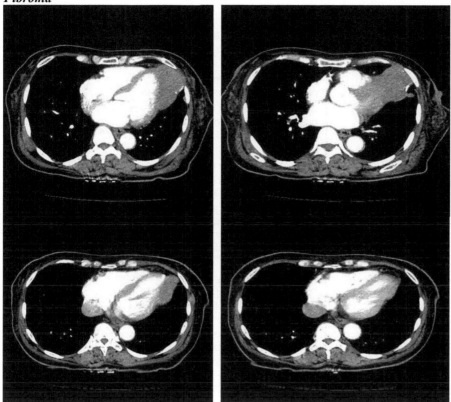

**FIG. 1.13**

Fibroma in a 4-year-old girl with large left ventricular mass that showed in thorax CT scan.

Fibromas are more prevalent in infants, are often located in the ventricle, and can be associated with a wider syndrome. In CT scan it is seen as a homogeneous mass with central calcification [23]. They are commonly located in the ventricular myocardium, usually in the left ventricular free wall or interventricular septum, and can often mimic hypertrophic cardiomyopathy [24]. They can be associated with familial adenomatous polyposis and Gorlin syndrome that usually originate from atriums. Although histologically benign patients may present with ventricular arrhythmias and sudden death secondary to interference with conduction pathways [25]. Large tumors can present with dyspnea [26].

## Malignant cardiac tumors

**Table 1.14** Histology of malignant primary cardiac tumors.

| Tumor | Histopathology | References |
|---|---|---|
| Angiosarcoma | Highly vascularized, myocardial pleomorphism, necrosis, and mitosis | [5,27] |
| Leiomyosarcoma | Compact bundles of spindled cells with blunt nuclei, regions of necrosis, and mitotic figures with epithelioid regions are often present | [7] |
| Rhabdomyosarcoma | Embryonal type with rhabdomyoblasts containing abundant glycogen and expressing desmin, myoglobin, and myogenin | [7] |
| Osteosarcoma | Histologically heterogeneous, most composed of spindle cell lesions or malignant fibrous histiocytoma with microscopic foci of osteosarcoma and chondrosarcoma in the spindle regions | [28,29] |
| Primary cardiac lymphoma | Diffuse large B-cell lymphoma is the most common subtype although Burkitt lymphoma, low-grade B-cell lymphoma, and T-cell lymphoma have also been described | [28,30] |
| Mesothelioma | Epithelioid (plump, rounded), sarcomatoid (spindled), or a combination of either | [31,32] |
| Metastasis | Largely dependent on primary tumor | [28,33] |

Malignant tumors are extremely rare and represent only 5%–6% of PCTs [34,35]. The most common are sarcomas (64.8%) followed by lymphomas (27%) and mesotheliomas (8%) [34]. Entity of rapid growth, local invasion, presence of feeding vessels, hemorrhage, or necrosis within the mass, involvement of >1 cardiac chamber, and pericardial effusion are all features suggestive of malignancy. However, no specific feature is both sensitive and specific [25,36]. As with benign cardiac tumors, the clinical presentation can vary but typically is dependent on the location of the tumor. Cardiac sarcomas represent more than two-thirds of all malignant primary tumors [34].

Compared with extracardiac soft tissue sarcomas, cardiac sarcomas are seen in younger patients in their 40s and who have worse prognosis with a 5-year survival rate of 14% [34]. Histopathological subtypes of primary cardiac sarcomas include angiosarcomas, leiomyosarcomas, liposarcomas, rhabdomyosarcomas, synovial sarcomas, myxofibrosarcomas, and undifferentiated pleomorphic sarcomas. Angiosarcomas followed by leiomyosarcomas are the most common differentiated sarcomas [37].

### *Angiosarcoma*

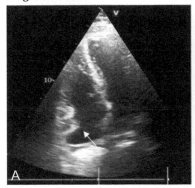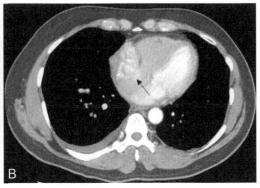

**FIG. 1.15**

Cardiac angiosarcoma with lung metastases in a 58-year-old man presenting with hemoptysis. (A) Heterogeneous irregular mass (*white arrow*) in the right atrium on echocardiography. (B) Mass involving the right atrium (*black arrow*), which is heterogeneous in appearance on enhanced cardiac CT with scattered areas of nonenhancing necrosis. Right-sided pleural effusion is present.

Angiosarcoma is an aggressive sarcoma that often originates in the right atrium and has a high possibility of metastases at the time of presentation. They preferentially affect men and have a peak incidence in the fourth decade of life. They are of right atrial origin in approximately 75% of cases and typically fill this chamber and then infiltrate into the pericardium, tricuspid valve, right ventricle, and right coronary artery [38].

### *leiomyosarcoma*

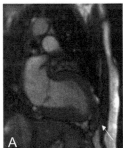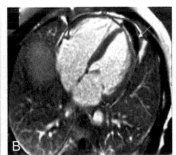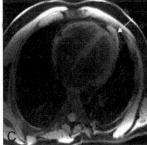

**FIG. 1.16**

Paracardiac leiomyosarcoma in a 42-year-old man presenting with chest pain.
(A) Paracardiac mass (*white arrow*) adjacent to the left ventricular apex that appears to be external to but closely adherent to the pericardium on SSFP imaging on CMR. (B) Paracardiac mass (*white arrow*) showing no late gadolinium enhancement on CMR. (C) Increased signal intensity on fat-water suppression imaging on CMR.

Leiomyosarcomas are rare but highly aggressive. They are usually only symptomatic once the tumor has reached an advanced stage. Leiomyosarcomas include 8%–9% of all cardiac sarcomas [39] and are a rare and highly aggressive cardiac sarcoma with no more than 200 cases reported in the literature [40]. These tumors are usually seen in the posterior left atrium and present as sessile masses that can have a mucoid appearance [41]. This tumor has also been described in all other cardiac chambers. The clinical presentation depends on the location and size of the tumor [42]; however, it is usually asymptomatic until it reaches an advanced stage. The tumors that infiltrate the myocardium are frequently associated with arrhythmias [42]. Other less common presentations include features of venous and intraaortic thrombosis [43].

### *Primary cardiac Lymphoma*

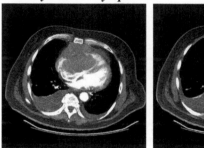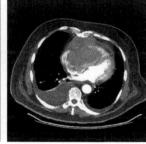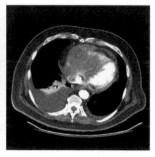

**FIG. 1.17**

Primary cardiac lymphoma in a 64-year-old man with weight loss presented with dyspnea and chest pain. The chest CT scan showed large right ventricular mass and right pleural effusion and also mild pericardial effusion was seen.

Primary cardiac lymphomas in immunocompetent patients are uncommon, accounting for 1.3% of PCTs [44], whereas cardiac metastases from extracardiac forms of lymphoma are more common (approximately 25% of patients with lymphoma have cardiac involvement). Almost all primary cardiac lymphomas are aggressive B-cell lymphomas, with an increasing incidence secondary to lymphoproliferative disorders related to Epstein–Barr virus in patients with AIDS and in patients who have received transplants. The mean age at diagnosis is 63 years of age [44]. They most commonly involve the right side of the heart, particularly the right atrium, but any chamber can be involved. There are frequently multiple lesions.

The symptoms of primary cardiac lymphoma are nonspecific. It can manifest as heart rhythm disturbances, including heart block, syncopal episodes, or even as a restrictive cardiomyopathy [45]. Constitutional complaints (fever, chills, sweats, and weight loss), chest pain, and dyspnea are also common. Approximately 20% of patients may develop acute heart failure before the presentation of other symptoms [46].

*Mesothelioma*

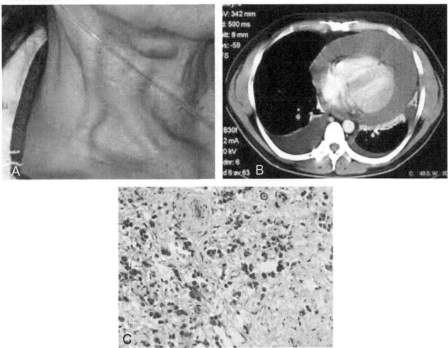

**FIG. 1.18**

Mesothelioma in a 68-year-old lady with dyspnea and chest pain. (A) Jugular vein distention (B). Thorax CT scan showed pericardial and right pleural effusion (C). Immunohistochemical staining for calretinin showing a biphasic mesothelioma (20×).

Mesothelioma is rare and commonly arises from pericardium. It often presents with a pericardial effusion with or without tamponade. It is a highly aggressive disease with an extremely poor prognosis, often treated palliatively only. Mesotheliomas consist of most of the cases of primary malignant pericardial tumors, and they arise from the pericardial mesothelial cell layer. Association with asbestos exposure is assumed, but a definitive causal relationship has not yet been established [27]. They are rare, accounting for <2% of all mesotheliomas. By definition, there must be a lack of pleural involvement or most of the tumor must be within the pericardial space [47].

## Secondary cardiac tumors

Cardiac metastases are 20–40 times more common than PCTs [27]. Up to 12% of oncology patients have metastases to the heart or pericardium at autopsy, although most remain clinically silent [48]. Melanomas have the greatest propensity for cardiac involvement [49], and also carcinomas of the thorax, including breast, lung, and esophageal, are the most common carcinomas that metastasize to the heart. The routes of metastasis include hematogenous, lymphatic, transvenous spread, or direct invasion [50]. Pericardial involvement may lead to pericardial effusion and tamponade [3,51]. Myocardial metastasis can result in conduction disturbances that trigger arrhythmias that may be resistant to standard antiarrhythmic medications [39,51]. Myocardial replacement with neoplastic cells may eventually lead to heart failure [3]. Intracavitary masses impede blood flow and cause valvular dysfunction [51]. Multiple masses or nodules are typical of metastases, although diffuse infiltration has also been recognized.

## References

[1] Reynen K. Frequency of primary tumors of the heart. Am J Cardiol 1996;77:107.

[2] Lam KY, Dickens P, Chan AC. Tumors of the heart. A 20-year experience with are view of 12,485 consecutive autopsies. Arch Pathol Lab Med 1993;117:1027.

[3] Vander Salm TJ. Unusual primary tumors of the heart. Semin Thorac Cardiovasc Surg 2000;12:89.

[4] Elbardissi AW, Dearani JA, Daly RC, et al. Embolic potential of cardiac tumors and outcome after resection: a case-control study. Stroke 2009;40:156.

[5] Basso C, Rizzo S, Valente M, Thiene G. Cardiac masses and tumors. Heart 2016;102:1230–45.

[6] Keeling IM, Oberwalder P, Anelli-Monti M, et al. Cardiac myxomas: 24 years of experience in 49 patients. Eur J Cardiothorac Surg 2002;22:971–7.

[7] Maleszewski JJ, Anavekar NS, Moynihan TJ, Klarich KW. Pathology, imaging, and treatment of cardiac tumors. Nat Rev Cardiol 2017;14:536–49.

[8] O'Donnell DH, Abbara S, Chaithiraphan V, et al. Cardiac tumors: optimal cardiac MR sequences and spectrum of imaging appearances. Am J Roentgenol 2009;193:377–87.

[9] Tamin SS, Maleszewski JJ, Scott CG, et al. Prognostic and bioepidemiologic implications of papillary fibroelastomas. J Am Coll Cardiol 2015;65:2420–9.

[10] Dujardin KS, Click RL, Oh JK. The role of intraoperative transesophageal echocardiography in patients undergoing cardiac mass removal. J Am Soc Echocardiogr 2000;13:1080–3.

[11] Wu HM, Chen Y, Xiao ZB, et al. Clinical and pathological characteristics of cardiac tumors: analyses of 689 cases at a single medical center. Chin J Pathol 2019;48:293–7.

[12] Habertheuer A, Laufer G, Wiedemann D, et al. Primary cardiac tumors on the verge of oblivion: a European experience over 15 years. J Cardiothorac Surg 2015;10:56.

[13] Ttirkmen N, Eren B, Fedakar R, Comunoglu N. An unusual cause of sudden death: cardiac myxoma. Adv Ther 2007;24:529–32.

[14] Freedom RM, Lee KJ, MacDonald C, Taylor G. Selected aspects of cardiac tumors in infancy and childhood. Pediatr Cardiol 2000;21:299–316.

[15] Grebenc ML, Green CE, Burke AP, Galvin JR. From the archives of the AFIP: cardiac myxoma: imaging features in 83 patients. Radiographies 2002;22:673–89.

[16] Rajiah P, Kanne JP, Kalahasti V, Schoenhagen P. Computed tomography of cardiac and pericardiac masses. J Cardiovasc Comput Tomogr 2011;5:16–29.

[17] Mankad R, Herrmann J. Cardiac tumors: echo assessment. Echo Res Pract 2016;3: R65–77.

[18] Zaragosa-Macias E, Chen MA, Gill EA. Real time three-dimensional echocardiography evaluation of intracardiac masses. Echocardiography 2012;29:207–19.

[19] Beroukhim RS, Prakash A, Buechel ER, et al. Characterization of cardiac tumors in children by cardiovascular magnetic resonance imaging: a multicenter experience. J Am Coll Cardiol 2011;58:1044–54.

[20] Parwani P, Co M, Ramesh T, et al. Differentiation of cardiac masses by cardiac magnetic resonance imaging. Curr Cardiovasc Imaging Rep 2020;13:1.

[21] Kocabaş A, Ekici F, Cetin II, et al. Cardiac rhabdomyomas associated with tuberous sclerosis complex in 11 children: presentation to outcome. Pediatr Hematol Oncol 2013;30:71–9.

[22] Tzani A, Doulamis IP, Mylonas KS, Avgerinos DV, Nasioudis D. Cardiac tumors in pediatric patients: a systematic review. World J Pediatr Congenit Heart Surg 2017;8:624–32.

[23] Araoz PA, Muvlagh SL, Julsrud PR, Breen JF. CT and MR imaging of benign primary cardiac neoplasms with echocardiographic correlation. Radiographies 2000;20:1303–9.

[24] Basso C, Buser PT, Rizzo S, Lombardi M, Thiene G. Benign cardiac tumours. In: Lombardi M, Plein S, Petersen S, et al., editors. The EACVI textbook of cardiovascular magnetic resonance. Oxford, UK: Oxford University Press; 2018. p. 469–73.

[25] Burke AP, Rosado-de-Christenson M, Templeton PA, Virmani R. Cardiac fibroma: clinicopathologic correlates and surgical treatment. J Thorac Cardiovasc Surg 1994;108:862–70.

[26] Agrawal SKB, Rakhit DJ, Livesey S, Pontefract D, Harden SP. Large intra-cardiac benign fibrous tumour presenting in an adult patient identified using MRI. Clin Radiol 2009;64:637–40.

[27] Butany J, Nair V, Naseemuddin A, Nair GM, Catton C, Yau T. Cardiac tumours: diagnosis and management. Lancet Oncol 2005;6:219–28.

[28] Hocy ETD, Mankad K, Puppala S, Gopalan D, Sivananthan MU. MRI and CT appearances of cardiac tumours in adults. Clin Radiol 2009;64:1214–30.

[29] Wang JG, Liu B, Gao H, Li YJ, Zhao P, Liu XP. Primary cardiac osteosarcoma. Heart Lung Circ 2016;25:698–704.

[30] Neragi-Miandoab S, Kim J, Vlahakes GJ. Malignant tumours of the heart: a review of tumour type, diagnosis and therapy. Clin Oncol 2007;19:748–56.

[31] Maleszewski JJ, Bois MC, Bois JP, Young PM, Stulak JM, Klarich KW. Neoplasia and the heart: pathological review of effects with clinical and radiological correlation. J Am Coll Cardiol 2018;72:202–27.

[32] Cao S, Jin S, Cao J, et al. Malignant pericardial mesothelioma: a systematic review of current practice. Herz 2018;43:61–8.

[33] Bussani R, De-Giorgio F, Abbate A, Silvestri F. Cardiac metastases. J Clin Pathol 2007;60:27–34.

[34] Cresti A, Chiavarelli M, Glauber M, et al. Incidence rate of primary cardiac tumors: a 14-year population study. J Cardiovasc Med 2016;17:37–43.

[35] Oliveira GH, Al-Kindi SG, Hoimes C, Park SJ. Characteristics and survival of malignant cardiac tumors a 40-year analysis of >500 patients. Circulation 2015;132:2395–402.

[36] Sparrow PJ, Kurian JB, Jones TR, Sivananthan MU. MR imaging of cardiac tumors. Radiographies 2005;25:1255–76.

[37] Ramlawi B, Leja MJ, Abu Saleh WK, et al. Surgical treatment of primary cardiac sarcomas: review of a single-institution experience. Ann Thorac Surg 2016;101:698–702.

[38] Best AK, Dobson RL, Ahmad AR. Best cases from the AFIP: cardiac angiosarcoma. Radiographies 2003;23, Sl415.

[39] Jellis C, Doyle J, Sutherland T, Gutman J, Macisaac A. Cardiac epithelioid leiomyosarcoma and the role of cardiac imaging in the differentiation of intracardiac masses. Clin Cardiol 2010;33:E69.

[40] Wang JG, Cui L, Jiang T, Li YJ, Wei ZM. Primary cardiac leiomyosarcoma: an analysis of clinical characteristics and outcome patterns. Asian Cardiovasc Thorac Ann 2015;23:623–30.

[41] Sarjeant JM, Butany J, Cusimano RJ. Cancer of the heart: epidemiology and management of primary tumors and metastases. Am J Cardiovasc Drugs 2003;3:407–21.

[42] Gierlak W, Syska-Suminska J, Zielinski P, Dlumiewski M, Sadowski J. Cardiac tumors: leiomyosarcoma—a case report. Kardiochir Torakochirurgia Pol 2015;12:251–4.

[43] Yoshida M, Ando SI, Naito Y, Yano H. Mediastinal leiomyosarcoma concurrent with intra-aortic thrombosis. BMJ Case Rep 2013;2013.

[44] Gowda RM, Khan IA. Clinical perspectives of primary cardiac lymphoma. Angiology 2003;54:599–604.

[45] Zhong L, Yang S, Lei K, Jia Y. Primary cardiac lymphoma: a case report and review of the literature. Chin Ger J Clin Oncol 2013;12:43–5.

[46] Carras S, Berger F, Chalabreysse L, et al. Primary cardiac lymphoma: diagnosis, treatment and outcome in a modern series. Hematol Oncol 2017;35:510–9.

[47] Burke A, Tavorn F. The 2015 WHO classification of tumors of the heart and pericardium. J Thorac Oncol 2016;11:441–52.

[48] Klatt EC, Heitz DR. Cardiac metastases. Cancer 1990;65:1456–9.

[49] Patel JK, Didolkar MS, Pickren JW, Moore RH. Metastatic pattern of malignant melanoma. A study of 216 autopsy cases. Am J Surg 1978;135:807–10.

[50] Goldberg AD, Blankstein R, Padera RF. Tumors metastatic to the heart. Circulation 2013;128:1790–4.

[51] Araoz PA, Eklund HE, Welch TJ, Breen JF. CT and MR imaging of primary cardiac malignancies. Radiographies 1999;19:1421–34.

# Multimodality imaging for diagnosis of cardiac masses

# 2

**Hamidreza Pouraliakbar**

*Department of Radiology, CardioOncology Research Center, Iran University of Medical Sciences, Rajaie Cardiovascular Medical and Research Center, Tehran, Iran*

## Key Points

- Cardiac tumors are being rare, but form an important component of cardio-oncology practice in which diagnosis and management are vital.
- Tumors encompass a broad set of lesions and/or masses that can be categorized as neoplastic or nonneoplastic.
- Neoplastic lesions can be further classified into primary and secondary tumors (i.e., metastasis to the heart).
- Up to 90% of primary neoplastic tumors are benign and may originate from the pericardium or myocardium.
- Compared with primary cardiac tumors, secondary cardiac tumors are 22–132 times more common and are by definition malignant.
- Transthoracic echocardiography is an appropriate initial imaging modality due to its wide availability and lack of radiation. Echocardiography (TTE and TEE) is a useful technique to diagnose intracardiac and extracardiac masses. Shape, size, location, and ultrasound features of the scanned mass can lead to correct diagnosis of the lesions (consist of thrombi, vegetation and benign masses, and malignant neoplasms).
- Cardiac magnetic resonance is the reference modality for the differentiation and characterization of cardiac masses. CMR is the most robust noninvasive imaging technique for cardiac masses. It provides a large field of view, multiplanar imaging along any axis, and high temporal and spatial resolution. Its tissue characterization capabilities are outstanding, even without intravenous contrast material, and CMR is the best of the noninvasive imaging techniques in this regard
- Multidetector CT has established a role in imaging cardiac tumors, due to its fast acquisition time, its high spatial resolution, and its incomparable ability to evaluate calcification.
- Positron emission tomography (PET) offers an accurate evaluation of the metabolic activity of tumors using fluorodeoxyglucose ($^{18}$F-FDG). FDG-PET is

**Multimodal Imaging Atlas of Cardiac Masses. https://doi.org/10.1016/B978-0-323-84906-7.00005-4**

**17**

helpful for staging malignancies while also revealing potential myocardial and pericardial involvement.

Cardiac masses may represent a spectrum of disorders from normal intracardiac structures to malignant processes.

The primary goal of noninvasive cardiac imaging modalities is to determine between benign and malignant diseases, in order to direct appropriate patient management.

Using four factors including age, location, epidemiologic likelihood, and tissue characterization, it is possible to determine the etiology of cardiac mass (Figs. 2.1 and 2.2) [1].

Multimodality imaging tools of choice for evaluating cardiac masses include echocardiography, cardiac magnetic resonance (CMR), cardiac computed tomography (CCT), and nuclear imaging [2,3].

The majority of patients with cardiac masses will come to attention following an echocardiogram.

The following paragraphs will describe these techniques and their advantages and limitations (Table 2.3) [4].

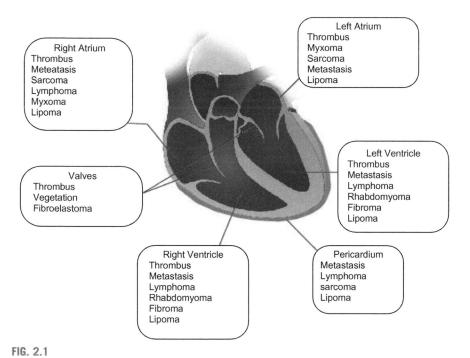

**FIG. 2.1**

The most typical locations of where different subtypes of cardiac masses are found. However, many cardiac tumours can occur in any chamber [1].

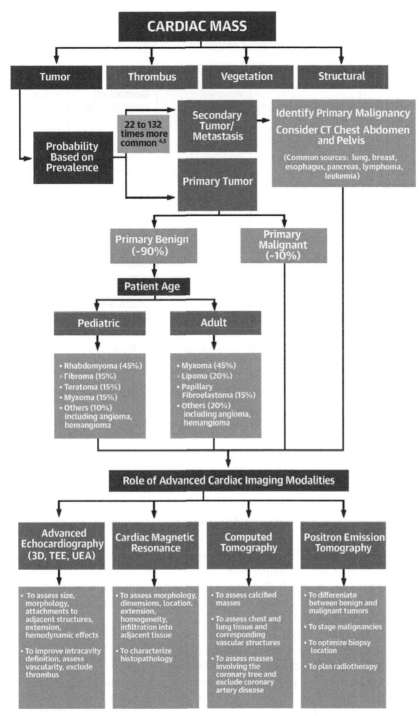

**FIG. 2.2**

Diagnostic approach when a cardiac mass is first identified. *3D*, 3-dimensional; *CT*, computed tomography; *TEE*, transesophageal echocardiography; *UEA*, ultrasound-enhancing agent.

**Table 2.3** Multimodality imaging assessment of cardiac and paracardiac masses.

|  | Echocardiography | Cardiac magnetic resonance | Computed tomography | Positron emission tomography |
|---|---|---|---|---|
| Advantage | Promptly available, no ionizing radiation, low cost, portable | No ionizing radiation, high contrast resolution, high temporal resolution, multiplanar imaging reconstruction, large field of view | Fast acquisition time, high spatial and temporal resolution, best modality for imaging of calcified lesion, multiplanar image reconstruction, evaluation of thoracic structures | High sensitivity of tumor detection, serial physiologic quantitative assessment of whole tumor mass |
| Disadvantage | Limited acoustic windows, operator dependent, limited tissue characterization | Long acquisition time, claustrophobia, contraindication in those with implanted magnetic devices | Ionizing radiation, iodinated contrast | Limited availability, limited spatial resolution, ionizing radiation |

## Echocardiography

Ultrasound is a safe and effective modality of evaluating both the anatomy and function of the heart.

Echocardiography (TTE and TEE) is a useful technique to diagnose intracardiac and extracardiac masses. Shape, size, location, and ultrasound features of the scanned mass associated with clinical and other instrumental data can lead to correct diagnosis of the lesions (consist of thrombi, vegetation and benign masses, and malignant neoplasms) [5,6].

The 3D TEE and newly intracardiac echocardiography with other proper multimodality imaging approach usually optimally and precisely define the nature and function of the mass and the best way for treatment.

Echocardiography can delineate multiple cardiac structures and characteristics of a mass such as its mobility, attachment, and potential hemodynamic consequences. It also allows for serial imaging over time without the need for radiation, iodine or gadolinium contrast agents [7].

However, echo contrast agents are useful to confirm the presence of an intracardiac mass and to characterize it further by virtue of the extent of contrast enhancement, which is a marker of vascularity.

Accordingly, malignant and highly vascular tumors demonstrate hyperenhancement with contrast, whereas thrombi do not appear to enhance at all; myxomas tend to be partially enhanced.

## Computed tomography

Multidetector CT has established a role in imaging cardiac tumors, due to its fast acquisition time, its high spatial resolution, and its incomparable ability to evaluate calcification. Depending on imaging parameters such as heart rate and mode of imaging, the entire heart can be imaged in as little as one heartbeat.

Submillimeter detector arrays provide spatial resolution superior to that of MRI. In addition, high spatial resolution in three planes (isovoxel) during image acquisition allows for post multiplanar reconstructions [8,9].

CT is the best imaging modality to demonstrate calcifications. The presence of calcification within a mass may provide important diagnostic information, and linear calcification in the myocardium indicative of earlier myocardial infarction can provide important information when thrombus is suspected.

Fat can also be readily identified on CT as low attenuation regions ($-30$ to $-100$ Hounsfield units) within cardiac masses [10].

Electrocardiogram (ECG) gating is essential to the use of CT to evaluate cardiac tumors. Not only does it eliminate blurring secondary to cardiac motion, but also it can provide functional analysis. If the heart is scanned retrospective ECG-gated such that the heart is effectively imaged throughout the entire cardiac cycle, an intracavitary mass can be depicted in both diastolic and systolic positions.

This is important when a mass is associated with or originating from a cardiac valve. Cardiac movement may display the pedunculated nature of the mass or assist in evaluating the site of origin or attachment. Finally, a high spatial resolution of cardiac CT, when combined with ECG gating, is an advantage of this modality over MRI [10].

Intravenous, nonionic contrast material is an important element of evaluating cardiac masses on CT. Opacification of the cardiac chamber helps to delineate the borders of an intracavitary mass. Contrast may also depict the differential enhancement of normal myocardium from an intramyocardial mass. The timing and composition of the contrast bolus are special considerations when performing cardiac CT. Configuring the contrast bolus is particularly challenging when evaluating a right atrial mass. Inflow of nonopacified contrast material from the inferior vena cava and coronary sinus and concentrated contrast material inflowing from the superior vena cava and causing beam-hardening artifact may obscure the borders of a mass. Accurate imaging may require injecting a dilute mix of contrast material and saline solution after the typical concentrated contrast bolus, or early delayed scans (90s) after injection of a large amount of contrast material to capture the second phase after systemic venous return. Injecting contrast material from a lower extremity vein may be considered when evaluating masses involving or near the inferior cavoatrial junction or when a mass has obstructed the superior vena cava [10].

When considering cardiac CT for the evaluation of myocardial masses, the examiner must be familiar with the limitations of this modality. Significant and persistent arrhythmias can make adequate ECG gating difficult or impossible. Similarly, high resting heart rates may limit the spatial resolution secondary to excessive motion artifact. Temporal resolution is lower in CT as compared with both echocardiography and MRI. With the exception of calcification, tissue characterization is inferior to that available with MRI. CT uses ionizing radiation, which is potentially hazardous. This factor is particularly important to consider when imaging young patients. Finally, cardiac CT almost always employs the use of intravenous contrast material, which is potentially nephrotoxic [10].

## Magnetic resonance imaging

CMR is the most robust of the noninvasive imaging technique for cardiac masses. It provides a large field of view, multiplanar imaging along any axis, and high temporal and spatial resolution. Its tissue characterization capabilities are outstanding, even without intravenous contrast material, and CMR is the best of the noninvasive imaging techniques in this regard. There are no problems related to acoustic windows, and no ionizing radiation or iodinated contrast material is used [11].

Anatomic definition and tissue characterization are evaluated using T1-weighted proton density and T2-weighted sequences. Cystic components and hemorrhage products can be distinguished using these sequences as elsewhere in the body. Gradient echo cine images provide wall motion and functional data and may demonstrate the dynamic interaction of a mass with cardiac valves. Early T1-based sequences and delayed enhancement sequences after gadolinium administration are usually employed both to evaluate enhancement and vascularity of the mass and to detect underlying myocardial scars when thrombus is suspected [10].

Gadolinium is an important component of the MRI evaluation of cardiac masses and should be used when possible. The principles of gadolinium enhancement were originally developed to evaluate myocardial infarction.

T1-weighted fast spin echo sequences are acquired before and after the administration of intravenous gadolinium to detect abnormal enhancement of the mass or to highlight the differential enhancement compared with normal myocardium. Cardiac masses may enhance after the administration of intravenous gadolinium by one mechanism or by a combination of several mechanisms. Gadolinium accumulates in the extracellular space. When cellular damage has occurred, such as in necrotic or fibrotic portions of a mass, gadolinium may enter the intracellular space and result in enhancement.

Another mechanism of gadolinium enhancement is its collection in a region of increased extracellular space, as in the case of myocardial edema. Local myocardial hyperemia incited by the presence of a mass may increase the delivery of gadolinium to the mass [10].

Cardiac MRI has a role not only in tumor characterization but also in differentiating mass from thrombus, an important and common clinical question when a mass is discovered. MRI has superior soft tissue resolution and better reproducibility than echocardiography. MRI is a valuable tool for both the diagnosis and follow-up imaging of intracavitary thrombus.

MRI is also useful for the determination of the degree of myocardial infiltration and pericardial involvement [10].

Limitation of CMR includes long imaging times, its limited availability, lack of portability, claustrophobia, greater complexity when scanning critically ill patients, exclusion of patients with certain cerebral aneurysm clips, and special precautions when scanning patients with permanent pacemakers or internal cardiac defibrillators. In addition, calcification is not well evaluated on MRI, an important component of tissue characterization best depicted on CT [4].

Nephrogenic systemic fibrosis, previously known as nephrogenic fibrosing dermopathy, is a disease characterized by fibrosis of the skin and internal organs that have been associated with gadolinium.

The relatively poor spatial resolution of cardiac MRI compared with echocardiography and CT limits its evaluation of very small masses, especially when associated with cardiac valves [10].

## Positron emission tomography

Positron emission tomography (PET) offers an accurate evaluation of the metabolic activity of tumors using fluorodeoxyglucose ($^{18}$F-FDG). FDG-PET is helpful for staging malignancies while also revealing potential myocardial and pericardial involvement. It is also useful in the evaluation of early responses to cancer therapy planning of radiation therapy and optimization of biopsy location [1].

The extent of FDG uptake by tumors is useful for differentiation between benign and malignant tumors; this is usually based on maximum standardized uptake value evaluation [12]. In a study of 20 patients who underwent hybrid magnetic resonance/PET scanning, $^{18}$F-FDG-PET scanning had a sensitivity of 100% and specificity of 92% for the differentiation of malignant cardiac masses versus benign cardiac masses [13]. Limitations included the need for dietary preparation, especially in patients with intramyocardial tumors and who had radiation exposure [14].

## References

[1] Tyebally S, Chen D, Bhattacharyya S, Mughrabi A, Hussain Z, Manisty C, Westwood M, Ghosh AK, Guha A. Cardiac tumors. JAC: CardioOncology 2020;2(2).

[2] Wintersperger B, Becker C, Gulbins H, et al. Tumors of the cardiac valves: imaging findings in magnetic resonance imaging, computed tomography, and echocardiography. Eur Radiol 2000;10:443–9.

[3] Araoz PA, Mulvagh SL, Tazelaar HD, Julsrud PR, Breen JF. CT and MR imaging of benign primary cardiac neoplasms with echocardiographic correlation. Radiographics 2000;20:1303–19.

 [4] Kramer CM. Multimodality imaging in cardiovascular medicine. Demos Medical Publishing; 2011.

 [5] Meng Q, Lai H, Lima J, et al. Echocardiographic and pathologic characteristics of primary cardiac tumors: a study of 149 cases. Int J Cardiol 2002;84:69–75.

 [6] Ragland M, Tak T. The role of echocardiography in diagnosing space-occupying lesions of the heart. Clin Med Res 2006;4:22–32.

 [7] Freedberg RS, Kronzon I, Rumancik WM, Liebeskind D. The contribution of magnetic resonance imaging to the evaluation of intracardiac tumors diagnosed by echocardiography. Circulation 1988;77:96–103.

 [8] Restrepo C, Largoza A, Lemos D, et al. CT and MR imaging findings of benign cardiac tumors. Curr Probl Diagn Radiol 2005;34:12–21.

 [9] Rienmuller R, Tiling R. MR and CT for detection of cardiac tumors. Thorac Cardiovasc Surg 1990;38(suppl 2):168–72.

[10] Abbara S, Kalva SP. Problem solving in radiology. Cardiovascular imaging; 2013. by Saunders, an imprint of Elsevier Inc.

[11] O'Donnell DH, Abbara S, Chaithiraphan V, et al. Cardiac tumors: optimal cardiac MR sequences and spectrum of imaging appearances. Am J Roentgenol 2009;193:377–87.

[12] Rahbar K, Seifarth H, Schäfers M, et al. Differentiation of malignant and benign cardiac tumors using 18F-FDG PET/CT. J Nucl Med 2012;53:856–63.

[13] Nensa F, Tezgah E, Poeppel TD, et al. Integrated 18F-FDG PET/MR imaging in the assessment of cardiac masses: a pilot study. J Nucl Med 2015;56:255–60.

[14] Osborne MT, Hulten EA, Murthy VL, et al. Patient preparation for cardiac fluorine-18 fluorodeoxyglucose positron emission tomography imaging of inflammation. J Nucl Cardiol 2017;24:86–99.

# Imaging pitfalls, artifacts, and normal variants mimicking cardiac masses

3

**Azin Alizadehasl[a], Majid Maleki[a], Kiara Rezaei-Kalantari[b], Feridoun Noohi[a], and Niloufar Akbari Parsa[c]**

[a]Cardio-Oncology Research Center, Rajaie Cardiovascular Medical and Research Center, Iran University of Medical Sciences, Tehran, Iran [b]Department of Radiology, CardioOncology Research Center, Iran University of Medical Sciences, Rajaie Cardiovascular Medical and Research Center, Tehran, Iran [c]Echocardiography Department, Guilan University of Medical Sciences, Rasht, Iran

## Key points

- Anatomic variants occurring in normal cardiac developments often simulate pathologic entities.
- Anatomic variants are particularly common in the right atrium.
- Due to the physical properties of ultrasound waves and specifics in ultrasound image reconstruction, cardiologists often encounter ultrasound image artifacts. It is particularly important to recognize such artifacts to avoid misdiagnosis of conditions ranging from aortic dissection to thrombosis and endocarditis.

**Table 3.1** Structures potentially mimicking cardiac masses in echocardiography.

| Structures potentially mimicking cardiac masses in echocardiography | | |
|---|---|---|
| Left ventricle webs, heartstrings, chords<br>Apical trabeculations<br>Dilated coronary sinus (PLAX view)<br>Dilated descending aorta (A4C view)<br>Multiple lobes of the left atrial appendage<br>Pectinate muscles of the right/left atrial appendage<br>Prominent moderator band<br>Prominent crista terminalis | Nodules of Arantius<br>Dystrophic calcification of the mitral valve<br>Noncompaction cardiomyopathy<br>Prominent papillary muscle<br>Lipomatous hypertrophy of the interatrial septum<br>Pacemaker wires<br>Central venous catheters<br>Valvular interventional devices | Near beam artifact<br>Reverberation<br>Enhancement<br>Refraction<br>Mirror image |

*Continued*

Multimodal Imaging Atlas of Cardiac Masses. https://doi.org/10.1016/B978-0-323-84906-7.00004-2

**Table 3.1** Structures potentially mimicking cardiac masses in echocardiography—Cont'd

| | | |
|---|---|---|
| Prominent Eustachian valve<br>Prominent Chiari network<br>Redundant mitral chordae or redundant leaflet tissue<br>Prominent epicardial fat pad<br>Apical hypertrophic cardiomyopathy<br>Interatrial septal aneurysm<br>Lambl's excrescence | Occluder interatrial/ interventricular devices | |

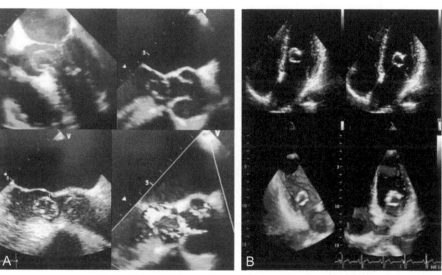

**FIG. 3.2**

The images depict the accessory mitral valve tissue. Transthoracic echocardiography of two patients (A and B) shows a round, cystic-like echo density attached to the anterior mitral valve leaflet and seen in the left ventricular outflow tract, compatible with accessory mitral valve tissue (Supplementary Video 3.1).

Accessory mitral valve tissue (AMWT) is a rare congenital cardiac anomaly sometimes responsible for left ventricular outflow tract (LVOT) obstruction. AMVT is most often associated with other cardiac and vascular congenital malformations such as septal defects and transposition of the great arteries (Supplementary Video 3.1 in the online version at https://doi.org/10.1016/B978-0-323-84906-7.00004-2).

Patients with AMVT may be asymptomatic with the presence of a murmur; none-theless, more frequently, they experience symptoms like dyspnea. Usually, patients become symptomatic when the mean gradient across the LVOT reaches 50 mmHg.

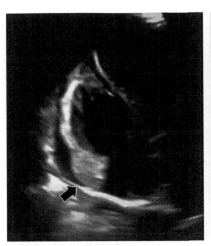 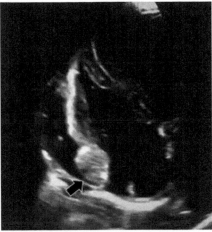

**FIG. 3.3**

The images illustrate lipomatous hypertrophy. Transthoracic echocardiography shows an incidental finding of a large mass at the lateral wall of the right ventricle (*black arrow*). This is lipomatous hypertrophy of the lateral part of the tricuspid annulus, which is a typical finding in the presence of pericardial fluid (Supplementary Video 3.2).

Signs of LVOT obstruction generally develop during the first decade of life in one-third of the patients and include typical symptoms. The current approach is intervention only for patients with significant LVOT obstruction (mean gradient $\geq 25\,mmHg$) and those undergoing correction of other congenital malformations or exploration of an intracardiac mass. For patients without significant LVOT obstruction, a follow-up with serial echocardiography to assess the progression of the gradient is indicated.

Benign lipomatous tumors of the heart are exceptionally rare. They encompass mainly lipoma and lipomatous hypertrophy of the atrial septum. Cardiac lipomatosis is characterized by the accumulation of nonencapsulated mature adipose tissue caused by hyperplasia of lipocytes. The etiology is unknown, but it may be associated with obesity and advancing age. The most frequent manifestation is lipomatous hypertrophy of the interatrial septum, but massive epicardial lipomatous hypertrophy is less well documented. Although histologically benign, it has been reported to cause cardiac tamponade, requiring decompressive pericardiectomy. Usually, lipomatosis remains asymptomatic and represents an incidental finding on echocardiography. Furthermore, it can be mistaken for other benign or malignant cardiac tumors, leading to unwarranted radical surgical resection (Supplementary Video 3.2 in the online version at https://doi.org/10.1016/B978-0-323-84906-7.00004-2).

The usual imaging to evaluate lipomatous hypertrophy is transthoracic and transesophageal echocardiography, where the septum appears unusually thick and spares the membrane of the fossa ovalis. Surgical resection is essentially not necessary and

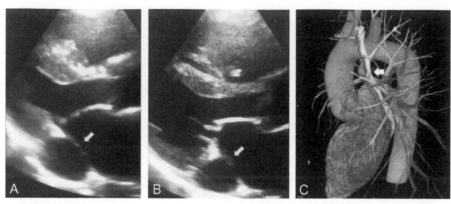

**FIG. 3.4**

The images demonstrated a dilated coronary sinus. Transthoracic echocardiography in the systole (A) and diastole (B) of a healthy man shows an incidental finding of a round, echo-free, well-defined, cystic-like mass posterior to the left atrium (*yellow arrows*). This finding is the typical appearance of a markedly dilated coronary sinus, which is mostly due to persistent left superior vena cava (PLSVC). (C) Computed tomography angiography 3D volume-rendered reconstruction shows PLSVC (*white arrow*), which drains into the coronary sinus.

should be reserved for patients who show evidence of right or left outflow obstruction or vena cava superior obstruction [1].

Persistent left superior vena cava (PLSVC) is a rare congenital anomaly; nevertheless, it is the most common abnormality of the thoracic venous system and the commonest cause of a dilated coronary sinus. Two types of PLSVC are known in the literature. In 92% of cases, PLSVC is connected to the right atrium through the coronary sinus without significant hemodynamic consequences, while in 8% of cases, PLSVC connects directly or through the pulmonary veins to the left atrium, causing a right-to-left shunt. It is most commonly an isolated finding but can be associated with other congenital heart defects. PLSVC should be suspected when a dilated coronary sinus is identified via echocardiography. This is often discovered incidentally during an echocardiographic examination or other cardiovascular imaging because it is almost always asymptomatic. Therefore the evidence of a dilated coronary sinus must always be investigated in search of a congenital malformation and especially PLSVC. Usually, agitated saline injected into the brachial left vein drains through the abnormal connection between the left-sided venous return and the coronary sinus, where the bubbles can be clearly seen first in the coronary sinus and the successive opacification of the right atrium. However, considering that physicians should attempt to rule out causes of right atrial pressure/volume overload such as atrial septal defect, coronary fistula, and other anomalous drainage patterns into the coronary sinus, nowadays, multislice computed tomography is more frequently applied by cardiologists and radiologists to visualize the coronary anatomy, coronary anomalies, and aortic pathology [2].

The Chiari network is an anomaly of the heart with a prevalence ranging from 1.3% to 4.0%. This anatomic variation, which is an embryologic remnant, is believed to be

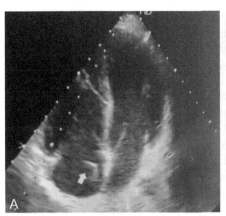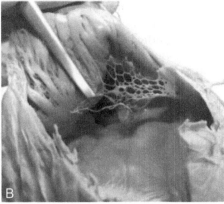

**FIG. 3.5**

The images demonstrate a prominent Chiari network. (A) The apical 4-chamber view of transthoracic echocardiography of a healthy man shows a hypermobile net-like mass floating freely in the right atrium. This finding favors a prominent Chiari network; however, pedunculated right atrial tumor, right atrial thrombus, tricuspid valve vegetation, and flail tricuspid valve are in the differential diagnosis. (B) Prominent Chiari network can be seen in the autopsy.

mostly clinically inapparent. Nevertheless, several cases have been described showing relevant pathophysiological consequences. Chang described a case of tricuspid valve regurgitation caused by a Chiari network and supraventricular fibrillations, demanding the surgical removal of the Chiari network. Atrial fibrillation and tricuspid valve regurgitation are relevant diseases; therefore, the presence of a Chiari network must be taken seriously. Further, the possibility of the presence of a Chiari network with or without a patent foramen ovale should be taken into consideration as a possible diagnosis for a patient suffering from embolism and infective endocarditis [3].

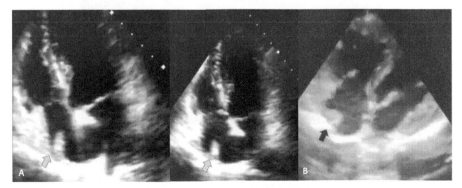

**FIG. 3.6**

The images depict a prominent crista terminalis. Transthoracic echocardiography of two different patients (A and B) with prominent crista terminalis is presented herein.

The crista terminalis is a landmark of the right atrium, extending along the posterolateral aspect of the right atrial wall. It is the fibromuscular ridge that begins at the upper portion of the septal surface and passes anteriorly to the opening of the superior vena cava and terminates at the lateral side of the entrance of the inferior vena cava. The differential diagnosis of the crista terminalis is particularly important, especially the mass in the right atrium, which is mostly detected by echocardiography except for the clinical manifestations of primary diseases. Tumors, thrombi, and vegetations constitute the commonest cardiac masses; accordingly, the early detection and accurate identification of these masses are of great significance in the diagnosis and prognosis. Except for these actual masses, several right atrial structures can mimic an abnormal mass and may not be shown well on routine standard views by echocardiography. These structures include the Eustachian valve, the Thebesian valve, the persistent sinus venosus, the Chiari network, and the crista terminalis.

Two-dimensional echocardiography can reveal the location, size, and mobility of the mass and differentiate it from extracardiac disease. Doppler echocardiography can evaluate the hemodynamic changes caused by cardiac masses, which are generally not needed in the atrium. Information required is the morphology of the mass and its relationship with the heart wall, as well as its activity, hardness, and echo intensity. Transesophageal echocardiography provides better spatial resolution and higher imaging quality and can be used to differentiate nonpathologic structures from pathologic ones in the right atrial structure [4,5].

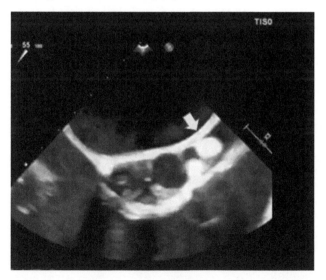

**FIG. 3.7**

The image illustrates a fat pad in the transverse sinus. Transesophageal echocardiography shows an incidental finding of a round, well-defined, echogenic mass in the transverse sinus. This finding is mostly the pericardial fat pad of a lymph node, although it might rarely be a thrombus. This case highlights the importance of understanding normal and variant anatomic relationships between the left atrial appendage and its surrounding structures to avoid the misrecognition of structures mimicking thrombi or tumors.

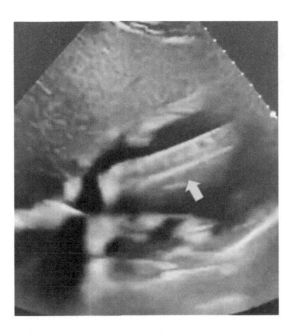

**FIG. 3.8**

The image demonstrates an iliac stent in the right ventricle. The subcostal view of transthoracic echocardiography of a patient with a history of iliac artery stenting shows a large, elongated echogenic mass floating freely in the right ventricle. The mass is the iliac stent, which has migrated upward and become lodged into the right ventricle.

The transverse sinus is a pericardial reflection between the arterial and venous mesocardium. The existence of an epicardial fat between the ascending aorta and the transverse sinus is a normal finding; however, the presence of a fat pad in the sinus adjacent to the left atrial appendage is rare and also may be misleading, not least before invasive procedures. Three-dimensional echocardiography allows a more comprehensive evaluation of the left atrial appendage anatomy and its nearby structures. The ability of 3D transesophageal echocardiography to differentiate the borders between the left atrial appendage and its adjacent structures makes it a feasible and reliable tool before invasive procedures such as left atrial appendage device closure [6,7].

Lambl's excrescences are asymptomatic and occur most commonly on aortic (ventricular surface) valves and less commonly on mitral valves (atrial side). They have been rarely described on native pulmonary, tricuspid valves, and prosthetic valves. A conglomeration of multiple Lambl's excrescences may detach from the cardiac valve and lead to peripheral embolization. Evidence suggests an association between Lambl's excrescences and embolic events and acute coronary syndromes. There have been case reports on giant Lambl's excrescence ($\geq 2\,cm$ in diameter) associated with ischemic stroke. However, no clear evidence has been found showing the correlation between the strand size and the potential risk of thromboembolic events. Ischemic events are more commonly observed in Lambl's excrescences of

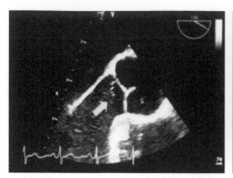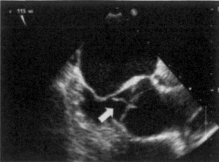

**FIG. 3.9**

The images depict a Lambl's excrescence. Transesophageal echocardiography of two different patients shows an incidental finding of a small filiform hypermobile mass on the aortic valve in the diastole (*yellow arrows*). This finding is compatible with a Lambl's excrescence.

the aortic valve. Some evidence suggests that physicians should consider Lambl's excrescences in the differential diagnosis for a patient with cryptogenic stroke. They recommend performing a transesophageal echocardiographic examination in this population, and if a Lambl's excrescence is present, treatment with dual antiplatelet therapy should be considered. Furthermore, if a recurrent ischemic event occurs while on this therapy, a trial of anticoagulation therapy should be considered before proceeding with the surgical resection of the Lambl's excrescence [8,9].

**Table 3.10** Differential diagnosis of the aortic valvular mass [10].

|  | Lambl's excrescence | Papillary fibroelastoma | Vegetation |
|---|---|---|---|
| Age | Elderly | Elderly in most cases | Variable |
| Fever, bacteremia | None | None | Present |
| Size | Thin (<1 mm) | 0.5–2 cm | Variable |
| Length | Long (about 10 mm) |  |  |
| Shape | Fine thread-like | Round | Irregular |
| Surface | Lint-like | Frond/jelly-like | Shaggy in fresh ones |
| Stalk | None | Short | None |
| Location | Valve closure line | Downstream | Upstream |
| Valve destruction | Minimal wearing | Minimal wearing | Significant |
| Significant valvular regurgitation | Rare | Rare | Common |

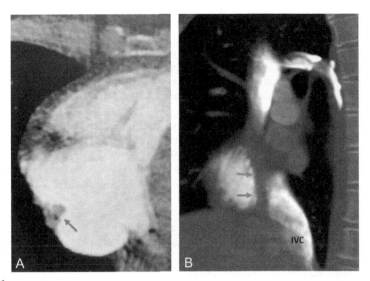

**FIG. 3.11**

Crista terminalis in a 55-year-old woman referred for further evaluation of a mass attached to the posterior wall of the left atrium on transthoracic echocardiogram. *Arrows* in axial (A) and sagittal (B) views of the cardiac CT demonstrate that the mentioned mass is actually a fibromuscular ridge which extends from upper portion of the septal surface to lateral side of the entrance of the inferior vena cava (IVC) consistent with a prominent crista terminalis.

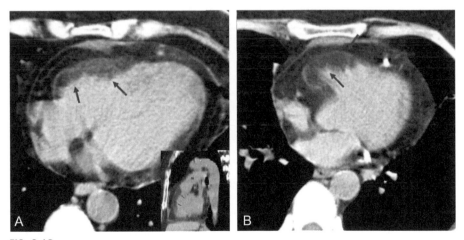

**FIG. 3.12**

A 61-year-old lady with ischemic cardiomyopathy and history of previous PCI on LAD and LCX. Transthoracic echocardiography was suspicious for clot at right ventricular free wall and outflow tract. (A and B) *Arrows* demonstrate the remarkable thickness of the epicardial fat and fatty of the RV free wall and RVOT.

## References

[1] L'Angiocola PD, Donati R. Cardiac masses in echocardiography: a pragmatic review. J Cardiovasc Echogr 2020;30(1):5–14. https://doi.org/10.4103/jcecho.jcecho_2_20.

[2] Bolognesi M. Dilated coronary sinus due to persistent left superior vena cava in a healthy athlete: a case report with brief review. J Integr Cardiol 2015;1. https://doi.org/10.15761/JIC.1000131.

[3] Schwimmer-Okike N, Niebuhr J, Schramek GGR. The presence of a large Chiari network in a patient with atrial fibrillation and stroke. Case Rep Cardiol 2016; 4839315. https://doi.org/10.1155/2016/4839315.

[4] Wang J, Wang G, Bi X, et al. An unusual presentation of prominent crista terminalis mimicking a right atrial mass: a case report. BMC Cardiovasc Disord 2018;18(210). https://doi.org/10.1186/s12872-018-0925-y.

[5] Alizadeasl A, Sadeghpour A, Kiyavar M. Transesophageal echocardiography bicaval view showing prominent crista terminalis. Anadolu Cardyol Derg 2013;13:E21–4.

[6] Mohseni-badalabadi R, Sahebjam M, Mohseni-badalabadi M. Epicardial and transverse sinus fat pad near left atrium appendage; role of 3D echocardiography. Clin Case Rep 2020. https://doi.org/10.1002/ccr3.3651.

[7] Alizadeasl A, Kaviani R, Noohi F, et al. A case report of left atrial appendage invagination in post operation setting. Multidiscip Cardiovasc Ann 2018;9(2). https://doi.org/10.5812/mca.69687, e69687.

[8] Kamran H, Patel N, Singh G, et al. Lambl's excrescences: a case report and review of the literature. Clin Case Rep Rev 2016;1. https://doi.org/10.15761/CCRR.1000254.

[9] Maleki M, Alizadehasl A, Haghjoo M. Practical cardiology. 2nd ed. Elsevier; 2021.

[10] Kim MJ, Jung HO. Anatomic variants mimicking pathology on echocardiography: differential diagnosis. J Cardiovasc Ultrasound 2013;21(3):103–12.

# Electrocardiography and cardio-oncology

**Majid Maleki**

*Cardio-Oncology Research Center, Rajaie Cardiovascular Medical and Research Center, Iran*
*University of Medical Sciences, Tehran, Iran*

## Key points

- Baseline ECG in any cardiac or extracardiac tumors is mandatory since therapeutic side effects of chemotherapy on heart are proven.
- Comprehensive understanding of the cardiac effect of anticancer agents is mandatory to predict side effects and prevent irreversible damage.

## Introduction

While life expectancy and quality of life have improved dramatically in this era of new oncology treatments, longer lifespan comes with its own set of issues and complications associated with new chemotherapy agents.

Although there are several techniques and modalities for detecting cardiac damage, such as echocardiography, nuclear medicine, and also measuring various biomarkers, the ECG is a simple, inexpensive, and rapid tool that can be used to diagnose clinical or subclinical cardiac damage prior to the progression of advanced cardiovascular disease. The electrocardiogram (ECG) can provide valuable information regarding the heart chambers, ischemia, and arrhythmia, among many other aspects. These alterations can be noticed prior to the onset of serious side effects from advanced treatment. For instance, anomalies in the left atrium caused by increased left ventricular end diastolic pressure (LVEDP) can be a prelude to atrial fibrillation (Fig. 4.1), while a prolonged QT interval can signal Torsade de points and other dangerous cardiac arrhythmias [1].

Atrial fibrillation after developing multiepisodes of frequent PACs and atrial tachycardia in a patient who receives anthracycline.

There are many clues to modify chemotherapy according to ECG. These ECG changes such as frequent premature atrial contraction (PAC) or premature ventricular contraction (PVC) may be signals of further atrial fibrillation or malignant ventricular arrhythmia, respectively, which will be relieved by reducing chemotherapy drug doses. Also agents such as 5 fluorouracil and interleukin can make coronary spasm with its own changes on ECG (Fig. 4.2).

Multimodal Imaging Atlas of Cardiac Masses. https://doi.org/10.1016/B978-0-323-84906-7.00015-7

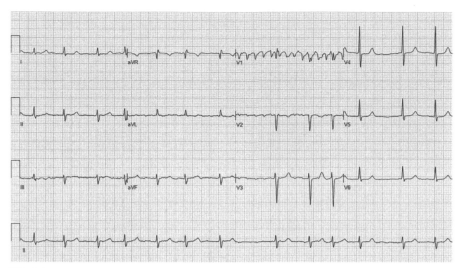

**FIG. 4.1**

Atrial fibrillation.

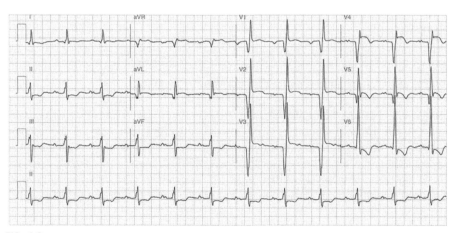

**FIG. 4.2**

Widespread ischemia after fluorouracil treatment.

## Baseline and follow-up ECG

I strongly advise taking an ECG prior to initiating any form of chemotherapy so that we can compare its alterations following treatment by an oncologist fellow. Many oncologists do not trust in ECGs, yet the processes underlying chemotherapy-induced arrhythmia have become obvious in recent years. Several of the most significant and well-known mechanisms include direct cardiac injury caused by chemotherapeutic agents, biomarker release as a result of the cancer process or treatment techniques, induced dilated cardiomyopathy, and elevated LVEDP. Additionally, other factors such as myocardial ischemia and spasm can result in a variety of arrhythmogenic mechanisms such as reentry induction or aberrant depolarization with late potentials (Fig. 4.3).

Effects on heart conduction system or ion channels effect with subsequent QT interval prolongation and all forms of bundle branch blocks, AV nodal or SA nodal disease are among well-known effects of chemotherapy agents. One of the common forms of these arrhythmias is sinus bradycardia which is known effect of taxanes plus its effects on other conduction system including right or left bundle branch and Purkinje system (Fig. 4.4).

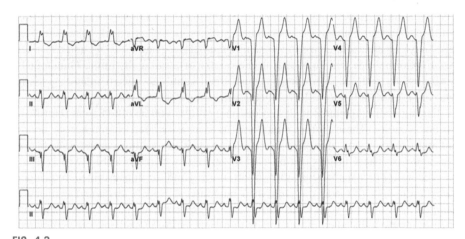

**FIG. 4.3**

Left bundle branch block in a patient on taxanes.

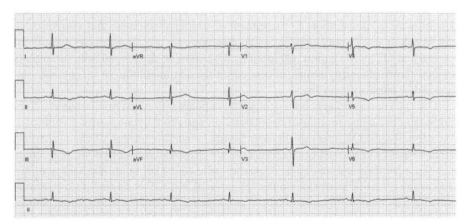

**FIG. 4.4**

Sinus bradycardia after taxane treatment which reversed spontaneously to normal sinus rhythm after 48 h.

Although conduction delay can progress after a few hours after initiation of some anticancer drugs, it can reverse within 48 h and both oncologist and cardiologist must be aware of this kind of complication for preventing further unnecessary action.

## Alkylating agents

By inducing ischemia as a result of coronary spasm, alkylating drugs such as cyclophosphamide or cisplatin might cause further cardiomyocyte damage. It is critical to assess individuals with atherosclerotic risk factors or a history of coronary artery disease for additional preventative measures against myocardial ischemia or infarction, which can further damage the heart muscle and reduce ejection fraction. Additionally, they can expand the size of the heart chambers, elevate LVEDP, and cause left atrial abnormalities with subsequent ventricular or atrial arrhythmia. Oncologists, cardiologists, and oncocardiologists must tread cautiously when treating patients who have heart failure or a lower ejection fraction (Table 4.5).

During visiting patients in cardio-oncology clinic you have to assess the risk of cardiac toxicity. These factors include the risk of associated chemotherapy and/or radiation therapy and also the risk related to their coexisting cardiac risk factor, age, and sex. These factors can be used to generate a risk score (Fig. 4.6) [2].

According to some studies, rates of atrial arrhythmias; nonsustained ventricular tachycardia (NSVT); and the combined outcome of NSVT, sustained ventricular tachycardia, and/or ventricular fibrillation are comparable in patients with chemotherapy-induced cardiomyopathy to patients with nonischemic cardiomyopathy (NICMO). In comparison to individuals with NICMO, those with ischemia cardiomyopathy (ICMO) had a higher rate of primary outcomes (Table 4.7) [4].

Electrolyte problems, low serum potassium levels, and a number of medications may all contribute to acquired QT prolongation. Cardiovascular monitoring; prudence in the administration or suspension of cancer medicines; and correction of any hypokalemia, hypocalcemia, or hypomagnesemia are all necessary treatments for marked QT prolongation. QT prolongation may be associated with potentially serious ventricular arrhythmias, necessitating the administration of magnesium sulfate and/or cardioversion [5].

The QT interval reflects both ventricular depolarization and repolarization. Chemotherapy can cause prolonged depolarization and repolarization of the ventricles. Occasionally, the QT interval surpasses 500 ms, signaling the end of chemotherapy. Other causes of prolonged QT intervals, such as hypokalemia or hypomagnesaemia, must be examined and treated as necessary prior to initiating chemotherapy drugs. Due to the effect of heart rate on the QT interval, the QT corrected (QTc) interval must be less than 460 ms. Although a prolonged QT interval greater than 500 ms increases the risk of malignant ventricular arrhythmia, it is recommended to consider a prolonged QT interval greater than 480 s as a red flag for discontinuing anticancer drugs, rather than 450 ms, due to the multifactor nature of the QT interval and to

**Table 4.5** Risk assessment with recommended test in patients on anticancer therapy [2].

| 1. Risk assessment | Tests: TTE with strain ECG, cTn |
|---|---|
| **Medication-related risk** | **Patient-related risk factors** |
| **High (risk score 4):** Anthracyclines, cyclophosphamide, ifosfamide, clofarabine, herceptin | • Cardiomyopathy or heart failure |
| **Intermediate (risk score 2):** Docetaxel, pertuzumab, sunitinib, sorafenib | • CAD or equivalent (incl. PAD) |
| **Low (risk score 1):** Bevacizumab, dasatinib, imatinib, lapatinib | • HTN |
| **Rare (risk score 0):** For example, etoposide, rituximab, thalidomide | • Diabetes mellitus |
|  | • Prior or concurrent anthracycline |
|  | • Prior or concurrent chest radiation |
|  | • Age $< 15$ or $> 65$ years |
|  | • Female gender |

**Overall risk by cardiotoxicity risk score (CRS)**
(risk categories by drug-related risk score plus number of patient-related risk factors: **CRS > 6**: very high, **5–6**: high, **3–4**: intermediate, **1–2**: low, **0**: very low)

**2. Monitoring recommendations**

**Very high cardiotoxicity risk:** TTE with strain before every (other) cycle, end, 3–6 months, and 1 year; optional ECG, cTn with TTE during chemotherapy

**High cardiotoxicity risk:** TTE with strain every 3 cycles, end, 3–6 months, and 1 year after chemotherapy; optional ECG, cTn with TTE during chemotherapy

**Intermediate cardiotoxicity risk:** TTE with strain midterm, end, and 3–6 months after chemotherapy; optional ECG, cTn midterm of chemotherapy

**Low cardiotoxicity risk:** Optional TTE with strain and/or ECG, cTn at the end of chemotherapy

**Very low cardiotoxicity risk:** None

**3. Management recommendations**

**Very high cardiotoxicity risk:** Initiate ACE-I/ARB, carvedilol, and statins, starting at lowest dose and start chemotherapy in 1 week from initiation to allow steady state, up-titrate as tolerated

**High cardiotoxicity risk:** Initiate ACE-I/ARB, carvedilol, and/or statins

**Intermediate cardiotoxicity risk:** Discuss risk and benefit of medications

**Low cardiotoxicity risk:** None, monitoring only

**Very low cardiotoxicity risk:** None, monitoring only

CAD, *coronary artery disease*; HTN, *hypertension*; PAD, *peripheral artery disease*; TTE, *transthoracic echocardiography*; cTn, *cardiac troponin*; ACE, *angiotensin-converting enzyme inhibitor*; ARB, *angiotensin receptor blocker*.

avoid patients stopping or discontinuing lifesaving chemotherapy agents. The QT interval can vary by up to 160 ms in oncologic patients, which is why we recommend continuing anticancer medications up to a QT interval of 480 ms [6].

Cardiac patients with a history of arrhythmia who are taking antiarrhythmia medications such as amiodarone, kinidin, and others may have an increased QT interval

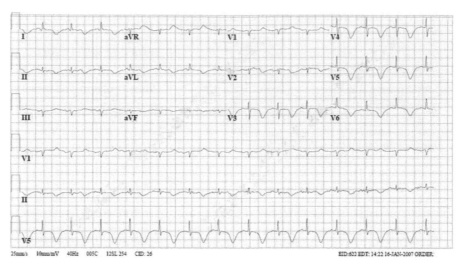

**FIG. 4.6**

Marked QT prolongation due to histone deacetylase inhibitors.

**Table 4.7** ECG changes by chemotherapeutic agents.

A. Antimetabolites
Drugs such as 5 fluorouracil can induce coronary spasm with clinical findings of chest pain, dyspnea, or aggravation of heart failure and ultimately ischemic cardiomyopathy. To relieve these complication calcium antagonists and nitrate can be prescribed in this group of patients (Fig. 4.2)

B. Histone deacetylase inhibitors
These groups of drugs are contraindicated in oncologic patients with preexisting long QT interval
(Fig. 4.6) because of probable induction of Torsade de pointes and malignant ventricular arrhythmia (Fig. 4.9)

C. Anthracyclines
The most common side effects of these drugs are reducing ejection fraction and to a lesser degree increased QT interval. Tyrosine kinase inhibitors can also increase QT interval but it usually does not induce Torsade de pointes. It should be mentioned that QT interval measurement is an easy and useful method which can be done by simple ECG tool (Fig. 4.8) [3]

and an increased risk of developing malignant ventricular arrhythmia as a result of drug interaction with anticancer agents that cause increased QT prolongation. Therefore it is critical to know the drug history of cardiac patients prior to initiating anticancer treatment. Reduced sum of absolute QRS amplitudes in six limb leads and an increase in corrected QT interval (QTC) are related with an increased risk of developing cardiomyopathy in children receiving anthracyclines. ECG may be a noninvasive risk assessment technique for anthracycline-induced cardiomyopathy prediction [7].

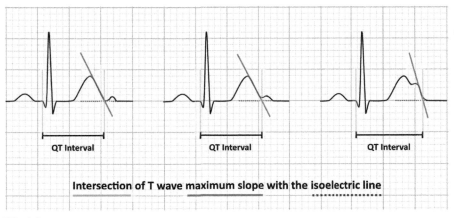

**FIG. 4.8**

Measurement of QT interval considering T wave maximum slope and isoelectric line.

## Ventricular Tachycardia Torsade de Pointes - EKG Reference

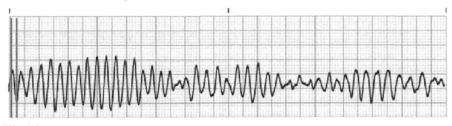

**FIG. 4.9**

Torsade de pointes in a patient with preexisting long QT syndrome who receives histone.

## Radiotherapy and ECG

Radiation to the mediastinum may raise the risk of coronary artery disease by accelerating the calcification of the aorta and great arteries, resulting in electrocardiographic alterations. Additionally, radiation can alter the electrocardiogram (ECG) due to pericarditis and various forms of cardiac autonomic dysfunction (see Fig. 4.10).

During all levels of activity, these patients may exhibit resting tachycardia and irregular heart rate recovery. It's worth noting that radiation side effects can manifest years after the original treatment. Additionally, it is associated with macro and microvascular illness, valvular heart disease (VHD), conduction abnormalities, and pericarditis. Acute pericarditis is uncommon nowadays due to decreased radiation doses and novel radiotherapy methods that shield the heart from the radiation field [7].

Diffuse PR depression and ST elevation following radiotherapy in a patient with history of breast cancer.

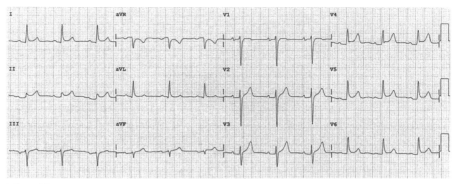

**FIG. 4.10**

ECG changes due to acute pericarditis after radiotherapy.

## Conclusion

Oncological treatment requires tight collaboration between cardiologists and oncologists, which is the primary reason that the specialty of oncocardiology is flourishing nowadays. Cardio-oncologists must be familiar with anticancer therapy techniques and their consequences on the cardiovascular system, particularly in patients who have prior cardiac issues or are taking cardiac medications. Cardio-oncologists must be conversant with the electrocardiogram (ECG), which is a basic technique that may be used at the bedside to assess the primary effects of cancer treatment on the heart. Additionally, they must be familiar with advanced echocardiography, speckle tracking, nuclear medicine, and MRI, among others. They should speak with both a cardiologist and an oncologist to get the best possible care and the fewest possible complications associated with cancer therapy. Cardio-oncologists must be well versed in anticancer medications, cardiac drugs, and all other therapeutic methods, as well as their effects on the circulatory system and the interplay of all necessary interventions. Additionally, oncologists, cardiologists, and cardio-oncologists must be completely aware of insignificant or subtle alterations that may occur during therapy and refrain from abruptly discontinuing lifesaving anticancer treatment.

Occasionally, nonsignificant atrial or ventricular arrhythmias, modest ST-T alterations, or mild QT interval prolongation occurs without clinical significance, and experienced clinicians can make the best option for the best outcome just by understanding the risks and benefits of any intervention.

## References

[1] Maleki M. Chapter 2—Evaluation of patient with cardiovascular problem. In: Maleki M, Alizadehasl A, Haghjoo M, editors. Practical cardiology. 2nd ed. Elsevier; 2022. p. 7–16. ISBN 9780323809153.

[2] Larsen CM, Mulvagh SL. Cardio-oncology: what you need to know now for clinical practice and echocardiography. Echo Res Pract 2017;4(1):R33–41. https:/doi.org/10.1530/ERP-17-0013.

[3] Desai L, Balmert L, Reichek J, Hauck A, Gambetta K, Webster G. Electrocardiograms for cardiomyopathy risk stratification in children with anthracycline exposure. Cardiooncology 2019;5:10. Published 2019 Aug 7 https:/doi.org/10.1186/s40959-019-0045-6.

[4] Fradley MG, Viganego F, Kip K, et al. Rates and risk of arrhythmias in cancer survivors with chemotherapy-induced cardiomyopathy compared with patients with other cardiomyopathies. Open Heart 2017;4(2), e000701. Published 2017 Dec 17 https:/doi.org/10.1136/openhrt-2017-000701.

[5] Coppola C, Rienzo A, Piscopo G, Barbieri A, Arra C, Maurea N. Management of QT prolongation induced by anti-cancer drugs: target therapy and old agents. Different algorithms for different drugs. Cancer Treat Rev 2018;63:135–43. https:/doi.org/10.1016/j.ctrv.2017.11.009.

[6] Chan A, Isbister GK, Kirkpatrick CMJ, Dufful SB. Drug-induced QT prolongation and torsades de pointes: evaluation of a QT nomogram. Int J Med 2007;100(10):609–15. https:/doi.org/10.1093/qjmed/hcm072.

[7] López-Fernández T, Martín García A, Santaballa Beltrán A, et al. Cardio-Oncohematology in clinical practice. Position paper and recommendations. Rev Esp Cardiol 2017;70(6):474–86. https:/doi.org/10.1016/j.rec.2016.12.041.

[8] Spînu Ş, Cismaru G, Boarescu PM, et al. ECG markers of cardiovascular toxicity in adult and pediatric cancer treatment. Dis Markers 2021;2021, 6653971. Published 2021 Jan 19 https:/doi.org/10.1155/2021/6653971.

# Angiographic clues for a cardiac mass

# 5

**Ata Firouzi and Ehsan Khalilipur**

*Cardiovascular Intervention Research Center, Rajaie Cardiovascular Medical and Research Center, Iran University of Medical Sciences, Tehran, Iran*

## Key points

- Most heart tumors are benign. Atrial myxomas make for 30%–50% of all primary cardiac tumors. (See Boxes 5.2 and 5.3.)
- Knowing the approximate position of a tumor in relation to its feeding vessel provides information for predicting the tumor's nature and behavior.
- Tumor blush is seen with benign atrial myxomas, hemangiomas, and rhabdomyomas, as well as malignant pheochromocytomas and angiosarcomas.

**Table 5.1** Scope of the problem.

It is widely known, particularly among surgical teams, that malignancies occasionally occur within the heart. Additionally, unlike general surgeons, many cardiac surgeons are unfamiliar with heart tumors [1]. The heart is primarily composed of mesenchymal tissues, with the exception of the endocardium and pericardium, which are epithelial structures. This requirement for carcinomas is a distinguishing factor that can distinguish the heart from other organs. It is possible that this requirement for carcinomas contributes to the widespread belief that malignancies of the heart are infrequent [2].

Heart neoplasms are classified histologically as benign or malignant. They are far less common than secondary neoplasms, occurring at a rate of 0.001%–0.03%. Diagnosis is usually difficult, as patients remain asymptomatic for extended periods of time and frequently present with nonspecific signs and symptoms that may mimic those of other cardiac disease types. Around 75% of all cardiac tumors are benign. Atrial myxomas account for between 30% and 50% of all primary cardiac tumors. Lipomas, papillary fibroelastomas, fibromas, rhabdomyomas, and hemangiomas are all benign tumors. Sarcomas include leiomyosarcomas, rhabdomyosarcomas, osteosarcomas, and lymphomas, as well as primitive neuroectodermal tumors (pheochromocytomas) [3].

Tumor neovascularization and angiogenesis are critical for tumor growth. Coronary angiography of malignancies frequently reveals late opacification of a well-vascularized heart tumor, referred to as "tumor blush." Certain cardiac neoplasms exhibit a distinctive "tumor blush": [1] benign myxomas, rhabdomyomas, and vascular malformations in the atrium and [2] malignant pheochromocytomas and angiosarcomas in the atrium [4,5]. The purpose of this chapter is to highlight the importance of coronary angiography in the workup of a cardiac tumor.

**Multimodal Imaging Atlas of Cardiac Masses. https://doi.org/10.1016/B978-0-323-84906-7.00028-5**

## Box 5.2 Coronary artery disease.

Coronary artery disease in cardiac tumors is determined by the patients' symptomatology. According to the most recent clinical guidelines, assessment of the coronary vasculature is suitable in a patient with typical symptoms suggestive of coronary artery disease [6]. On the other hand, many heart team approaches prefer to visualize coronary artery anatomy prior to surgical care in patients older than 40 years of age in order to diagnose and treat preclinical coronary artery disease concurrently with the operation [7,8]

## Box 5.3 Tumor feeding vessel.

The imaging of the feeding arteries by angiogram has a number of clinical and therapeutic implications. The placement of these vessels may alter the surgical strategy in cases where evidence of blood shunting exists, either as a result of fistula formation or spurting from the tumor surface. This may be the catalyst for many surgeons to ligate these feeding vessels during surgery in order to avert this problem [9]. Separately, the proximity of a vascular supply to the tumor was associated with unusual clinical manifestations such as angina and sick sinus syndrome caused by blood shunting and subsequent myocardial and nodal ischemia [10,11]. In cases when differentiating cardiac tumor from thrombus is difficult, the angiographic detection of neovessels favors the diagnosis of cardiac tumor over thrombi, which are frequently nonvascularized [12]. Detection of a heart tumor's blood supply also has therapeutic implications, as removing the feeding channel may impair tumor growth [4,13]. Additionally, knowing the approximate position of a tumor in relation to its feeding channel provides information for predicting the tumor's nature and behavior (Table 5.1) [14,15]

**Table 5.4** Location of common cardiac neoplasm.

| Type of tumor | Left atrium | Right atrium | Left ventricle | Right ventricle | Valve | Pericardium |
|---|---|---|---|---|---|---|
| Myxoma | 90% | 10% | Rare | Rare | Rare | 0 |
| Sarcoma | 46%[a] | 26% | 21% (right or left)[b] | b | 0 | 7% |
| Fibroma | Rare | Rare | 80% (majority in IVS) | 20% | 0 | 0 |
| Papillary fibroelastoma | 2% | c | 10% | 3% (right heart)[c] | 85% (AV, MV) | 0 |
| Rhabdomyoma[d] | 0 | 30% (atrium or ventricle)[e] | 70% (and ventricular septum) | c | 0 | 0 |
| Lipoma (LI)/ lipomatous hypertrophy (LM) | 0 | Majority LH | Epicardial surface (LI) | Epicardial surface (LI) | 0 | 0 |
| Angioma | Any location | Any location | Any location | Any location | Varix | 0 |

AV, aortic valve; MV, mitral valve; IVS, interventricular septum.
[a]Angiosarcoma predominantly in right atrium.
[b]Right or left.
[c]Right heart.
[d]90% multiple and rare in adults.
[e]Atrium or ventricle.

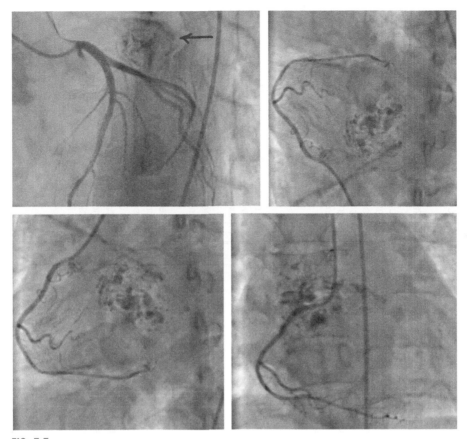

**FIG. 5.5**

Tumor blush in a cardiac mass. Coronary angiography may be used to determine whether contrast enhancement or "tumor blush" is present. Neovascularization of tumors is essential for tumors to grow in size. The appearance of a flushed tumor has been observed in a few, but not all, cardiac neoplasms, most notably benign atrial myxomas, hemangiomas, and rhabdomyomas, as well as malignant pheochromocytomas and angiosarcomas [4,16,17] (Fig. 1).

**Table 5.6** Clinicopathologic characteristics of tumors demonstrating tumor blush on coronary angiography.

| Type of tumor | Epidemiological features | Typical tumor location | Blood supply/tumor blush | Additional features | Common clinical presentation |
|---|---|---|---|---|---|
| Myxomas | Most common benign cardiac neoplasm. 30–50 y/o, F > M 1.7–4:1; rarely affects children | Endocardial surface of interatrial septum with 75% LA, 20% RA, rarely in the ventricles | Tumor blush emanating from RCA > LCx > dual coronary blood supply | Endocardial masses, pedunculated solitary masses. Surgical excision, excellent prognosis, low recurrence | Obstructive symptoms, embolic phenomena, rhythm disturbances, and systemic symptoms. Twenty percent of patients are asymptomatic |
| Rhabdomyomas | Most common primary benign neoplasm in children, represents fetal hamartoma | Ventricles > atria | Tumor blush emanating from LAD | Well circumscribed, firm white/yellow tumors, 1 mm to 9 cm in size, appear more echodense than fibromas | 50% are associated with tuberous sclerosis. Almost complete regression, overall prognosis is excellent |
| Hemangioma | Most common benign vascular tumor. Occurs in all ages, M = F | Lateral wall of the left ventricle and on the anterior wall of the right ventricle | Tumor blush emanating from RCA > LAD > LCx > dual blood supply | Present as well-circumscribed soft masses and can occur as a cavernous, capillary, or arteriovenous neoplasm | Associated with extracardiac hemangiomas in the GIT and Kasabach–Merritt syndrome. Symptoms are related to obstruction, embolization, and rhythm disturbances |

**Table 5.6** Clinicopathologic characteristics of tumors demonstrating tumor blush on coronary angiography—*Cont'd*

| Type of tumor | Epidemiological features | Typical tumor location | Blood supply/tumor blush | Additional features | Common clinical presentation |
|---|---|---|---|---|---|
| Paragangliomas | Benign tumors arising from chromaffin cells—pheochromocytomas. Occurs in all ages, M = F | Epicardial surface in the roof of left atrium, interatrial septum, rarely in left ventricle | Tumor blush emanating from LCx | Extremely rare neoplasms arise from intrinsic cardiac paraganglial (chromaffin) cells | Catecholamine producing tumors. Symptoms may include HTN, headaches, palpitations, and flushing. Elevated levels of urinary and plasma norepinephrine and vanillylmandelic acid |
| Angiosarcomas | Most common malignant primary cardiac sarcoma in adults. 30–50 y/o, M > F | 80% arise as mural masses in the right atrium | Tumor blush emanating from right coronary artery | Composed of endothelial and mesenchymal cells. Tumors often invade SVC and TV and have poorly defined borders with areas of hemorrhage | Patients typically present with advanced disease, with 70% of patients presenting with evidence of metastatic disease at the time of diagnosis |

M, *male*; F, *female*; LA, *left atrium*; RA, *right atrium*; RCA, *right coronary artery*; LCx, *left circumflex*; LAD, *left anterior descending*; SVC, *superior vena cava*; TV, *tricuspid valve*; GIT, *GI tract*; HTN, *hypertension*.

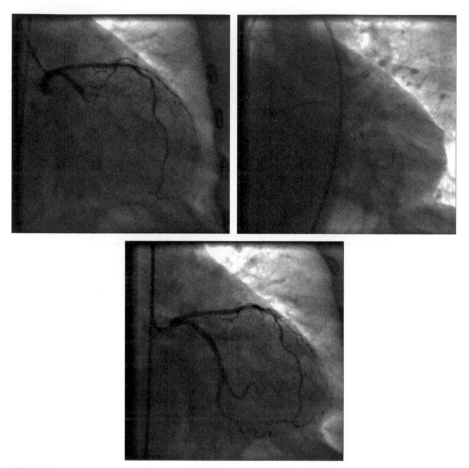

**FIG. 5.7**

Acute coronary syndrome because of embolization of thrombus from a cardiac mass to left coronary system subsequently treated with manual thrombus aspiration. The atrial myxoma was diagnosed subsequently with transthoracic echocardiography and patient underwent surgical resection.

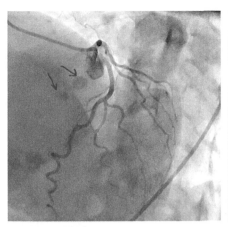
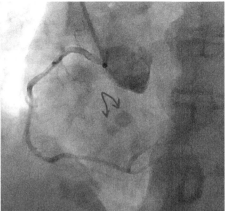

**FIG. 5.8**

Cardiac thrombus visualization. When a cardiac tumor presents, thrombus formation occurs, which may result in a mobile particle passing over the cardiac mass or, in more severe cases, embolization of the thrombus to the distal vascular bed or even to the coronary arteries, resulting in acute cerebrovascular ischemia, acute limb ischemia, or acute coronary syndrome (Figs. 2 and 3) [18,19]. In rare scenarios, at the time of coronary angiography, intracardiac thrombus enhances with contrast because of tumor feeding vessel late venous phase and gives us the proof for a cardiac mass.

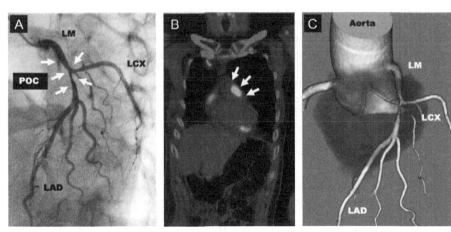

**FIG. 5.9**

Tumor compressive effect on coronary arteries: (A) coronary angiography demonstrating severe stenosis at the polygon of confluence (POC) (*white arrows*). (B) Fluorine-18-fluorodeoxyglucose positron emission tomographic (PET) picture showing positive cardiac uptake, suggesting a metastatic area (*white arrows*). (C) Computed tomographic angiographic (CTA)/PET 3-dimensional fusion picture shows the metastatic tumor concentrated around the compressed POC [19].

# References

[1] Committee for Scientific Affairs, The Japanese Association for Thoracic Surgery, Masuda M, Okumura M, Doki Y, Endo S, Hirata Y, Kobayashi J, Kuwano H, Motomura N, Nishida H, Saiki Y, Saito A, Shimizu H, Tanaka F, Tanemoto K, Toh Y, Tsukihara H, Wakui S, Yokomise H. Thoracic and cardiovascular surgery in Japan during 2014: annual report by The Japanese Association for Thoracic Surgery. Gen Thorac Cardiovasc Surg 2016;64(11):665–97. https://doi.org/10.1007/s11748-016-0695-3. 27590348. PMC5069321.

[2] Hoffmeier A, Sindermann JR, Scheld HH, Martens S. Cardiac tumors—diagnosis and surgical treatment. Dtsch Arztebl Int 2014;111(12):205–11. https://doi.org/10.3238/arztebl.2014.0205. 24717305. PMC3983698.

[3] Amano J, Nakayama J, Yoshimura Y, Ikeda U. Clinical classification of cardiovascular tumors and tumor-like lesions, and its incidences. Gen Thorac Cardiovasc Surg 2013;61 (8):435–47. https://doi.org/10.1007/s11748-013-0214-8. Epub 2013 Mar 5. Erratum in: Gen Thorac Cardiovasc Surg. 2013 Aug;61(8):448 23460447. PMC3732772.

[4] Marok R, Klein LW. Tumor blush in primary cardiac tumors. J Invasive Cardiol 2012;24 (3):139–40. 22388311.

[5] Parikh SS, Li F, Fong MW. Cardiac arteriovenous malformation. J Am Coll Cardiol 2010;55(16). https://doi.org/10.1016/j.jacc.2009.11.078, e133. 20394866.

[6] Abu Daya H, Hage FG. Guidelines in review: ACC/AATS/AHA/ASE/ASNC/SCAI/ SCCT/STS 2017 appropriate use criteria for coronary revascularization in patients with stable ischemic heart disease. J Nucl Cardiol 2017;24(5):1793–9. https://doi.org/ 10.1007/s12350-017-1017-6. Epub 2017 Aug 23 28836156.

[7] Rahmanian PB, Castillo JG, Sanz J, Adams DH, Filsoufi F. Cardiac myxoma: preoperative diagnosis using a multimodal imaging approach and surgical outcome in a large contemporary series. Interact Cardiovasc Thorac Surg 2007;6(4):479–83. https://doi.org/10.1510/icvts.2007.154096. Epub 2007 May 30 17669910.

[8] Li AH, Liau CS, Wu CC, Chien KL, Ho YL, Huang CH, Chen MF, Lee YT. Role of coronary angiography in myxoma patients: a 14-year experience in one medical center. Cardiology 1999;92(4):232–5. https://doi.org/10.1159/000006979. 10844382.

[9] Roth JE, Conner WC, Porisch ME, Shry E. Sinoatrial nodal artery to right atrium fistula after myxoma excision. Ann Thorac Surg 2006;82(3):1106–7. https://doi.org/10.1016/j.athoracsur.2006.01.067. 16928553.

[10] Burns AC, Osula S, Harley A, Rashid A. Left circumflex coronary artery to left atrial fistula in a patient with mitral regurgitation after excision of a left atrial myxoma. Ann Thorac Surg 2001;72(5):1732–3. https://doi.org/10.1016/s0003-4975(01)02613-3. 11722076.

[11] Bayramoğlu Z, Caynak B, Oral K, Erdim R, Teyyareci Y, Akpınar B. Left atrial myxoma with neovascularization presenting as a sick sinus syndrome. Heart Surg Forum 2012;15 (4):E200–3. https://doi.org/10.1532/HSF98.20111180. 22917824.

[12] Kono T, Koide N, Hama Y, Kitahara H, Nakano H, Suzuki J, Isobe M, Amano J. Expression of vascular endothelial growth factor and angiogenesis in cardiac myxoma: a study of fifteen patients. J Thorac Cardiovasc Surg 2000;119(1):101–7. https://doi.org/ 10.1016/s0022-5223(00)70223-6. 10612767.

[13] Fitzgerald PJ, Ports TA, Cheitlin MD, Magilligan DJ, Tyrrell JB. Intracardiac pheochromocytoma with dual coronary blood supply: case report and literature review. Cardiovasc Surg 1995;3(5):557–61. https://doi.org/10.1016/0967-2109(95)94459-a. 8574544.

[14] Burke A, Tavora F. The 2015 WHO classification of tumors of the heart and pericardium. J Thorac Oncol 2016;11(4):441–52. https://doi.org/10.1016/j.jtho.2015.11.009. Epub 2015 Dec 25 26725181.

[15] Ladich E, Virmani R. Chapter 19—Tumors of the cardiovascular system: heart and blood vessels. In: Buja LM, Butany J, editors. Cardiovascular pathology. 4th ed. Academic Press; 2016. p. 735–72.

[16] Brizard C, Latremouille C, Jebara VA, Acar C, Fabiani JN, Deloche A, Carpentier AF. Cardiac hemangiomas. Ann Thorac Surg 1993;56(2):390–4. https://doi.org/10.1016/0003-4975(93)91193-q. 8347036.

[17] Krasuski RA, Hesselson AB, Landolfo KP, Ellington KJ, Bashore TM. Cardiac rhabdomyoma in an adult patient presenting with ventricular arrhythmia. Chest 2000;118(4):1217–21. https://doi.org/10.1378/chest.118.4.1217. 11035702.

[18] Maleszewski JJ, Anavekar NS, Moynihan TJ, Klarich KW. Pathology, imaging, and treatment of cardiac tumours. Nat Rev Cardiol 2017;14(9):536–49. https://doi.org/10.1038/nrcardio.2017.47. Epub 2017 Apr 24 28436488.

[19] Uetani T, Inaba S, Nishiyama H, Yamaguchi O. Metastatic cardiac tumor-induced acute coronary syndrome. JACC Cardiovasc Interv 2020;13(20):e179–80. https://doi.org/10.1016/j.jcin.2020.08.016. Epub 2020 Sep 30 33011140.

# Cardiac thrombi and imaging modalities (diagnosis, approach, and follow-up)

**Feridoun Noohi[a], Hamidreza Pouraliakbar[b], Azin Alizadehasl[a], Kiara Rezaei-Kalantari[b], and Sheikh Mohammed Shariful Islam[c]**

*[a]Cardio-Oncology Research Center, Rajaie Cardiovascular Medical and Research Center, Iran University of Medical Sciences, Tehran, Iran [b]Department of Radiology, CardioOncology Research Center, Iran University of Medical Sciences, Rajaie Cardiovascular Medical and Research Center, Tehran, Iran [c]Institute for Physical Activity and Nutrition, School of Exercise and Nutrition Sciences, Deakin University, Melbourne, VIC, Australia*

## Key points

- Intracardiac thrombi constitute an important clinical condition because of their potential complications.
- Detection of ventricular thrombi is generally performed by transthoracic echocardiography, while atrial thrombi are generally evaluated by transesophageal echocardiography.
- Contrast-enhanced computerized tomography is more sensitive for detecting ventricular and atrial thrombi than transthoracic echocardiography, but the technique has been demonstrated to be inferior to transesophageal echocardiography for displaying atrial thrombi.
- Cardiac magnetic resonance imaging provides superior specificity for the evaluation of tissue characteristics and helps differentiate thrombi from other masses (Table 6.1).

Multimodal Imaging Atlas of Cardiac Masses. https://doi.org/10.1016/B978-0-323-84906-7.00030-3

**Table 6.1** Differentiating intracardiac thrombi from cardiac tumors [1].

| Differentiating intracardiac thrombi from cardiac tumors | | |
| --- | --- | --- |
| **Imaging feature** | **Intracardiac thrombus** | **Intracardiac mass** |
| Location | Left heart is more common | Right heart is more common |
| Morphology | Intrachamber masses<br>Rarely sessile | Infiltrative masses<br>Multiple masses |
| Appearance | Usually homogeneous | Usually heterogeneous |
| MRI | T2 hypointense when chronic | T2 hyperintense |
| Enhancement | No internal enhancement<br>Rarely peripheral pseudoenhancement when chronic | Often enhancing |
| Gadolinium-enhanced MRI | Progressively hypointense on contrast-enhanced inversion time scout sequence | Avid first-pass perfusion<br>Late gadolinium enhancement |
| Other discriminators | Pericardial disease is not directly associated<br>Left atrial enlargement or left ventricular infarction | Pericardial effusion is most common<br>Extracardiac cancer |

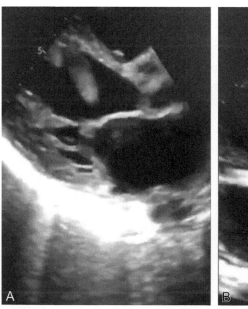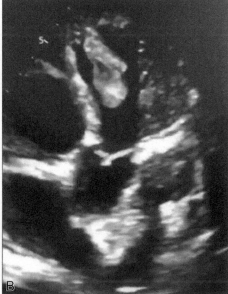

**FIG. 6.2**

Transthoracic echocardiography of a patient with anterior ST-elevation myocardial infarction shows apical left ventricular mobile thrombosis in the parasternal long-axis (A) and apical 4-chamber (B) views.

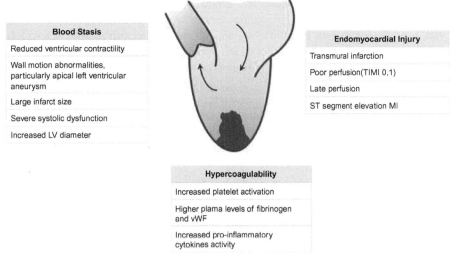

| **Blood Stasis** |
| --- |
| Reduced ventricular contractility |
| Wall motion abnormalities, particularly apical left ventricular aneurysm |
| Large infarct size |
| Severe systolic dysfunction |
| Increased LV diameter |

| **Endomyocardial Injury** |
| --- |
| Transmural infarction |
| Poor perfusion(TIMI 0,1) |
| Late perfusion |
| ST segment elevation MI |

| **Hypercoagulability** |
| --- |
| Increased platelet activation |
| Higher plama levels of fibrinogen and vWF |
| Increased pro-inflammatory cytokines activity |

**FIG. 6.3**

Pathophysiologic factors involved in left ventricular thrombosis formation are presented herein. *LV*, left ventricle; *TIMI*, thrombolysis in myocardial infarction; *MI*, myocardial infarction; *vWF*, von Willebrand factor.

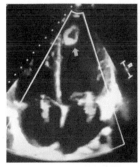
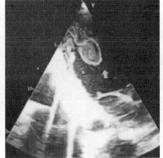
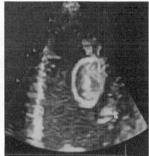

**FIG. 6.4**

Transthoracic echocardiography of a patient with regional wall motion abnormalities in the left ventricular apical segments shows a large, round hypermobile thrombus with central liquefaction mimicking a cystic mass.

Cystic masses of the left ventricle are rare. The differential diagnosis includes epithelial-lined cystic tumors, intracardiac teratomas, benign blood cysts, pericardial cysts, bronchogenic cysts, hydatid cysts, and thrombi. Echocardiography is a widely applied technique for the estimation of left ventricular masses; however, CMR has evolved to confer the capability for imaging cardiac masses and in some cases may offer additive information to echocardiography because of its high spatial accuracy and expanded possibilities for tissue characterization. Spontaneous clot dissolution can begin soon after its formation, and clot lysis is an integral part of this process. Be that as it may, a more rapid resolution has rarely been reported.

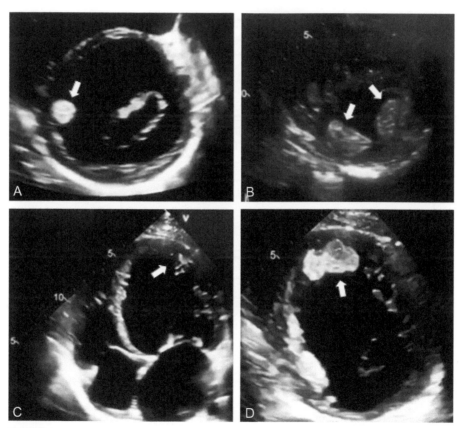

**FIG. 6.5**

The images demonstrate multiple left ventricular clots in the transthoracic echocardiographic examination of a patient with metastatic lung cancer. The parasternal short-axis view at the mitral valve level (A) shows a bright homogeneous echo density attached to the base of the interventricular septum (*white arrow*), suggestive of a thrombus. Two similar echo densities are depicted at the mid-ventricular level of the parasternal short-axis view (B, *white arrows*). The apical 4-chamber view (C) shows a small bright echo density attached to the apical segment of the lateral wall (*white arrow*), which is adjacent to another large thrombus in the left ventricular apex, which is best shown in the off-axis apical 2-chamber view (D) (Supplementary Video 6.1).

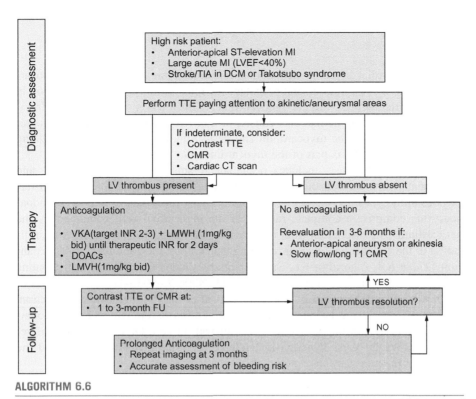

**ALGORITHM 6.6**

The image depicts the proposed algorithm for the diagnosis, management, and follow-up of LV thrombi [3]. *MI*, myocardial infarction; *LVEF*, left ventricular ejection fraction; *TIA*, transient ischemic attack; *DCM*, dilated cardiomyopathy; *TTE*, transthoracic echocardiography; *CMR*, cardiac magnetic resonance; *CT*, computed tomography; *LV*, left ventricle; *VKA*, vitamin K antagonist; *INR*, international normalized ratio; *LMWH*, low molecular weight heparin; *DOAC*, direct acting oral anticoagulant; *FU*, follow up.

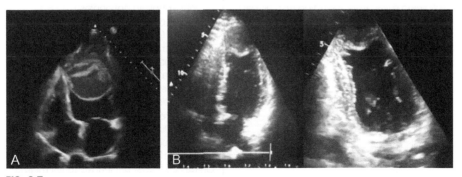

**FIG. 6.7**

The images depict intramyocardial dissecting hematomas in the transthoracic echocardiographic examination of two patients (A and B) after anterior myocardial infarction. Large echolucent cavitation almost occupies the akinetic left ventricular apex, surrounded by a thin and mobile endomyocardial border and filled with fresh thrombi and bulges into the left ventricle in the systole. The finding demonstrates intramyocardial dissecting hematomas.

Intramyocardial dissecting hematomas constitute a rare complication of myocardial infarction, chest trauma, and percutaneous interventions. They can develop in the left ventricular free wall, the right ventricle, or the interventricular septum. Intramyocardial dissecting hematomas consist of a cavity filled with blood. The outer wall of the cavity is the myocardium and pericardium, and the inner wall, facing the ventricular cavity, is part of the myocardium and the endocardium.

Differential diagnosis includes pseudoaneurysms, intracavitary thrombi, and prominent ventricular trabeculations. Establishing the integrity of epicardium differentiates intramyocardial dissecting hematomas from pseudoaneurysms, as pseudoaneurysms comprise a complete rupture of the myocardial wall contained by the pericardium. The distinction from intracavitary thrombi relies on the clear identification of the endocardial layer surrounding the neoformation and its systolic expansion (Table 6.8, Algorithm 6.6, Supplementary Videos 6.1 and 6.2 in the online version at https://doi.org/10.1016/B978-0-323-84906-7.00030-3).

In more than 90% of cases, rupture occurs after the first myocardial infarction, and it has a strong correlation with single-vessel disease, reflecting a lack of collateral circulation. Risk factors include anterior wall infarct, large transmural infarction, age over 60 years, hypertension, female sex, single-vessel disease, and the absence of previous cardiac events.

**Table 6.8** Predisposing conditions for left ventricular thrombi [2].

| Predisposing conditions for left ventricular thrombi | |
|---|---|
| **Left ventricular thrombi with impaired left ventricular function (more common)** | **Left ventricular thrombi with preserved left ventricular function (extremely rare)** |
| Left ventricular apical aneurysms<br>Following myocardial infarction with apical akinesia<br>Following myocardial infarction in segments other than the left anterior descending territory<br>Left ventricular pseudoaneurysms<br>Dilated cardiomyopathy<br>Apical ballooning (Takotsubo) syndrome | Hypercoagulable states<br>Antiphospholipid antibodies<br>Protein C deficiency<br>Myeloproliferative disorders<br>Essential thrombocythemia<br>Myelofibrosis<br>Salmonella septicemia<br>Cardiac trauma<br>Eosinophilic endocarditis<br>Connective tissue disease<br>Systemic lupus erythematosus<br>Behçet disease<br>On the surface of left ventricular tumors<br>On device leads that inadvertently migrate to the left ventricle<br>Administration of large doses of erythropoietin |

Echocardiographic features of intramyocardial dissecting hematomas include the formation of 1 or more neocavitations within the tissue with an echolucent center, a thinned and mobile endomyocardial border surrounding the cavitary defect, ventricular myocardium identified in the regions outside of the cystic areas, and changes in the echogenicity of the neocavitation, suggesting blood content.

The management of intramyocardial dissecting hematomas depends on multiple factors, including the patient's age, hemodynamic stability, the size of the hematoma, the presence of ventricular septal defects, left ventricular function, and pericardial effusion. Intramyocardial dissecting hematomas limited to the apex have a high probability of spontaneous reabsorption, and an initial conservative approach may be reasonable. Patients with the expansion of dissection on serial echocardiography, ventricular septal defects, compromised hemodynamics, and low ejection fractions in the anterior wall myocardial infarction should undergo surgery [4].

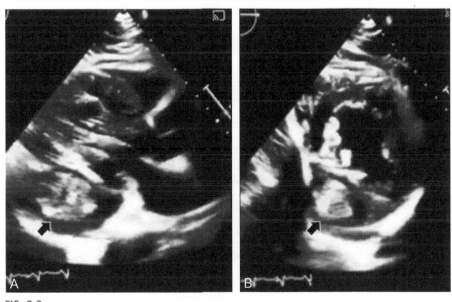

**FIG. 6.9**

The images illustrate a large thrombus in a left ventricular pseudoaneurysm in the transthoracic echocardiographic examination of a patient with a history of old inferoposterior myocardial infarction in (A) the parasternal long-axis view and (B) the parasternal short-axis view. The images demonstrate a large, echo-free space attached to the posterior wall of the left ventricle with a narrow neck, containing a large heterogeneous mass (*black arrow*). All the earlier mentioned findings are in favor of a large left ventricular pseudoaneurysm with an organized clot (Supplementary Video 6.2).

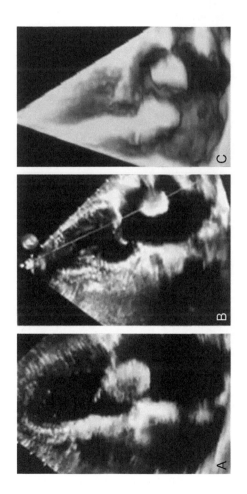

**FIG. 6.10**

The images present a left atrial thrombus in the transthoracic echocardiographic examination of a patient with severe mitral stenosis. A free-floating thrombus in the left atrium is visualized. (A) The apical 4-chamber view shows the protrusion of the left atrial thrombus into the mitral inflow. (B) The apical 2-chamber view reveals the left atrial thrombus in the middle of the left atrial cavity. (C) Live 3D acquisition of the left atrial thrombus is shown herein.

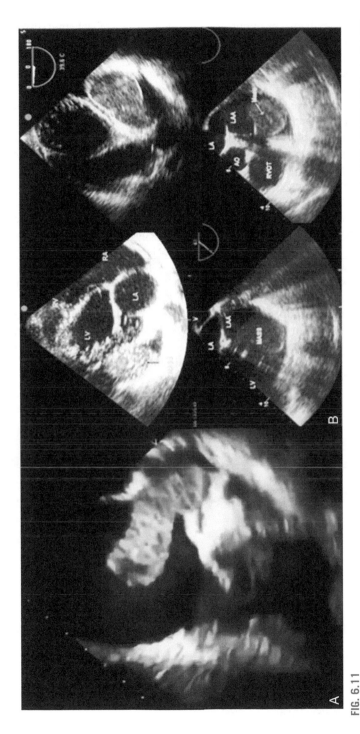

**FIG. 6.11**

(A) The transesophageal echocardiographic examination of a patient with rheumatic mitral stenosis shows a large, oval-shaped mobile clot in the LAA protruding into the LA (Supplementary Video 6.3). (B) The upper panel presents transthoracic echocardiography and the lower panel transesophageal echocardiography. The image reveals a huge LAA aneurysm or diverticulum with a large, heterogeneous well-defined mass (*arrow*), measuring 5.5 cm × 4.5 cm, attached to the body of the LAA. The mass is suggestive of a thrombus or a primary tumor. The patient underwent surgery, and the pathology results revealed a fresh thrombus. *LA*, left atrium; *LAA*, left atrial appendage.

Cardiac thromboemboli may be implicated in more than 15% of ischemic strokes, and the left atrial appendage may be the site of more than 90% of thrombi originating in the left atrium. Fifty percent of left atrial thrombi occur in patients with rheumatic valvular disease, and nearly 90% of left atrial thrombi in patients with nonvalvular atrial fibrillation are limited to the left atrial appendage. TEE findings associated with the increased risk of thromboembolism include left atrial and left atrial appendage smoke, decreased left atrial appendage emptying velocity, left atrial enlargement, increased severity of mitral stenosis, and multiple left atrial appendage lobes. A left atrial appendage emptying velocity of less than 40 cm/s is associated with the increased risk of spontaneous echo contrast. As this velocity decreases below 20 cm/s, there is an even greater risk of visual left atrial appendage and thromboembolism. Patients with mitral stenosis in sinus rhythm should be treated with anticoagulation therapy if they have a history of paroxysmal atrial fibrillation, left atrial appendage thrombi, previous embolism, spontaneous echo contrast seen on TEE, or a left atrial diameter of greater than 50 mm [5].

The terms "left atrial diverticulum" and "accessory left atrial appendage" have both been used to describe structures protruding from the left atrium that have normal myocytes and are clearly different from a left atrial aneurysm. The incidence rate of left atrial diverticulum/accessory appendage is between 10% and 23%. This condition is thought to be associated with ectopic foci that initiate atrial fibrillation, incomplete ablation lines on the left atrial roof, and potential complications such as thrombus formation and cardiac tamponade during atrial fibrillation ablation [6] (Supplementary Video 6.3 in the online version at https://doi.org/10.1016/B978-0-323-84906-7.00030-3).

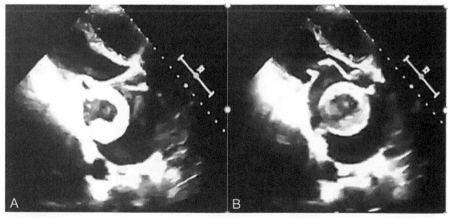

**FIG. 6.12**

The images demonstrate a ball valve left atrial thrombus in the transthoracic echocardiographic examination of a patient with a history of severe rheumatic mitral stenosis. The large ball valve thrombosis, which floats freely in the left atrium with central liquefaction, is demonstrated in the systole (A) and the diastole (B).

Left atrial ball thrombi appear to be an unusual occurrence in mitral stenosis. Symptoms are dyspnea, syncope, peripheral arterial embolism, and sudden cardiac death. The physical examination is the same as that for mitral stenosis. TEE has been recommended as the best choice for identifying the presence of left atrial thrombi and for guiding further therapy designed to reduce the thromboembolic risk. The presence of free-floating thrombi may be expected to indicate a higher embolic potential. Anticoagulation and thrombolytic therapies do not appear to have a role in the acute management of left atrial ball thrombi, although the importance of anticoagulation in the prevention of recurrence is obvious. Surgical removal of the thrombus with the simultaneous treatment of the underlying cause is the first choice treatment with good results in most cases (Tables 6.13 and 6.14).

**Table 6.13** Welch diagnostic criteria for ball valve thrombosis.

| Welch diagnostic criteria for ball valve thrombosis |
| --- |
| 1. Entire absence of the attachment of the thrombus with consequent free mobility |
| 2. Imprisonment in consequence of an excess in the diameter of the first narrowing in the circulatory passage ahead of it |

**Table 6.14** Classification of left atrial thrombi [7].

| Classification of left atrial thrombi |
| --- |
| Ia: Thrombi confined to the left atrial appendage |
| Ib: Thrombi in the left atrial appendage protruding into the left atrial cavity |
| IIa: Thrombi attached to the left atrial roof but above the plane of the fossa ovalis |
| IIb: Thrombi reaching below the plane of the fossa ovalis |
| III: Thrombi attached to the interatrial septum |
| IV: Mobile thrombi with attachment to the interatrial septum or the left atrial wall |
| V: Ball valve thrombosis |

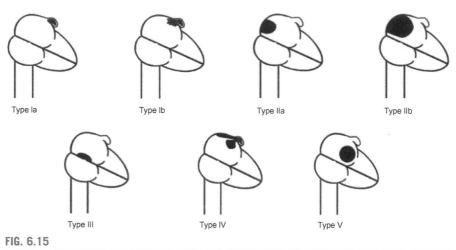

**FIG. 6.15**

The images depict the classification of left atrial thrombi.

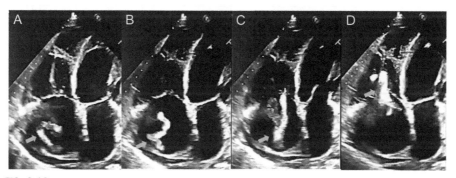

**FIG. 6.16**

The images illustrate a worm-shaped right atrial thrombus. The orange arrows point to a large, elongated, worm-shaped, highly mobile mass in the right atrium in the systole (A and B) that protrudes into the right ventricle in the diastole (C and D). Enlargement of the right and left ventricles is suggestive of hemodynamically significant pulmonary emboli (Supplementary Video 6.4).

Right heart thrombi comprise an uncommon condition found in about 4% of patients with pulmonary emboli. They are often found in transit, originating from a systemic vein source; nonetheless, they may also form within the cardiac chambers from primary processes such as atrial fibrillation. Right heart thrombi are associated with significantly increased mortality, with rates reported to range from 27% to 45% despite treatment and rates approaching 100% in untreated patients. The treatment options include anticoagulation, thrombolysis, and surgical thrombectomy [8] (Tables 6.17 and 6.18, Supplementary Video 6.4 in the online version at https://doi.org/10.1016/B978-0-323-84906-7.00030-3).

**Table 6.17** Right heart thrombus morphology [2].

| Right heart thrombus morphology | | | |
|---|---|---|---|
| **Characteristics** | **Type A** | **Neither (AB)** | **Type B** |
| Shape | Worm-like | Mixed | Round |
| Mobility | +++ | +/++ | −/+ |
| Deep vein thrombosis | Likely | Unknown | Rare |
| Right heart pathology | Absent | Unknown | Present |
| Pulmonary emboli (any) | 100% | Unknown | 40% |
| Pulmonary emboli (fatal) | 27% | | 0% |

**Table 6.18** Risk factors for right heart thrombi [2].

| **Patients** | **Diseases** | **Devices** | **Drugs** |
|---|---|---|---|
| Hypercoagulable state (protein C/S deficiency) Age at thrombophilia (≥65 y) Male Trauma/surgery Obesity Immobility Pregnancy | Cardiomyopathy Congestive heart failure Malignancy Atrial fibrillation/flutter Right ventricular infarct Hemodialysis Chronic obstructive pulmonary disease Arrhythmogenic right ventricular dysplasia/cardiomyopathy Cor pulmonale Inflammatory bowel disease Behçet | Central venous catheters (size, type) Pacemaker (especially temporary) Peripheral catheters size Internal jugular location Subclavian location Duration (>6 d) Distal position Multiple peripheral or central lines | Amphotericin B Total parenteral nutrition No prophylaxis Cigarettes Contraceptives |

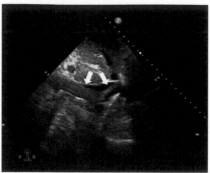
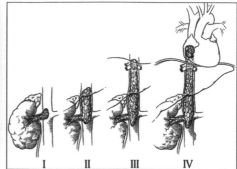

**FIG. 6.19**

The images demonstrate a snake thrombus in the inferior vena cava in the transthoracic echocardiographic examination of a patient with renal cell carcinoma. The subcostal view (*left*) reveals a large snake-like thrombus extending from the inferior vena cava to the right atrium (*white arrows*). The schematic illustration of the tumor in the inferior vena cava (*right*) shows the four categories of tumor thrombi based on the surgical technique and the dissection extent needed to remove the thrombi [9].

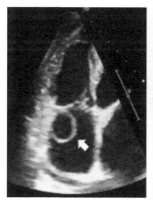
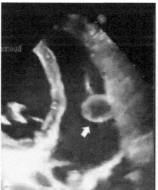
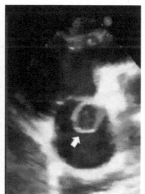

**FIG. 6.20**

The images depict a right atrial thrombus with central necrosis in transthoracic echocardiography. A round, semimobile, well-defined cystic mass (*white arrow*) is attached to the atrial side of the base of the anterior leaflet of the tricuspid valve. The mass is a right atrium thrombus with central vacuolization in an atypical site.

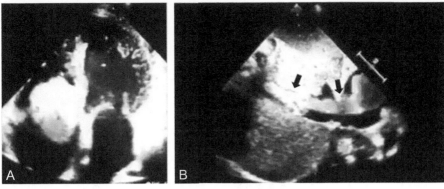

**FIG. 6.21**

The images reveal an extensive tumor thrombus in the transthoracic echocardiographic examination of a patient with prostate cancer. The subcostal view (B) shows a large thrombus extending from the inferior vena cava to the right atrium (*black arrows*). The apical 4-chamber view (A) shows the free-floating part of the thrombus in the right atrium. Given the significant risk of pulmonary thromboemboli, the patient was scheduled for surgery.

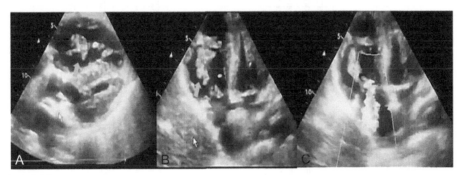

**FIG. 6.22**

(A and B) Transthoracic echocardiography shows a large, heterogeneous irregular mass in a dilated right ventricle, indicative of a thrombus in the setting of massive pulmonary emboli. (C) Moderate tricuspid regurgitation is visualized.

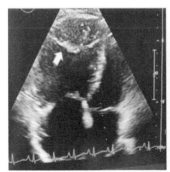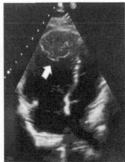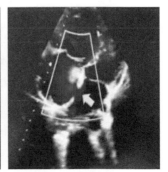

**FIG. 6.23**

The images demonstrate a right ventricular apex thrombus in the transthoracic echocardiographic examination of a 27-year-old woman presenting with dyspnea on exertion of long duration. The images show a secundum type atrial septal defect (*yellow arrow*), severe right ventricular dilation, severe right ventricular dysfunction, and severe pulmonary hypertension. The important and unusual finding is a large right ventricular apical clot (*white arrow*).

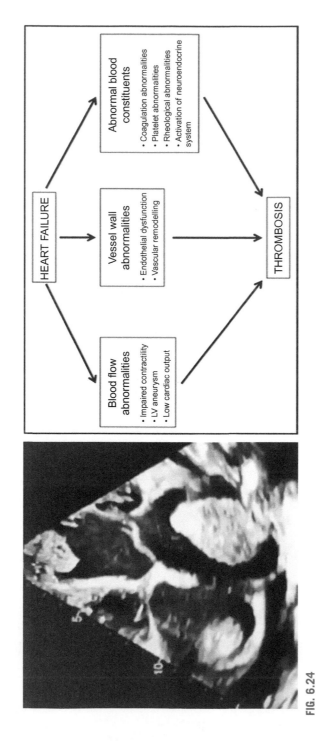

**FIG. 6.24**

The image reveals multiple large clots in end-stage cardiomyopathy in the transthoracic echocardiographic examination of a patient with end-stage cardiomyopathy with severely reduced left and right ventricular dysfunction. Severe spontaneous echo contrast is visualized in all cardiac chambers with multiple clots. The algorithm (*right*) shows the assumed pathophysiology in the development of cardiac thrombi during heart failure [10].

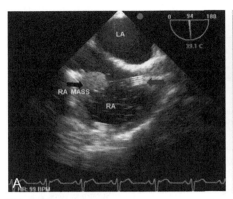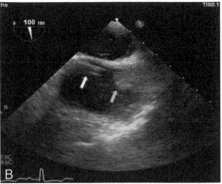

**FIG. 6.25**

The images illustrate a device/catheter-associated RA thrombus. (A) The transesophageal echocardiographic examination of a patient with cancer shows a round, well-defined mass in the RA (*black arrow*) on the tip of the chemotherapy catheter (*red arrow*), which is a thrombus. (B) The transesophageal echocardiographic examination of a 32-year-old woman on hemodialysis with the catheter in the superior vena cava, performed after insufficiency of the catheter, shows complete occlusion in the superior vena cava by thrombosis, which is extended into the RA. The white arrow points to another dialysis catheter, implanted from the femoral vein into the inferior vena cava and the RA. *LA*, left atrium; *RA*, right atrium.

Central venous catheters are frequently used in patients with end-stage renal disease or cancer. The reported incidence rate for catheter-associated right atrial thrombosis varies between 2% and 29%. Potential mortality associated with catheter-associated right atrial thrombosis has been reported to be as high as 18% in hemodialysis patients and greater than 40% in nonhemodialysis patients. There are 2 types of catheter-associated right atrial thrombosis: type A and type B. Type A is mobile, is thromboembolic in nature, and has a high incidence of emboli as well as a high mortality rate by comparison with type B. Type B forms around foreign bodies in the right atrium. The pathogenesis for type B catheter-associated right atrial thrombosis includes mechanical irritation of the right atrial wall, intraluminal clot elongation, hypercoagulability in patients on hemodialysis, and fluid dynamics of the right atrium.

Catheter-associated right atrial thrombosis is an underreported phenomenon because not only are some patients entirely asymptomatic at presentation but also the diagnostic accuracy of TEE may be limited if the catheter tip is proximal in the superior vena cava. In suspected cases, TEE and CMR with gadolinium contrast can also be useful tools for diagnosis and tissue characterization.

Oral/systemic anticoagulation, surgical thrombectomy (open-heart, percutaneous), and thrombolysis are reported treatment options for catheter-associated right atrial thrombosis. All modalities should be combined with the removal of central venous catheters after an initial period of anticoagulation [11] (Algorithm 6.26, Supplementary Video 6.5 in the online version at https://doi.org/10.1016/B978-0-323-84906-7.00030-3).

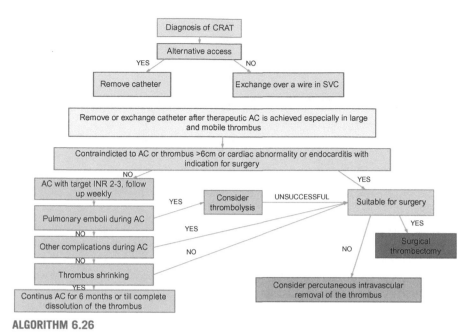

**ALGORITHM 6.26**

The image presents the management algorithm in CRAT. *CRAT*, catheter-associated right atrial thrombosis; *SVC*, superior vena cava; *AC*, anticoagulant; *INR*, international normalized ratio.

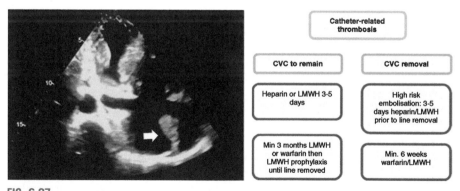

**FIG. 6.27**

The image demonstrates catheter-related thrombosis in the transthoracic echocardiographic examination of a patient early after valvular surgery. The right ventricular inflow view (*left*) shows a large, worm-like thrombus extending from the superior vena cava to the right atrium (*white arrow*). The proposed algorithm for the approach to catheter-related thrombosis (*right*) based on the choice between catheter removal and nonremoval is presented herein (Supplementary Video 6.5) [12,13]. *CVC*, central venous catheter; *LMWH*, low molecular weight heparin.

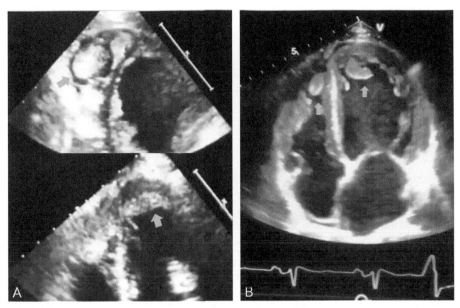

**FIG. 6.28**

The images reveal biventricular thrombi in the transthoracic echocardiographic examination of two patients with simultaneous right and left ventricular apical thrombi. (A) The patient presented with right ventricular infarction and a history of previous anterior infarction. Akinetic and thin walls are visualized in the left anterior descending artery and the right coronary artery territories. Echocardiography shows multiple clots in the right and left ventricles apex (*arrows*). (B) The patient has biventricular severe systolic dysfunction and multiple biventricular apical thrombi (*arrows*).

Biventricular thrombi complicating acute myocardial infarction are rare and are generally seen in patients with a prothrombotic state like antiphospholipid antibody syndrome, heparin-induced thrombocytopenia-induced thrombosis, and hypereosinophilic syndrome. Cases of biventricular thrombi in association with peripartum cardiomyopathy, nonischemic cardiomyopathy, dilated cardiomyopathy, myocarditis, and human immunodeficiency virus infection-induced dilated cardiomyopathy have been reported [14].

The detection of ventricular thrombi using echocardiography is sometimes difficult, as is its treatment strategy. The majority of intracardiac thrombi are detected on TTE, which is low in cost and widely available. The distinguishing characteristics of thrombi include (1) a mass with margins distinct from the endocardium; (2) a mass noted throughout the cardiac cycle and visualized in at least two orthogonal views; (3) a mass distinguishable from the papillary muscles, chordae, trabeculations, and technical artifacts; (4) characteristics consistent with avascular tissue; and (5) potential regional wall motion abnormalities.

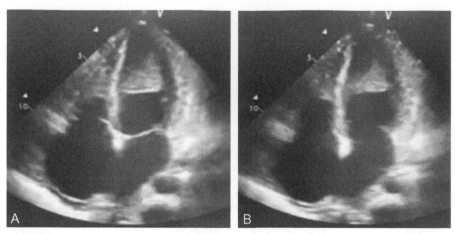

**FIG. 6.29**

The images present Löffler's syndrome. The apical 4-chamber view of transthoracic echocardiography on a patient with significant eosinophilia shows that the apices of both ventricles are filled by large thrombosis that occupies almost half the ventricles (panel A in the systole and panel B in the diastole). The most relevant differential diagnosis of this echocardiographic finding in the setting of eosinophilia is endomyocardial fibrosis (Löffler's syndrome).

The use of contrast can help nearly double the sensitivity of thrombus detection on echocardiography. In a study, the sensitivity of left ventricular thrombus detection with TTE was improved from 35% to 64% with the use of contrast. CMR is another useful tool in the diagnosis of thrombi and the most sensitive diagnostic imaging modality. There are several options for the treatment of intracardiac thrombi such as anticoagulation, thrombolysis, percutaneous retrieval, and surgical intervention [15,16].

Löffler's endocarditis is commonly characterized as a rare complication of hypereosinophilic syndrome. However, any condition causing an eosinophilic state can make patients susceptible to this condition. Eosinophil-associated cardiac injury is described as having three stages. The first stage is associated with eosinophilic infiltration, resulting in the formation of toxic cationic proteins and causing acute necrosis. This stage is mostly asymptomatic. The second stage is associated with thrombus formation. The final stage is characterized by fibrosis, resulting in restrictive cardiomyopathy. Patients with eosinophil-associated endocarditis can present with a wide array of symptoms, including dyspnea, chest pain, cough, congestive heart failure, and valvular involvement. The most involved cardiac valve is the mitral valve, resulting in mitral valve insufficiency in almost 42% of cases. It can also result in the involvement of the aortic valve, causing aortic valve stenosis and regurgitation in 4% of cases.

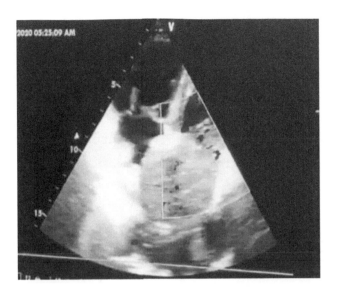

**FIG. 6.30**

The image depicts a left atrial thrombus in a patient with COVID-19. Transthoracic echocardiography shows a dilated left atrium completely occupied by thrombosis.

Echocardiographic findings suggestive of Löffler's endocarditis include endomyocardial thickening, apical thrombi, left ventricular hypertrophy, and the involvement of the mitral valve cusp, causing mitral valve regurgitation. CMR can identify injured myocardial tissue and differentiate between inflammation and fibrosis by analyzing the difference between early and late contrast enhancements. Late contrast gadolinium enhancement is pathognomonic of Löffler's endocarditis. In addition, it is more sensitive in detecting early changes in cardiac function and structure and helps identify changes that may be missed on echocardiography [17,18].

Multiple studies have proven the relationship between COVID-19 infection and coagulopathy with unknown causes. The main cause of mortality after acute respiratory distress syndrome is cardiac cavity thrombosis. The most frequent cause of thrombi in these patients can be pulmonary embolism. Hypercoagulability parameters (D-dimer and fibrinogen) are shown to be highest in most patients, reflecting hypercoagulable status in patients with COVID-19 infection.

Routine bedside TTE and a multidisciplinary approach could be sensitive in the early detection of heart thrombi, which could improve the diagnostic and therapeutic process at the right time and identify the risk of systemic or pulmonary embolism for the better management of patients with COVID-19 infection. Anticoagulation with unfractionated heparin seems to be the reasonable treatment for this rare cardiac complication of COVID-19 infection after eliminating any contraindications; additionally, it helps avoid the risk of bleeding following the use of these anticoagulants [19].

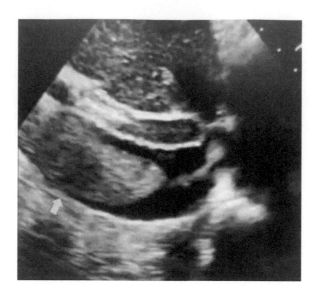

**FIG. 6.31**

The subcostal view of transthoracic echocardiography on a patient hospitalized with COVID-19 shows a plethoric inferior vena cava with a large heterogeneous mass almost extending into the right atrium, indicative of a thrombus (*yellow arrow*).

## Thrombus on cardiac computed tomography (CT)

Thrombus is the most common intracardiac mass and is caused by hypercoagulable states, wall motion abnormalities, artificial devices, or atrial fibrillation [20].

On CT imaging with contrast, thrombi appear as a filling defect within the cardiac chamber, which remains with delayed postcontrast imaging (Fig. 6.32). Left atrial thrombus appears as a round or oval filling defect, most commonly located in the atrial appendage. Pseudo-filling defects can occur with circulatory stasis because of incomplete mixing of contrast material and blood. The ratio of left atrial appendage attenuation to that of the ascending aorta of <0.75 has high sensitivity for prediction of thrombus or stasis and a ratio >0.75 has 100% negative-predictive value [21]. Although thrombi persist in early and late-phase images, pseudo-filling defects are present only on early phase images. Although there is no significant difference of the ratio of left atrial appendage attenuation to that of the ascending aorta between thrombus and stasis in the early phase, the ratio is significantly lower for thrombus ($0.29 \pm 12$) than for slow flow ($0.85 \pm 12$) in the delayed phase [22]. In the ventricles, thrombus manifests as a crescent-shaped filling defect adjacent to infarcted or dyskinetic areas (30% of patients with myocardial infarction) with attenuation less than that of the myocardium. In dilated cardiomyopathy, thrombus more often develop in the left ventricular apex. Attachment may be broad based with little to no motion on cine images [23].

Cardiac thrombus on cardiac magnetic resonance imaging (MRI)

MRI has a great potential in the diagnosis of suspected cardiac thrombi (Fig. 6.33). The signal intensity characteristics of thrombus vary at MR imaging depending on the age of the thrombus. An acute thrombus usually has intermediate signal intensity on both T1- and T2-weighted images because the hemoglobin content is still in the oxygenated state. In subacute thrombus, the hemoglobin has been metabolized to methemoglobin, which has a different paramagnetic effect (shorter T1 and T2 relaxation times), leading to a lower T1-weighted signal intensity, but T2-weighted signal intensity is usually increased due to the higher water content from lysed red blood cells (Table 6.34) [24]. Over a greater time period, thrombus becomes water depleted and the cellular debris containing

**Thrombus on cardiac computed tomography (CT)—Cont'd**

methemoglobin is replaced by fibrous tissue. This change in macromolecular composition with greater fibrin content leads to a lower signal intensity on both T1- and T2-weighted images in chronic organized thrombus (Table 6.34) [25]. Contrast-enhanced MR imaging with first-pass perfusion, EGE, or LGE imaging enables clear differentiation of, and hence characterized by an absence of contrast material uptake—rarely very chronic, organized thrombus may enhance peripherally due to its fibrous content [24,26–29].

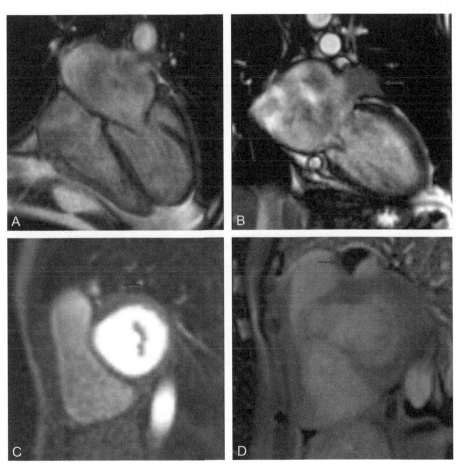

**FIG. 6.32**

A 42-year-old man with rheumatic mitral valve and reduced ejection fraction. (A and B) CMR SSFP sequence in four (A) and two (B) chamber view represents the thickened restricted mitral valve with accompanied left atrial (LA) enlargement and internal flow stagnation demonstrated as inhomogeneous signal intensity. Hypointensity (*arrow*) in LA raises suspicion for an obscured LA appendage (LAA) thrombus. (C) First-pass perfusion in short-axis view shows a filling defect in LAA. Late gadolinium enhancement sequence with high time of inversion (high TI, 600 ms) confirms the presence of a nonenhancing clot in LAA.

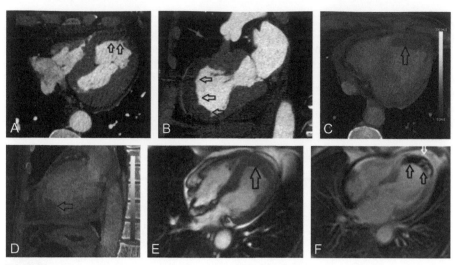

**FIG. 6.33**

Cardiac CT angiography with dual-phase and dual-energy acquisition technique. Prospective ECG-gated cardiac CT angiography (A and B) reveals aneurysmal dilatation of left ventricle apex with filling defect (*arrow*) which is isodense to myocardium. Non-ECG-gated dual-energy cardiac CT (C and D) acquisition by dual source machine demonstrates hypodense nonenhancing mass (*arrow*) in LV apex and thin wall LV apex. (E and F) Cardiac magnetic resonance (CMR). Four-chamber cine SSFP sequence (E) represents dilatation of apex and low signal mass in apex (*black arrow*). Four-chamber late gadolinium enhancement (LGE) sequence (F) displays low signal mass in LV apex (*black arrow*) and transmural LGE (*white arrow*) due to myocardial infarction [Movie Online].

**Table 6.34** Cardiac MR imaging signal intensity characteristics for thrombus.

| Age of thrombus | T1-w signal intensity | T2-w signal intensity | Late gadolinium enhancement |
|---|---|---|---|
| Acute | High | High | No enhancement |
| Subacute | High | Low | No enhancement |
| Chronic | Low | Low | No enhancement or may reveal peripheral enhancement in chronic organized thrombus |

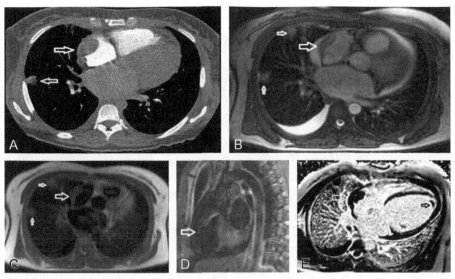

**FIG. 6.35**

This figure shows subacute thrombosis of right atrium. The patient had a history of malignancy and a chief complaint of chest pain admitted to the emergency department. Echocardiography showed a mass lesion in the right atrium. (A) Cardiac CT image demonstrated hypodense lesion in posterolateral wall of RA and without enhancement (*white arrow*). Peripheral opacities are seen in the right lung (*yellow arrows*), suggestive for pulmonary infarction. Cardiac magnetic resonance images displayed: Cine SSFP sequence (B) image showed an isolow signal mass lesion in RA. Images reveal an isohigh signal mass in T1 W sequence (C) and low signal mass in STIR sequence (D) image in RA. Late gadolinium enhancement sequence (E) with TI: 500 demonstrated a low signal mass in RA (*white arrow*) and apex of LV (*black arrow*) [Movie Online].

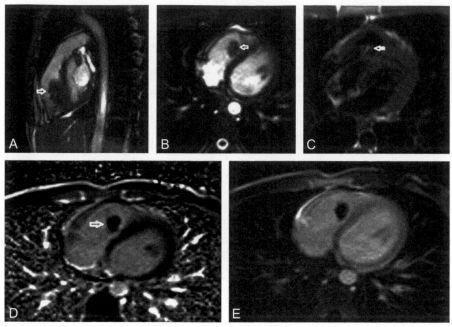

**FIG. 6.36**

CMR displays right ventricular thrombi (arrows) in a middle-aged patient. (A and B) Cine SSFP sequence shows iso signal filling defect in RV cavity and RVOT in a 4-chamber view. (C) Four-chamber view T1-W sequence, iso to hyper signal filling defect in RV cavity. (D) Four-chamber view PSIR late gadolinium enhancement (LGE) sequence, low signal filling defect in RV cavity without enhancement [Movie Online].

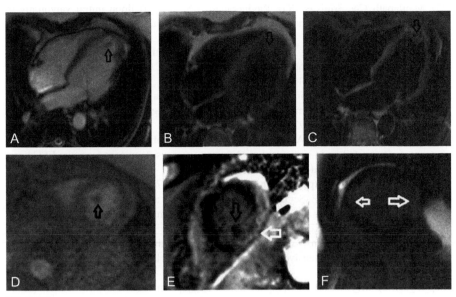

**FIG. 6.37**

Cardiac magnetic resonance imaging shows left ventricular thrombosis (*black arrow*) in a patient with history of coronary artery disease. (A) Iso to low signal filling defect in cavity, axial cine SSFP sequence. (B) Iso to high signal filling defect, axial T1-w sequence. (C) Iso signal filling defect, axial STIR sequence. (D) Low signal lesion in perfusion sequence. (E and F) Low signal intracavity lesion (*black arrow*), short-axis late gadolinium enhancement (LGE) sequence. Transmural and subendocardial LGE in apicoseptal and apicolateral segments of LV due to myocardial infarction.

## References

[1] Lichtenberger JP, Reynolds DA, Keung J, et al. Metastasis to the heart: a radiologic approach to diagnosis with pathologic correlation. Am J Roentgenol 2016;207. https://doi.org/10.2214/AJR.16.16148.

[2] Yingchoncharoen T, Klein AL. Introduction to echocardiographic assessment of cardiac tumors and masses, https://thoracickey.com.

[3] Massussi M, Scotti A, Lip G, et al. Left ventricular thrombosis: new perspectives on an old problem. Eur Heart J 2021;7(2):158–67. https://doi.org/10.1093/ehjcvp/pvaa066.

[4] Agarwal G, Kumar V, Srinivas KH, et al. Left ventricular intramyocardial dissecting hematomas. JACC Case Rep 2021;3(1):94–8. https://doi.org/10.1016/j.jaccas.2020.07.038.

[5] Gorbaty BJ, Perelman S, Applebaum RM. Left atrial appendage thrombus formation after perioperative cardioversion in the setting of severe rheumatic mitral stenosis. J Cardiothorac Vasc Anesth 2020. https://doi.org/10.1053/j.jvca.2020.04.027.

[6] Nagai T, Fujii A, Nishimura K, et al. Large thrombus originating from left atrial diverticulum, a new concern for catheter ablation of atrial fibrillation. Circulation 2011;124: 1086–8. https://doi.org/10.1161/CIRCULATIONAHA.110.000315Circulation.

[7] Manjunath CN, Srinivasa KH, Ravindranath KS, et al. Balloon mitral valvotomy in patients with mitral stenosis and left atrial thrombus. Catheter Cardiovasc Interv 2009;74:653–61.

[8] Lai E, Alishetti S, Wong JM, et al. Right ventricular thrombus in transit: raising the stakes in the management of pulmonary embolism. CASE 2019;3(6):272–6. https://doi.org/10.1016/j.case.2019.05.006.

[9] Nesbitt JC, Soltero ER, Dinney CPN, et al. Surgical management of renal cell carcinoma with inferior vena cava tumor thrombus. Ann Thorac Surg 1997;63(6):1592–600. https://doi.org/10.1016/S0003-4975(97)00329-9.

[10] Lip GYH, Ponikowski P, Andreotti F, et al. Thrombo-embolism and antithrombotic therapy for heart failure in sinus rhythm. A joint consensus document from the ESC heart failure association and the ESC working group on thrombosis. Eur J Heart Fail 2012;14(7):681–95. https://doi.org/10.1093/eurjhf/hfs073.

[11] Hussain N, Shattuck PE, Senussi MH, et al. Large right atrial Thrombus associated with central venous catheter requiring open heart surgery. In: Hindawi case reports in medicine; 2012. https://doi.org/10.1155/2012/501303.

[12] Algorithm adapted from Wall C, Moore J, Thachil J. Catheter-related thrombosis: a practical approach. J Intensive Care Soc 2016;17(2):160–7. https://doi.org/10.1177/1751143715618683.

[13] Ziyaeifard M, Alizadehasl A, Aghdaii N, et al. Heparinized and saline solutions in the maintenance of arterial and central venous catheters after cardiac surgery. Anesth Pain Med 2015;5(4). https://doi.org/10.5812/aapm28056. PMID: 26478866; PMCID: PMC4604422, e28056.

[14] Sanghvi S, Baroopal A, Sardac P. Biventricular thrombi complicating acute myocardial infarction. Indian Heart J 2016;68(Suppl. 2):S102–4. https://doi.org/10.1016/j.ihj.2016.02.020.

[15] Jacobson AM, Darrah JR. Biventricular thrombi in substance-induced dilated cardiomyopathy. CASE 2020;4(3):170–4. https://doi.org/10.1016/j.case.2020.01.007.

[16] Sadeghpour A, Alizaeasl A. The right ventricle: a comprehensive review from anatomy, physiology, and mechanics to hemodynamic, functional, and imaging evaluation. Arch Cardiovasc Imaging 2015;3:4. https://doi.org/10.5812/acvi.35717.

[17] Afzal S, Ahmed T, Saleem T, et al. Loeffler's endocarditis and the diagnostic utility of multimodality imaging. Cureus 2020;12(8). https://doi.org/10.7759/cureus.10061, e10061.

[18] Maleki M, Alizadehasl A, Haghjoo M. Practical cardiology. 2nd ed. Elsevier; 2021.

[19] Aidouni GE, Merbouh M, Aabdi M, et al. Intra cardiac thrombus in critically ill patient with coronavirus disease 2019: case report. Ann Med Surg 2021;66. https://doi.org/10.1016/j.amsu.2021.102434, 102434.

[20] Rajiah P, Kanne JP, Kalahasti V, et al. Computed tomography of cardiac and pericardiac masses. J Cardiovasc Comput Tomogr 2011;5:16–2911.

[21] Patel A, Au E, Donegan K, et al. Multi-detector row computed tomography for identification of left atrial appendage filling defects in patients undergoing pulmonary vein isolation for treatment of atrial fibrillation; comparison with transesophageal echocardiography. Heart Rhythm 2008;5:253–60.

[22] Hur J, Kim JY, Lee HJ, et al. Left atrial appendage thrombi in stroke patients: detection with two-phase cardiac CT angiography versus transesophageal echocardiography. Radiology 2009;251:683–90.

[23] Tatlli S, Lipton MJ. CT for intracardiac thrombi and tumors. Int J Cardiovasc Imaging 2005;21:115–31.

[24] Paydarfar D, Krieger D, Dib N, et al. In vivo magnetic resonance imaging and surgical histopathology of intracardiac masses: distinct features of subacute thrombi. Cardiology 2001;95(1):40–7.

[25] Motwani M, Kidambi A, Herzog BA, et al. MR imaging of cardiac tumors and masses: a review of methods and clinical applications. Radiology 2013;268(1).

[26] Mollet NR, Dymarkowski S, Volders W, et al. Visualization of ventricular thrombi with contrast-enhanced magnetic resonance imaging in patients with ischemic heart disease. Circulation 2002;106(23):2873–6.

[27] Alizadehasl A, Parsa NA, Azarfarin R, et al. Innovations in cardiovascular imaging. Trends Cardiovasc Med 2021;3. https://doi.org/10.1016/j.tcm.2021.01.007. S1050-1738(21)00014-1.

[28] Rezaei-Kalantari K, Saedi S, Alizadeasl A, et al. Left ventricular intra-myocardial dissection after myocardial infarction. Echocardiography 2020. https://doi.org/10.1111/echo.14843.

[29] Naghavi B, Alizadehasl A, Sadeghipour P, et al. Clinical and imaging predictors of recovery in patient with pulmonary emboli. Eur Heart J 2020;41. https://doi.org/10.1093/ehjci/chaa946.2249, chaa946.2249.

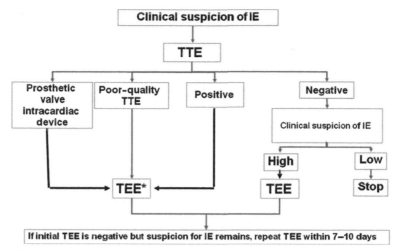

**ALGORITHM 7.1**

The image depicts the approach to IE [1]. *IE*, infective endocarditis; *TTE*, transthoracic echocardiography; *TEE*, transesophageal echocardiography.

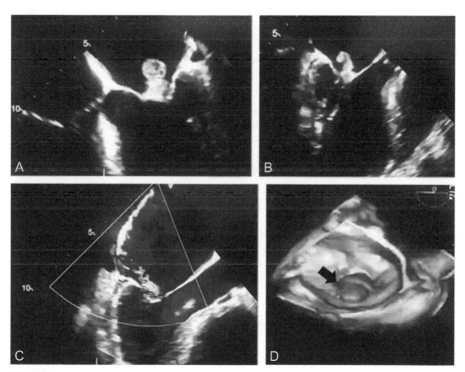

**FIG. 7.2**

Transesophageal echocardiography in a patient with mitral valve endocarditis shows a large, mobile, shaggy, bizarre-shaped mass on the anterior mitral valve leaflet (A and B), which has resulted in the malapposition of the leaflets and a severe, eccentric-jet, posterolaterally directed mitral regurgitation (C). A 3D zoom reconstruction of the mitral valve mass is depicted in section (D, *black arrow*). The mass characteristics and clinical findings are compatible with infective endocarditis, as documented by *Staphylococcus aureus* growth in postsurgical specimen growth.

# Infectious lesions mimicking cardiac masses

7

**Azin Alizadehasl[a], Kiara Rezaei-Kalantari[b], and Shirin Habibi Khorasani[a]**

[a]*Cardio-Oncology Research Center, Rajaie Cardiovascular Medical and Research Center, Iran University of Medical Sciences, Tehran, Iran* [b]*Department of Radiology, CardioOncology Research Center, Iran University of Medical Sciences, Rajaie Cardiovascular Medical and Research Center, Tehran, Iran*

## Key points

- Vegetations are oscillating or nonoscillating intracardiac masses on the valves or other endocardial structures or intracardiac implanted materials.
- Vegetations are typically located on the upstream side of the valves, are usually irregularly and grotesquely shaped, and exhibit disordered motions that are not in pattern with the excursion of the valve leaflets.
- Abscesses are thick, nonhomogeneous, echolucent, or echodense perivalvular areas.
- Three echocardiographic findings are considered to be major criteria for the diagnosis of endocarditis: (1) the presence of vegetations, (2) the presence of abscesses, and (3) the presence of new dehiscence in a valvular prosthesis (Algorithm 7.1, Figs. 7.2–7.4, Tables 7.5 and 7.6, Figs. 7.7–7.9, Table 7.10).
- Any component of the heart is vulnerable to be involved by hydatid cysts, with the presentation depending on the location, size, and integrity of the cyst (Figs. 7.11–7.18, Tables 7.19–7.21).

Multimodal Imaging Atlas of Cardiac Masses. https://doi.org/10.1016/B978-0-323-84906-7.00006-6

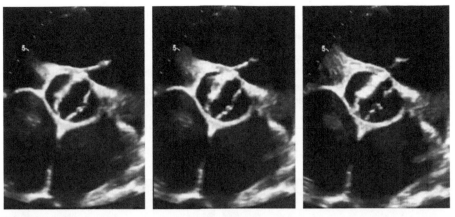

**FIG. 7.3**

The image illustrates the transesophageal echocardiographic examination of a patient with a bicuspid aortic valve (mediolateral orientation). There is a shaggy, semimobile echodensity attached to the tip of the medial leaflet (B, *white arrow*). The valve is destructed with the perforation and flail of the lateral leaflet (C, *white arrow*).

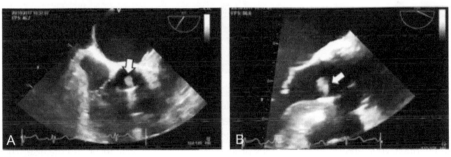

**FIG. 7.4**

Transesophageal echocardiography in a patient with aortic bioprosthesis shows a large, semimobile, oval-shaped echodensity on the right cusp of the aortic bioprosthesis *(white arrows)*. The postsurgical specimen confirmed fungal endocarditis with *Candida albicans* [2].

**Table 7.5** Risk factors for fungal endocarditis.

| Risk factors for fungal endocarditis |
| --- |
| Intravenous drug abuse |
| Prolonged antibiotic therapy |
| Prolonged indwelling central venous catheter |
| Prosthetic heart valve |
| Previous history of endocarditis |
| Parenteral nutrition |
| Neutropenia |
| Diabetes mellitus |

**Table 7.6** Clinical significance of fungal endocarditis.

**Clinical significance of fungal endocarditis**

Fungal endocarditis is a very devastating disease

Timely diagnosis is the key, because it presents mostly with general constitutional symptoms; high index of suspicion is required for early diagnosis. Induction treatment followed by suppressive therapy (in selected patients) is key to management

Surgical replacement of the infected valve is a class I recommendation

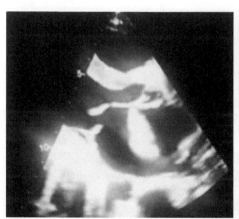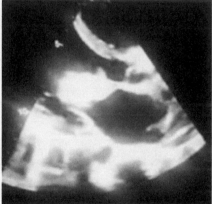

**FIG. 7.7**

Transthoracic echocardiography in the parasternal long-axis view shows a large, hypermobile, oval-shaped, hyper echo mass attached to the atrial side of the base of the anterior mitral valve leaflet, which protrudes into the left ventricle in the diastole. The mass is a large fungal vegetation in an intravenous drug abuser presenting with fever and malaise. The mass has a high probability for endocarditis complications, including valve destruction, mitral stenosis, regurgitation, abscess formation, and systemic embolism (Supplementary Video 7. S1 in the online version at https://doi.org/10.1016/B978-0-323-84906-7.00006-6). Fungi account for fewer than 10% of infective endocarditis cases, with native valve fungal endocarditis being even less common. Approximately, 24% of fungal endocarditis cases are caused by *Candida albicans*. It is usually seen in patients with valvular disease, intravenous drug use, indwelling vascular lines, or immunocompromised states. Echocardiography cannot distinguish fungal vegetations from other microorganisms definitely; nevertheless, a dense, hyperechoic, large mass ($\approx$ 2 cm) in the relevant clinical setting can be in favor of a fungal vegetation. Overall, patients with fungal endocarditis have a poor prognosis, and left-sided fungal endocarditis, acute heart failure, and exclusive medical treatment are independent risk factors for mortality [3].

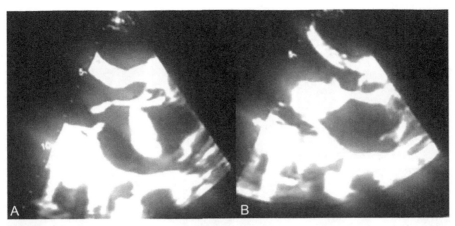

**FIG. 7.8**

The figures reveal tricuspid valve infective endocarditis in transthoracic echocardiography. (A) Echocardiography in the apical 4-chamber view in a 38-year-old woman on hemodialysis presenting with prolonged fever shows a shaggy, mobile vegetation on the tricuspid valve oscillating between the right ventricle and the right atrium. (B) Echocardiography in the parasternal short-axis view in a young intravenous drug abuser reveals tricuspid valve vegetations. The differential diagnosis of these vegetations is the tricuspid valve tumor.

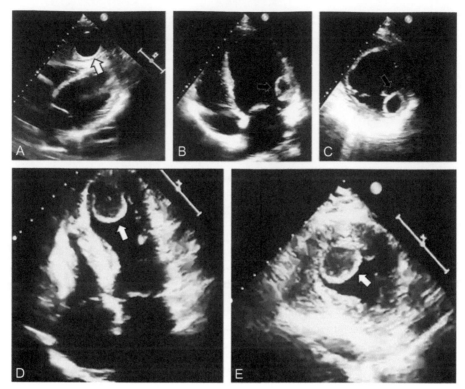

**FIG. 7.9**

Transesophageal echocardiography in 2 patients with hydatid cysts. There is a large, round-shaped cystic mass, with an echolucent center attached to the base of the left ventricular lateral wall (B and C, *black arrows*). This mass is accompanied by a similar lesion in the liver (A, *white arrow*), which suggests cardiac and hepatic hydatid cysts. A large, globular cystic lesion with a central opacity is seen attached to the left ventricular apicoseptal segment, in favor of a hydatid cyst with a daughter cyst within it. Cardiac hydatid cysts are uncommon, with the dominant involvement of the left ventricle. The cysts may grow and lead to compression effects on the adjacent myocardium, resulting in coronary vessel involvement, rhythm disturbances, and interference with valvular and ventricular function. Echocardiography is the method of choice for the assessment of cardiac hydatidosis [4].

**Table 7.10** Localization of cardiac hydatid cysts (%).

| Localization of cardiac hydatid cysts (%) | |
| --- | --- |
| Left ventricle | 60 |
| Right ventricle | 10 |
| Pericardium | 7 |
| Left atrium | 6–8 |
| Right atrium | 3–4 |
| Interventricular septum | 4 |

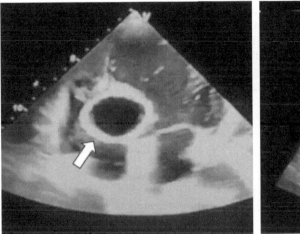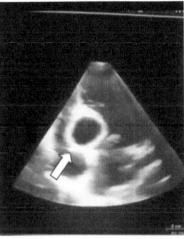

**FIG. 7.11**

The images demonstrate hydatid cysts in the upper interventricular septum. Transthoracic echocardiography in a patient with a hydatid cyst in the upper interventricular septum. There is a large, round-shaped cystic mass, with an echolucent center attached to the base of the interventricular septum *(white arrows)*. The initial manifestation of this patient was a complete heart block, which is one of the rare complications of the interventricular septum hydatid cyst. Echocardiography is a preferred and effective modality for the diagnosis of cardiac hydatidosis. This modality shows the cysts, their locations in the interventricular septum, their number, and their size, as well as the hemodynamic compromise and eventual complications such as pericardial effusion. The coronary circulation is the main pathway by which the parasitic larvae reach the heart. Cardiac involvement through the pulmonary veins has also been reported. Due to the rich coronary blood supply, the left ventricular wall is the most common cardiac location (60%), followed by the right ventricle (10%), the pericardium (7%), the left atrium (6%–8%), and the right atrium (3%–4%). The interventricular septum is less frequently involved. It is reported in just 4% of cardiac cases [5].

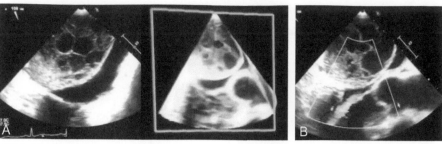

**FIG. 7.12**

The images depict a large left atrial hydatid cyst visualized by transesophageal echocardiography (109°) in a 61-year-old male traveler presenting with chest pain and dyspnea on exertion. (A) Studies in 2D and 3D reveal a large, round, spongy mass in the left atrium consisting of multiple echolucent, round components. The feature is typical of a large hydatid cyst, confirmed by pathology. (B) Diastolic turbulence over the mitral valve is indicative of the compressive effect of the mass, resulting in functional mitral stenosis, the most probable reason for the patient's symptoms (Supplementary Video 7.S2 in the online version at https://doi.org/10.1016/B978-0-323-84906-7.00006-6).

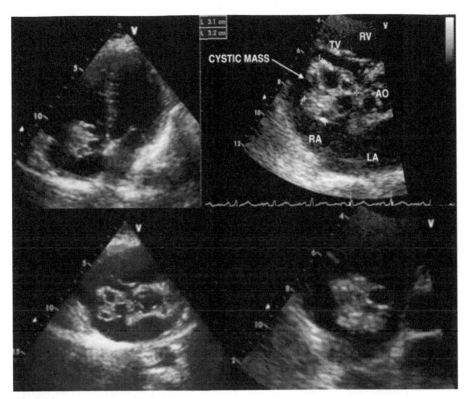

**FIG. 7.13**

The images present a hydatid cyst in the right ventricle. Transesophageal echocardiography shows a large cystic mass in the right ventricle in a 51-year-old woman presenting with dyspnea. The mass measures 3.1 cm × 3.2 cm in size and is located adjacent to the tricuspid valve. It protrudes into the right ventricle in the diastole, resulting in tricuspid regurgitation and moderate pulmonary hypertension. The feature of the mass is suggestive of cardiac hydatidosis (confirmed by pathology).

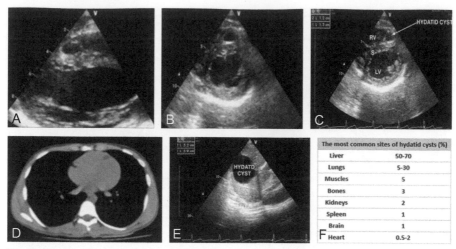

| The most common sites of hydatid cysts (%) | |
| --- | --- |
| Liver | 50-70 |
| Lungs | 5-30 |
| Muscles | 5 |
| Bones | 3 |
| Kidneys | 2 |
| Spleen | 1 |
| Brain | 1 |
| Heart | 0.5-2 |

**FIG. 7.14**

The images depict a hydatid cyst in the right ventricle (A, B, and C). The apical long-axis and apical short-axis views of transthoracic echocardiography in a patient show a solitary, round, echolucent cystic mass in the right ventricular apex, suggestive of a hydatid cyst. The mass measures 1.2 cm × 1.3 cm in size. (D) Thoracic computed tomography scan confirms the cystic mass of the right ventricular apex. (E) The interrogation of the liver shows an associated finding: a large, hepatic hydatid cyst, which is a supporting finding for the cardiac finding of a hydatid cyst. (F) The most common sites of hydatid cysts are the liver (50%–70%), lungs (5%–30%), muscles (5%), bones (3%), kidneys (2%), spleen (1%), and brain (1%). Cardiac echinococcosis is an uncommon disease, with an estimated prevalence ranging from 0.5% to 2% [5].

Two-dimensional echocardiography is the first-line test of choice to make the diagnosis of a cardiac hydatid cyst, with greater than 90% sensitivity. It is a quick, highly sensitive, noninvasive imaging modality that can demonstrate the presence of cardiac masses and characterize cysts using ultrasound. The use of an ultrasound-enhancing agent may be helpful to clearly delineate the location and size of the mass. Furthermore, it can determine whether the cyst is enclosed or ruptured, whether it is communicating with the blood supply within the heart, and whether it is vascularized. Patients with exposure to or the presence of echinococcosis in any part of the body should undergo assessment using echocardiography of their heart and major vessels [6].

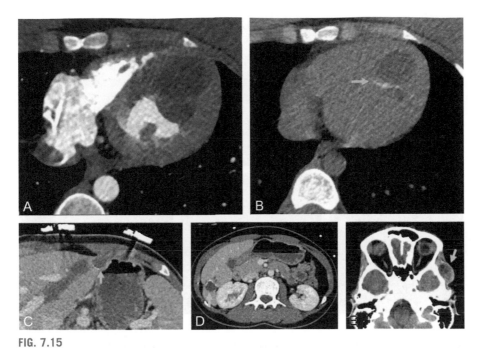

**FIG. 7.15**

A 21-year-old female with a bilobed cystic lesion in left ventricular cavity (A). Unenhanced CT (B) depicts the partial faint calcification of the cyst wall, characteristic for hydatid cyst. Abdominal (C and D) and brain CT scan reveal other lesion *(arrows)* with the same feature scattered in liver and subcutaneous temporal fossa.

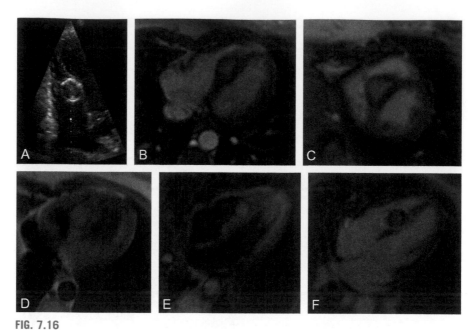

**FIG. 7.16**

A 42-year-old female for whom echocardiography (A) reported a round interventricular septum mass with peripheral echogenic wall bulging toward the right ventricular cavity suggestive of a hydatid cyst. Steady-state free precession (SSFP) sequence of the CMR demonstrates the well-defined somewhat thick-wall cystic lesion with homogeneous internal material which show high T1-weighted (D) and STIR (E) intensity likely due to the high proteinaceous content. The ring-like reactive capsular peripheral of the lesion in late gadolinium enhancement (LGE) sequence (F) is compatible with the diagnosis of hydatid cyst.

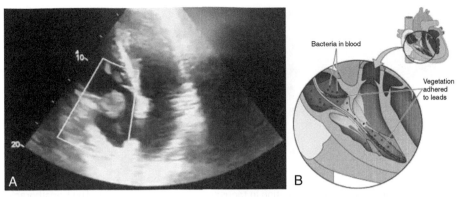

**FIG. 7.17**

The image presents permanent pacemaker-associated infective endocarditis.
(A) Transthoracic echocardiography in the apical 4-chamber view in a patient with a history of permanent pacemaker implantation presenting with long-standing fever after COVID-19 infection shows a round, heterogeneous mass attached to the right ventricular lead of the permanent pacemaker. Given the patient's history, the echocardiographic finding is mostly a large vegetation, but thrombosis is the differential diagnosis. (B) A schematic figure of the vegetations on the right ventricular and right atrial leads is presented herein.

Transesophageal echocardiography is most often required to detect lead vegetations. Mostly, local pocket infections have smaller vegetations, whereas larger vegetations are more commonly associated with the signs of systemic illness. The guidelines of the American Heart Association and the Heart Rhythm Society recommend complete device removal with a prolonged course of antibiotics in any patient with cardiac implantable electronic device infection. Lead removal can be accomplished in most cases via percutaneous techniques. Clinically significant pulmonary emboli secondary to percutaneous extraction are rare. This is even true for patients with large vegetations seen on echocardiography. An open surgical approach is usually reserved for patients with concomitant valvular endocarditis or extremely large vegetations (generally > 3 cm) [7,8].

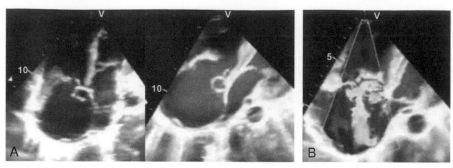

**FIG. 7.18**

The images illustrate abscess formation in tricuspid valve endocarditis. (A) The transthoracic echocardiographic examination of a patient presenting with fever, fatigue, and weight loss shows severe dilation in the right ventricle and the right atrium, together with a round cystic mass at the atrial side of the base of the septal leaflet of the tricuspid valve. The *left* and *right panels* show the mass in the systole and the diastole, respectively. (B) Color Doppler study shows fistulization in the cystic mass into the right ventricular outflow tract. Considering the patient's clinical status and laboratory findings, the diagnosis is complicated infective endocarditis, a tricuspid valve abscess with a fistula into the right ventricular outflow tract, and septic pulmonary embolism, resulting in the hemodynamic compromise of the right heart.

The tricuspid valve is involved in 90% of right-sided infective endocarditis cases mostly related to intravenous drug use. The frequency of specific complications depends on variables such as the infecting pathogen, the duration of the disease before therapy, and the type of treatment. Congestive heart failure is the most important complication of infective endocarditis, and it has the greatest impact on the prognosis. Periannular abscesses are a relatively common complication of infective endocarditis (42%–85% of cases during surgery or at autopsy, respectively), associated with higher morbidity and mortality. Patients who develop abscesses are more likely to undergo surgery than those who do not (84%–91% vs 36%), and also their in-hospital mortality rate is higher (19% vs 11%). The prompt detection of complications often allows an earlier surgical treatment, which represents the best way to improve the outcome [9–12].

**Table 7.19** Structural complications of infective endocarditis [13].

| Structural complications of infectious endocarditis |
|---|
| Cusp or leaflet rupture (flail leaflets) |
| Perforation |
| Abscess formation |
| Aneurysms or pseudoaneurysms |
| Fistula |
| Dehiscence of prosthetic valves |
| Formation of intracardiac shunts |
| Embolization (systemic, cerebral, pulmonary) |

**Table 7.20** Factors associated with a poor prognosis in right-sided infective endocarditis.

| Factors associated with poor prognosis in right-sided infective endocarditis |
|---|
| Persistent infection that does not respond to antibiotic therapy |
| Patients with worsening tricuspid regurgitation contributing to deteriorating right heart failure |
| Increase in vegetation size despite antibiotic treatment |
| Fungal etiology |
| Recurrent septic pulmonary emboli |
| Septic shock |
| Multivalvular involvement |

**Table 7.21** Indications for surgical interventions for right-sided infective endocarditis.

| Indications for surgical interventions for right-sided infective endocarditis |
|---|
| Microorganisms difficult to eradicate (e.g., persistent fungi) |
| Large, persistent tricuspid valve vegetations (>20 mm) |
| Right heart failure secondary to severe tricuspid regurgitation |
| Persistent bacteremia for >7 d (e.g., *Staphylococcus aureus*, *Pseudomonas aeruginosa*) despite adequate antimicrobial therapy |
| Recurrent pulmonary emboli with or without concomitant right heart failure |
| Abscess (more common in the setting of prosthetic valve) |

## Appendix: Supplementary material

Supplementary material related to this chapter can be found on the accompanying CD or online at https://doi.org/10.1016/B978-0-323-84906-7.00006-6.

## References

[1] Habib G, Badano L, Tribouilloy C, et al. Recommendations for the practice of echocardiography in infective endocarditis. Eur J Echocardiogr 2010;11:202–19. https://doi.org/10.1093/ejechocard/jeq004.

[2] Pasha AK, Lee JZ, Low SW, Desai H, Lee KS, Al Mohajer M. Fungal endocarditis: update on diagnosis and management. Am J Med 2016;129(10):1037–43. https://doi.org/10.1016/j.amjmed.2016.05.012.

[3] Salmi D, Bhat A, Corman L, et al. Diagnostic challenges in native valve fungal endocarditis producing a massive septic pulmonary embolus. Jpn J Med Mycol 2010;51:207–10.

[4] Firouzi A, Neshati Pir Borj M, Alizadeh Ghavidel A. Cardiac hydatid cyst: a rare presentation of echinococcal infection. J Cardiovasc Thorac Res 2019;11(1):75–7. https://doi.org/10.15171/jcvtr.2019.13.

[5] Yaman ND, Sirlak M. Cardiac hydatid cysts—review of recent literature. J Vet Med Res 2017;4(8):1102.

[6] Mir H, McClure A, Thampinathan B, et al. Echocardiographic features of cardiac echinococcal infection. CASE 2020;5:26–32. https://doi.org/10.1016/j.case.2020.10.002.

[7] Greenspon AJ, Le KY, Prutkin JM. Influence of vegetation size on the clinical presentation and outcome of lead-associated endocarditis: results from the MEDIC registry. J Am Coll Cardiol Img 2014;7(6):541–9.

[8] Ziyaeifard M, Alizadehasl A, Aghdaii N, et al. Heparinized and saline solutions in the maintenance of arterial and central venous catheters after cardiac surgery. Anesth Pain Med 2015;5(4). https://doi.org/10.5812/aapm28056, e28056. 26478866.

[9] Mocchegiani R, Natalon M. Complications of infective endocarditis. Cardiovasc Hematol Disord Drug Targets 2009;9:240–8. https://doi.org/10.2174/1871529X10909040240.

[10] Shmueli H, Thomas F, Flint N, et al. Right-sided infective endocarditis 2020: challenges and updates in diagnosis and treatment. J Am Heart Assoc 2020;9(15):e017293. https://doi.org/10.1161/JAHA.120.017293.

[11] Maleki M, Alizadehasl A, Haghjoo M. Practical cardiology. 2nd ed. Elsevier; 2021.

[12] Alizadehasl A, Parsa NA, Azarfarin R, et al. Innovations in cardiovascular imaging. Trends Cardiovasc Med 2021;3. https://doi.org/10.1016/j.tcm.2021.01.007.

[13] Alizadehasl A, Roudbari S, Salehi P, et al. Infectious endocarditis of the prosthetic mitral valve after COVID-19 infection. Eur Heart J 2020;41(48):4604. https://doi.org/10.1093/eurheartj/ehaa852.

# Echocardiography in benign cardiac tumors (diagnosis, approach, and follow-up)

**Azin Alizadehasl and Majid Maleki**

*Cardio-Oncology Research Center, Rajaie Cardiovascular Medical and Research Center, Iran University of Medical Sciences, Tehran, Iran*

## Key points

- The most common benign cardiac tumors are myxomas. Arising from a stalk attached to the fossa ovalis membrane, myxomas are generally found in the left atrium.
- The most common primary cardiac tumors in children are rhabdomyomas and fibromas, both of which are benign. Rhabdomyomas usually decrease in size with age.
- The most common cardiac tumors involving valves are papillary fibroelastomas.
- Transthoracic echocardiography can evaluate the location and morphology of the mass as well as its hemodynamic effect.
- Transesophageal echocardiography has increased spatial and temporal resolution; hence, it is superior in depicting small, highly mobile masses.
- Cardiac magnetic resonance and cardiac computed tomography are complementary in that they provide tissue characterization.

**Table 8.1** WHO classification of benign cardiac tumors.

| WHO classification of benign cardiac tumors |
| --- |
| Cardiac myxomas |
| Rhabdomyomas |
| Papillary fibroelastomas |
| Lipomas |
| Cardiac fibromas |
| Hemangiomas |
| Histiocytoid cardiomyopathies |
| Hamartomas of mature cardiac myocytes |
| Adult cellular rhabdomyomas |
| Inflammatory myofibroblastic tumors |
| Cystic tumors of the atrioventricular nodes |

**Multimodal Imaging Atlas of Cardiac Masses.** https://doi.org/10.1016/B978-0-323-84906-7.00012-1

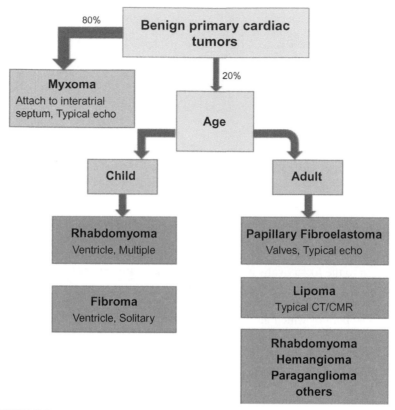

**ALGORITHM 8.2**

The image depicts the diagnostic algorithm for the evaluation of benign primary cardiac tumors. *CT*, cardiac tomography; *CMR*, cardiac magnetic resonance [1].

**Table 8.3** Advantages and limitations of cardiac imaging modalities for the diagnosis of cardiac myxomas.

|  | Advantages | Limitations |
|---|---|---|
| Echocardiography | Easily available<br>High spatial resolution (TEE > TTE)<br>Detection of small masses<br>High temporal resolution<br>Functional and hemodynamic repercussions<br>Detection of underlying heart diseases | Patient dependent (echogenicity)<br>Restricted field of view<br>Poor tissue characterization |
| CMR | 3D visualization<br>Tissue characterization (differential diagnosis)<br>Large field of view<br>Moderate temporal resolution | Limited availability<br>Average spatial resolution<br>Reduced ability to characterize small and highly mobile masses<br>Long examination time<br>Patient dependent (rhythm and collaboration)<br>Contraindications (e.g., metal implants and renal failure) |
| CT | 3D visualization<br>Fast acquisition<br>Easy available<br>Spatial resolution<br>Chest wall (robotic surgery) | Radiation exposure, even more, when ECG gated<br>Low temporal resolution<br>Average tissue characterization, except for fat and calcification<br>Contraindications (renal failure) |
| 18F-FDG PET/CT | Large field of view<br>Exclusion of secondary malignant tumors | Limited availability<br>Poor spatial and temporal resolution<br>Limited ability to differentiate other diseases (pseudotumors, benign tumors, or infectious/inflammatory tumors) |

TEE, *transesophageal echocardiography;* TTE, *transthoracic echocardiography;* CMR, *cardiac magnetic resonance;* CT, *computed tomography;* ECG, *electrocardiography;* [18]F-FDG, *[18]F-fluorodeoxyglucose;* PET, *positron emission tomography.*

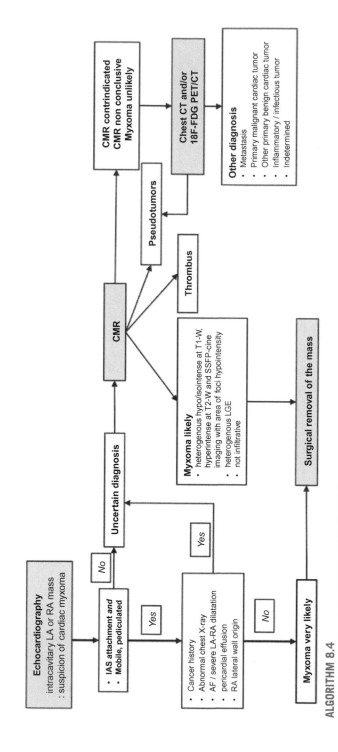

**ALGORITHM 8.4.**

The image depicts the proposed diagnostic imaging algorithm for suspicion of cardiac myxomas [2].

## Differential diagnosis of cardiac myxoma with interatrial septum attachment

**Lipomatous hyperplasia of the interatrial septum**
- Typically elderly population
- Dumbbell shaped appearance
- Signal characteristics at CMR, attenuation characteristic at CT

**Thrombi**
- Context: atrial (severe) dilatation, atrial fibrillation, deep venous line or pacemaker
- Very rarely attached to the IAS
- CMR: low signal at T2-weighted imaging; signal characteristics at LGE imaging

**Metastasis**
- Context of known malignancy often present
- Very rarely attached to the IAS
- CMR presentation depends on malignance etiology

**Lymphoma/ chloroma**
- Location often not limited to the IAS with extending to the atrioventricular grooves; sometimes extending through more diffusely in the LA wall
- Infiltrative>nodular, not mobile
- CMR: homogenous>heterogeneous; isointense at T2-weighted imaging
- PET: often high 18F-FDG uptake (lymphoma)

**Infectious/inflammatory disease (tuberculosis, granulomatosis with polyangiitis)**
- Infiltrative>nodular, not mobile
- Pericardial enhancement / involvement
- CMR: high enhancement at perfusion imaging
- PET: often high 18F-FDG uptake

**Pheochromocytoma-paraganglioma**
- No intracavitary but extracardiac mass often located at the roof of IAS/LA
- 123I-MIBG uptake

**Lipoma**
- Rounded appearance
- Typical signal characteristics at CMR

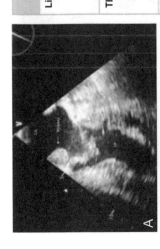

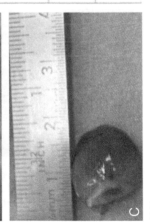

**FIG. 8.5**

(A) Transesophageal echocardiography shows a round, heterogeneous mass attached to the left atrial side of the interatrial septum, suggestive of a myxoma. (B) Cardiac catheterization demonstrates the typical appearance of tumor blush at the level of the left atrium after contrast injection in the left coronary artery, indicative of the vascular support of the tumor (arrows). (C) The excised cardiac myxoma with a gelatinous appearance is presented herein.

**Table 8.6** Diagnostic triad in the presentation of atrial myxomas [3].

| Diagnostic triad in the presentation of atrial myxomas | | |
|---|---|---|
| **Features** | **Manifestations** | **Frequency (%) of patients** |
| Obstructive symptoms | Heart failure, dyspnea, syncope, and sudden death (rare) | 54–95 |
| Constitutional symptoms | They may mimic autoimmune disease or vasculitis (e.g., myalgia, arthralgia, weight loss, fatigue, fever, Raynaud's phenomenon, and finger clubbing). | 34–90 |
| Embolic phenomena | Emboli may travel to any organ, but 73% reach the central nervous system, including the spinal cord | 10–45 |

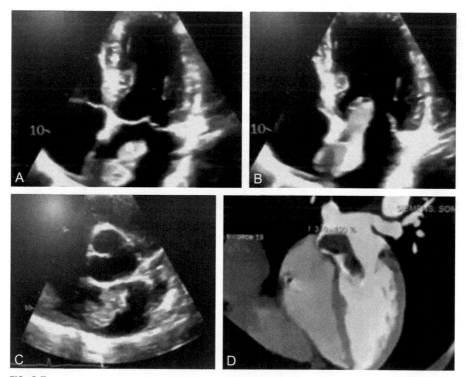

**FIG. 8.7**

The images illustrate a left atrial myxoma. (A and B) The 4-chamber view of transthoracic echocardiography demonstrates a large semimobile heterogeneous mass, which is attached to the left atrial side of the interatrial septum and protrudes into the left ventricle in the diastole, suggestive of a large left atrial myxoma. (C) The same mass is visualized in the short-axis view at the level of the aortic valve. (D) Cardiac magnetic resonance confirms the left atrial myxoma.

Transthoracic and transesophageal echocardiographic examinations can be used in combination to assess the size, shape, morphology, and hemodynamic effects of the tumor. Cardiac myxomas are usually attached with a stalk to the atrial septum in the fossa ovalis and have lobulated margins. Their range of movement is dependent on the length, size, and morphology of the stalk. Cardiac myxomas are better visualized with the use of echocardiography contrast. On computed tomography, a myxoma appears as a well-defined, ovoid, intracavitary mass with lobulated contours, and the contrast helps to delineate the mass as a low-attenuation lesion surrounded by enhanced intracardiac blood. On cardiac magnetic resonance images, cardiac myxomas appear isointense on T1-weighted sequences and have higher signal intensity on T2-weighted sequences owing to the high extracellular water content. Regions of acute hemorrhage appear hypointense on both T1-weighted and T2-weighted images and can subsequently become hyperintense as hemoglobin in the blood is progressively oxidized. Steady-state free precession imaging can reveal the stalk-like attachment and the mobile nature of these masses, as well as prolapse across the valves. Internally, myxomas may contain cysts, regions of necrosis, fibrosis, hemorrhage, and calcification, leading to a typically heterogeneous appearance at contrast enhancement. Postcontrast delayed imaging typically shows a heterogeneous enhancement pattern, with many myxomas having a layer of surface thrombus with low signal intensity. [4].

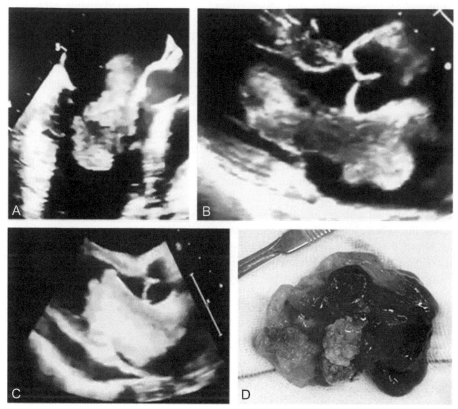

**FIG. 8.8**

The images show a left atrial myxoma. The results of the transthoracic (B and C) and transesophageal (A) echocardiographic examinations of a patient with a left atrial myxoma are illustrated herein. Myxomas are described as nonhomogeneous, well-circumscribed echodensities that may have a globular structure. The left atrium is the most common site of myxomas ($\approx$75%). Large left atrial myxomas may cause mitral inflow obstruction (i.e., functional mitral stenosis), significant mitral regurgitation (interference with mitral valve coaptation), and subsequent pulmonary hypertension [5].

Mitral valve obstruction caused by atrial myxomas represents an important hemodynamic consequence, leading to symptoms of congestive heart failure and pulmonary hypertension, as well as syncope and even sudden death. Mitral stenotic effects usually occur when the tumor diameter exceeds 5 cm. Echo Doppler studies are the most important method for the differential diagnosis with primary valve disease since they can estimate the transvalvular gradient. Chest X-rays may reveal enlargement in the left atrium and some signs of pulmonary hypertension and congestion [6].

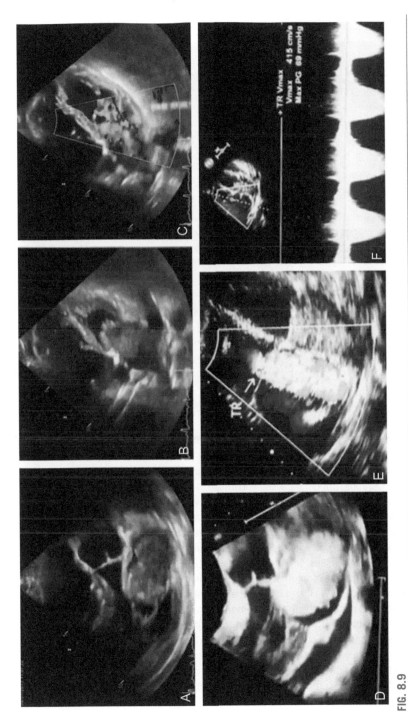

**FIG. 8.9**

The images demonstrate a huge left atrial myxoma. (A, B, and D) Transthoracic echocardiography in two different patients shows huge left atrial myxomas obstructing the mitral valve flow (C) and mimicking mitral stenosis hemodynamics. The consequence is severe tricuspid valve regurgitation (E) and pulmonary hypertension (F).

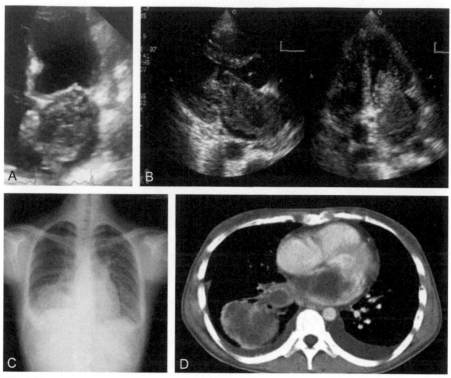

**FIG. 8.10**

The images illustrate a left atrial myxoma and a left atrial myxosarcoma. (A and B) Transthoracic echocardiography in two different patients presenting with dyspnea on exertion shows a giant heterogeneous mass in the left atrium involving the right pulmonary veins with a similar echocardiographic appearance. (A) The image shows that the giant left atrial myxoma had entered the right pulmonary vein (Supplementary Video 8.1). (B–D) The primary myxosarcoma of the right inferior pulmonary vein presents clinically as a benign left atrial myxoma with a concurrent right lower lung tumor in the chest X-ray and the thoracic computed tomography scan. These images indicate the importance of pulmonary vein involvement in left atrial masses. Myxomas are usually attached with a stalk to the cardiac wall, most often the interatrial septum and, in descending order of frequency, the posterior atrial wall, the anterior atrial wall, and the atrial appendage. Other findings are suggestive of malignancy. Such findings include the involvement of the tumor in the pulmonary vein or the vena cava, the infiltration of the myocardium or the adjacent cardiac anatomy or organs, a broad attachment, a nonseptal origin, and the presence of pericardial effusion. In the second case, the tumor lacks any definite attachment to the interatrial septum; in addition, the chest computed tomography shows the extension of the tumor into the pulmonary vein and a concurrent right lower lung tumor. These findings are crucial in differentiating a malignant tumor from a myxoma [7].

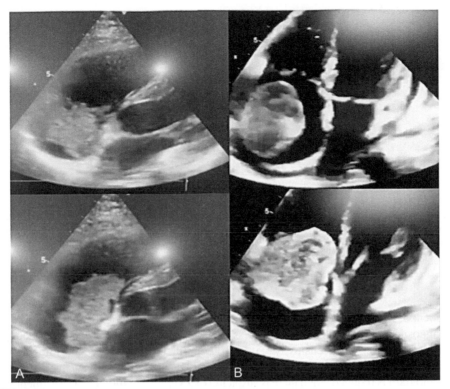

**FIG. 8.11**

The images illustrate a right atrial myxoma. (A) Transthoracic echocardiography shows a giant right atrial villous myxoma with simultaneous pulmonary embolism considering the dilation in the right ventricle. Right atrial villous myxomas comprise a rare subtype in an unusual location with the high potential of pulmonary embolism (Supplementary Video 8.2). (B) The image demonstrates a very hypermobile right atrial myxoma protruding into the right ventricle in the diastole.

A low incidence rate has been reported for right atrial myxomas. They usually originate in the fossa ovalis or the base of the interatrial septum. The signs and symptoms of right atrial myxomas are atypical and highly variable, depending on the size, position, and mobility of the tumor, and are modified according to the physical activity and body position of the patient. Right atrial myxomas may remain asymptomatic or eventually cause constitutional signs and symptoms, including fever, weight loss, arthralgia, Raynaud's phenomenon, anemia, hypergammaglobulinemia, and an increased erythrocyte sedimentation rate due to the production of interleukin-6. These symptoms disappear after the tumor is removed. Patients may also present with atypical chest pain, syncope, lethargy, malaise, palpitation, peripheral edema, pulmonary embolism, and hemoptysis. Nevertheless, the most common manifestation is dyspnea (in 80% of

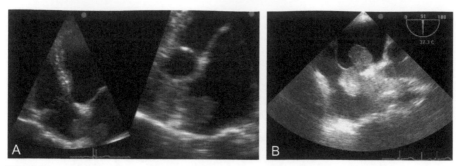

**FIG. 8.12**

The images illustrate a biatrial myxoma. Transthoracic (A) and transesophageal (B) echocardiographic examinations of a 53-year-old man with a history of a recent cerebrovascular event show a large, mobile, homogeneous mass in the right atrium attached to the interatrial septum with a broad base (2.9 cm × 2 cm). The mass protrudes into the left atrium across a patent foramen ovale. The patient underwent surgery, and the pathology results showed a biatrial myxoma.

patients), and right heart failure has been reported. Echocardiography remains the best diagnostic method for locating and assessing the extent of myxomas and for detecting their recurrence, with a sensitivity of up to 100%. Still, transthoracic echocardiography may fail to identify tumors smaller than 5 mm in diameter, and a transesophageal echocardiogram is required when there is suspicion of a very small tumor. The treatment of choice for myxomas is surgical removal, and the recurrence rate of sporadic tumors is very low (between 1% and 3%) [8] (Supplementary Videos 8.1 and 8.2 in the online version at https://doi.org/10.1016/B978-0-323-84906-7.00012-1).

A dumbbell or butterfly wing or so-called biatrial myxoma or interatrial septal myxoma with a biatrial extension usually arises from the left atrial side of the fossa ovalis and prolapses into the right atrium through the foramen ovale. Its incidence is less than 1%–5% of all intracardiac myxomas. A close differential diagnosis is a biatrial thrombus crossing a patent foramen ovale; nonetheless, either a biatrial myxoma or a straddling thrombus through the foramen ovale is a rare diagnosis. Thrombi in this situation may have identifiable causes such as deep vein thrombosis, metastasis, and mitral stenosis. Thrombi are more irregular in shape. Intracardiac thrombi are more fragile, and they usually present with evidence of pulmonary, systemic, or coronary embolism. They should be removed by wide-base resection as soon as possible because of the higher frequency of embolization. Echocardiography yields a significant number of clues such as polypoid or smooth surface myxomas, the site of origin, the satellite focus, and the diastolic blockage of the mitral or tricuspid inflow, which almost support the provisional diagnosis of a cardiac myxoma [9].

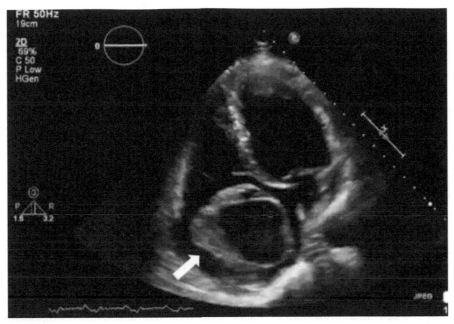

**FIG. 8.13**

The image depicts a right atrial myxoma with central necrosis. Transthoracic echocardiography shows a large, round mass in a dilated right atrium (*arrow*). The pathology results confirmed a myxoma with central necrosis.

Most myxomas appear as round and solid masses without cystic architecture or cavitation. Although several cases of cystic myxomas that had serous fluid or hemorrhage within the cyst have been reported, histological examinations are usually needed to confirm the diagnosis, especially in cases with a multicystic or multiseptated nature. The differential diagnosis of intracardiac cystic masses should include thrombi, hydatid cysts, intracardiac varices, and bronchogenic cysts [10].

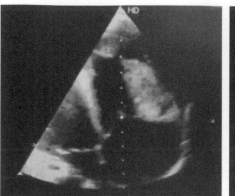 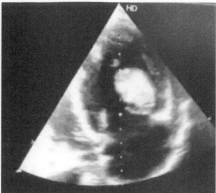

**FIG. 8.14**

The images demonstrate a right ventricular myxoma. Transthoracic echocardiography shows a large, heterogeneous mass in the right ventricle attached to the lateral wall from the anterior tricuspid valve leaflet to the near apex. The pathology results showed a right ventricular myxoma.

Only 5% of cardiac myxomas are found in the right ventricle. Tumors originating from the right ventricular outflow tract present unusual diagnostic and therapeutic challenges. The symptoms are dependent on the size and location of the tumor. Such tumors are capable of generating major clinical consequences, including arrhythmias, pulmonary emboli, and sudden death. Once the diagnosis of the tumor obstructing the right ventricular outflow tract is confirmed, immediate surgery is indicated. The risk of life-threatening complications indicates the importance of early diagnosis and prompt surgical resection. One of the main concerns is the risk of tumor embolization and pulmonary obstruction during anesthesia induction or at any stage thereafter. Hemodynamic instability and the inconvenient manipulation of the tumor and the heart must be avoided to prevent these complications. Femoral arterial–venous cannulation can be performed for cardiopulmonary bypass initiation in the case of complete right ventricular outflow tract obstruction with a hemodynamic collapse. Several surgical techniques have been suggested. In each case, however, it depends on the site of the tumor. Follow-ups for a recurrent myxoma in an uncommon location are recommended [11].

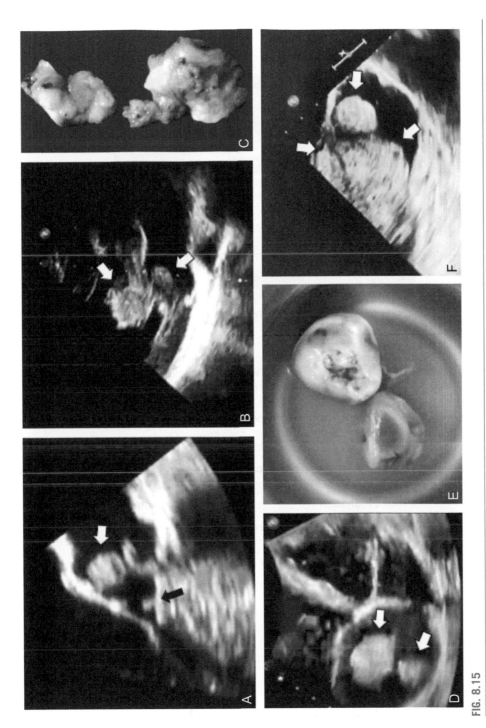

**FIG. 8.15**

The images illustrate myxomas with atypical locations in 4 different patients. A subaortic membrane with severe obstruction (A, *black arrow*) and a round, well-defined echodensity on the left coronary cusp of the aortic valve can be seen (myxomas) (A, *white arrow*). Mitral valve myxomas (B and C), involving both leaflets and the subvalvular apparatus, are presented herein. Large, multilobulated, well-circumscribed masses can be observed in the right atrium (D and E). They were attached to the interatrial septum and diagnosed as myxomas based on the postoperative specimen pathology. A giant right atrial villous myxoma is seen (F) with simultaneous pulmonary embolism, prompting urgent surgery.

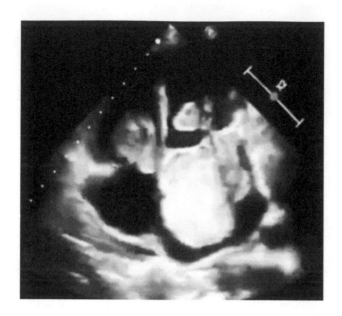

**FIG. 8.16**

The image depicts the Carney complex. Multiple cardiac myxomas are visualized in a patient with the presentation of the Carney complex. The Carney complex is described as a rare, autosomal dominant syndrome presenting with pigmented lesions of the skin and mucosae, accompanied by cardiac, endocrine, cutaneous, and neural myxomatous tumors. In 70% of cases, mutations in the *PRKAR1A* gene have been identified. The Table 8.18 presents the known manifestations in affected individuals with their prevalence [12].

**Table 8.17** Manifestations of the Carney complex.

| Manifestations of Carney complex in affected individual | Percentage |
|---|---|
| Primary pigmented nodular adrenal cortical disease (PPNAD) | 25–60 |
| Cardiac myxoma | 30–60 |
| Skin myxoma | 20–63 |
| Lentiginosis | 60–70 |
| Multiple blue nevus | |
| Breast ductal adenoma | 25 |
| Testicular tumors | 33–56 |
| Ovarian cyst | 20–67 |
| Acromegaly | 10 |
| Thyroid tumor | 10–25 |
| Melanotic schwannoma | 8–18 |
| Osteochondrotic myxoma | <10 |

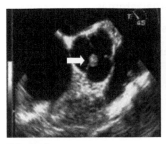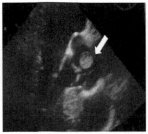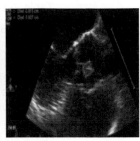

**FIG. 8.18**

The images demonstrate aortic valve papillary fibroelastomas. Transesophageal echocardiography shows a well-defined, round mass (0.9 cm × 0.9 cm) on the arterial side of the aortic valve (arrow). The pathology results confirmed aortic valve papillary fibroelastomas. The Table 8.20 shows the distribution of this benign tumor in the heart, with the aortic valve being the most common location (Supplementary Video 8.3).

Papillary fibroelastomas account for 7%–8% of cardiac tumors. They are usually discovered postmortem, although their premorbid detection rate is rising with the increasing use of echocardiography. While they are usually found in patients older than 60 years of age, they have also been reported in younger patients. The clinical manifestations include cerebral embolism, myocardial infarction, pulmonary embolism, syncope, and sudden death. Surgical excision is generally recommended. Mobile tumors have been suggested to be independent predictors of the occurrence of death or nonfatal embolization. The echocardiographic features of papillary fibroelastomas are their small size, with independent motion and attachment to an endocardial surface. On transesophageal echocardiography, the borders may appear slightly stippled or shimmering, which is due to vibration at the tumor–blood interface because of its finger-like projection. Transesophageal echocardiography is more sensitive in identifying papillary fibroelastomas than transthoracic echocardiography because of the typically small size of these tumors, which reinforces the role of transesophageal echocardiography in the evaluation of an embolic event. Surgical excision is recommended for larger (≥1 cm) left-sided papillary fibroelastomas in patients who are deemed appropriate surgical candidates with low risk or at the time of cardiac surgery for another cardiovascular condition. This dramatically reduces the risk of stroke [13] (Supplementary Videos 8.3 and 8.4 in the online version at https:/doi.org/10.1016/B978-0-323-84906-7.00012-1).

**Table 8.19** Locations of papillary fibroelastomas.

| Locations of papillary fibroelastoma | |
|---|---|
| **Location** | **% present** |
| Aortic valve | 44 |
| Mitral valve | 35 |
| Tricuspid valve | 15 |
| Pulmonary valve | 8 |
| Left ventricle | 9 |
| Left atrium | <2 |
| Atrial septum | |
| Right ventricle | |

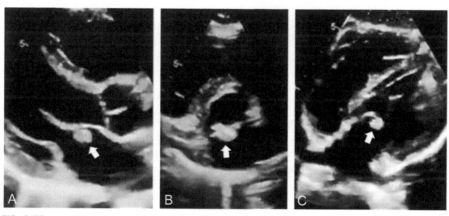

**FIG. 8.20**

The images illustrate a mitral valve papillary fibroelastoma. Transthoracic echocardiography in a patient with papillary fibroelastoma shows a well-defined, heterogeneous mass with a small stalk attached to the atrial aspect of the anterior mitral valve leaflet (*white arrows*). Papillary fibroelastomas are rare primary cardiac tumors that mainly involve the heart valves (most common on the aortic valve, followed by the mitral valve). They are usually asymptomatic and found incidentally. Echocardiography is the most sensitive and reliable modality to establish the diagnosis, to determine the presence or absence of multiple lesions, and to plan the best surgical approach [14].

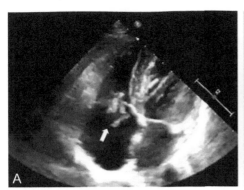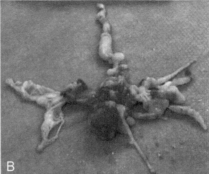

**FIG. 8.21**

The images demonstrate a tricuspid valve papillary fibroelastoma. Transthoracic echocardiography in a patient shows a large, semimobile, multilobulated, heterogeneous mass (A, *white arrow*) attached to the anterior leaflet with extension to the chordae and the septal leaflets. The gross appearance of the tumor is depicted after surgical removal (B). Right-sided papillary fibroelastomas might be a potentially fatal cause of syncope, chest pain, and sudden cardiac death. Despite their slow growth, their tendency to accumulate superficial thrombi and embolize into the distal pulmonary vasculature or paradoxically to the left sided circulation is noteworthy [15].

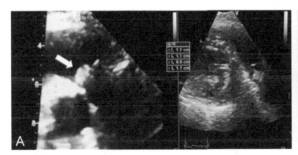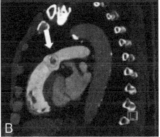

**FIG. 8.22**

The images illustrate pulmonary valve papillary fibroelastomas. (A) Transthoracic echocardiography shows a round, well-defined mass ($\approx 1\,cm \times 1\,cm$) on the arterial side of the pulmonary valve, suggestive of a pulmonary valve fibroelastoma. (B) Cardiac magnetic resonance shows the tumor (*arrow*).

The pulmonary valve is rarely involved by papillary fibroelastomas, with only 8% of the tumors described on it. They may project into the ventricular or arterial lumen. Among the extremely rare cases of pulmonary papillary fibroelastomas reported in the literature, there is no correlation between them and symptoms. Right-sided papillary fibroelastomas are usually managed conservatively unless they are associated with a hemodynamically significant obstruction or the risk of paradoxical embolism (e.g., in cases of intracardiac shunts) [13].

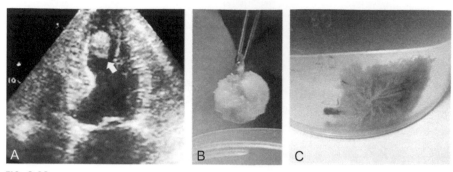

**FIG. 8.23**

The images depict a left ventricular apical fibroelastoma. Transthoracic echocardiography in a patient shows a left ventricular papillary fibroelastoma (A, *white arrow*). This neoplasm is generally asymptomatic; however, in some cases, the patient may present with syncope and chest pain due to the most feared complication of fibroelastoma: embolism. Embolic events to the circulation of both the brain and the coronary arteries may lead to fatal complications. Given the mentioned risks, the surgical excision of the tumor is the treatment of choice (Supplementary Video 8.4) [15,16].

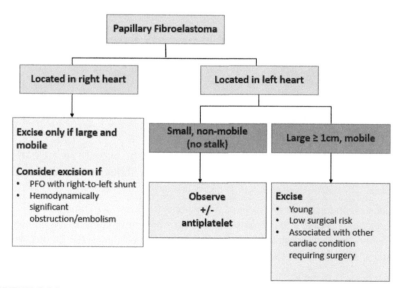

**ALGORITHM 8.24**

The proposed management of papillary fibroelastomas based on echocardiographic findings is shown herein.

*Adapted from [1].*

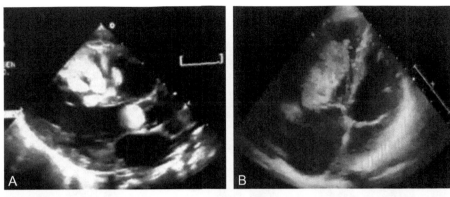

**FIG. 8.25**

The images show 2 cases of cardiac rhabdomyomas. (A) Transthoracic echocardiography in a 19-year-old man presenting with dyspnea shows multiple hyperechoic masses on the interventricular septum and in the left ventricular outflow tract with obstructive effects on the aortic valve flow. (B) Transthoracic echocardiography in a 15-year-old boy with new-onset murmurs and complaints of decreased exercise tolerance when playing football demonstrates a large mass almost filling the right ventricle with obstructive effects on the tricuspid valve.

Cardiac rhabdomyomas constitute rare and benign mesenchymal tumors of striated muscle origins. They most commonly involve the head and the neck. Most cardiac rhabdomyomas are associated with tuberous sclerosis and appear in the ventricular myocardium, the atria, the cavoatrial junction, or the epicardial surface. Most cardiac rhabdomyomas are multiple and pursue a course of spontaneous regression. Surgical resection is not advisable unless the patient is symptomatic. The symptoms develop as a result of the obstruction of the blood inflow or outflow, resulting in congestive heart failure. Arrhythmias can also occur ranging from bradycardia secondary to sinus or atrioventricular node dysfunction to atrial/ventricular tachycardia, atrioventricular node reentrant tachycardia, or ventricular preexcitation https://doi.org/10.1016/B978-0-323-84906-7.00012-1

The imaging modality of choice for rhabdomyomas is echocardiography. Cardiac rhabdomyomas present as multiple, echogenic, nodular masses in the ventricular myocardium. Cardiac rhabdomyomas can also protrude into the ventricular cavity. They are more homogeneous and hyperechoic than the normal myocardium. Magnetic resonance imaging confers a better delineation of the tumor and can be very helpful in cases of planned surgical resection. It also provides a more reliable estimate of the ventricular systolic function [17].

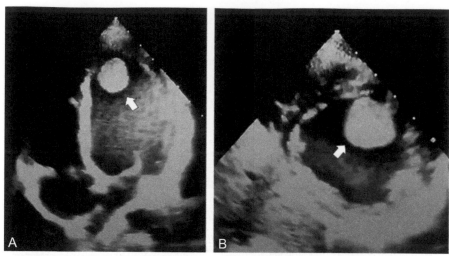

**FIG. 8.26**

The images demonstrate a cardiac rhabdomyoma. Transthoracic echocardiography in a patient shows a left ventricular rhabdomyoma. A large, round, well-defined, semimobile mass (*white arrows*) is seen attached to the left ventricular apex. This lesion is a rare hamartoma-type tumor that arises from striated cardiac muscle fibers. They are mostly associated with tuberous sclerosis and may be detected in the ventricular myocardium, the atria, the cavoatrial junction, or the epicardial surface. As cardiac rhabdomyomas usually regress spontaneously, surgical resection is not recommended unless the patient is symptomatic. The symptoms include the obstruction of the blood inflow or outflow and subsequent congestive heart failure, tachy- and bradyarrhythmia [17].

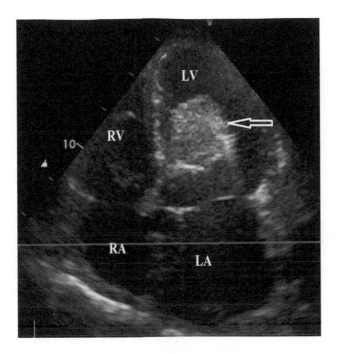

**FIG. 8.27**

The image depicts a lipoma. Transthoracic echocardiography in the apical 4-chamber view shows a benign tumor in the LV (*arrow*). The pathology results reported a lipoma. *LV*, left ventricle; *RV*, right ventricle; *RA*, right atrium; *LA*, left atrium.

Lipomas are rare and mostly sporadic benign cardiac tumors. They comprise only 3% of all benign tumors. Lipomas tend to occur in the right atrium but may be found anywhere in the heart, as well as the pericardium. Lipomas are associated with older age, increased body mass, and the female sex. The echocardiographic appearance of lipomas varies with their location. Lipomas in the pericardial space may be completely hypoechoic, have hypoechoic regions, or be completely echogenic, whereas intracavitary lipomas are homogeneous and hyperechoic. A computed tomography scan can provide better tissue characterization because cardiac lipomas display a low-attenuation signal similar to subcutaneous or mediastinal fat. On cardiac magnetic resonance, these lesions have signal intensity similar to that in the surrounding fat on the chest wall on T1-weighted and T2-weighted images. Homogeneous high-signal intensity relative to the myocardium on T1-weighted images that is markedly suppressed with the application of fat saturation prepulses is indicative of the presence of a lipoma. Given their avascularity, these lesions do not enhance on delayed postcontrast imaging.

The differential diagnosis with lipomatous hypertrophy is crucial. Septal thickening is usually limited to the limbus of the fossa ovalis. Lipomatous hypertrophy, histologically, is a nonencapsulated lesion that contains 3 elements: mature fat, immature fat, and atrial myocytes. In lipomas, areas of degeneration and extensive radiographically apparent calcification may be present [4].

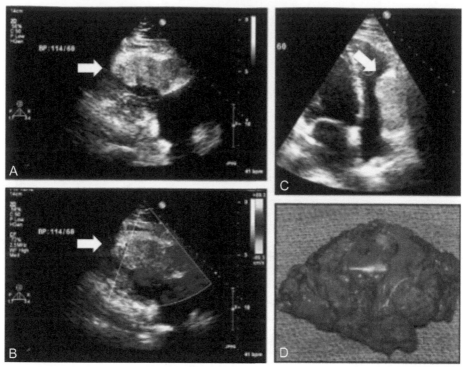

**FIG. 8.28**

The images demonstrate a hemangioma. A hemangioma is found in a 46-year-old man presenting with palpitations. (A and B) Transthoracic echocardiography shows a large, fixed mass in the left ventricle (*arrow*). (C) Color Doppler studies illustrate vascularity in the mass. (D) The surgical specimen is presented herein [18].

Cardiac hemangiomas represent rare nonmyxomatous benign tumors of the heart. They are more frequently located into the anterior wall of the right ventricle and are less likely to be found on the lateral wall of the left ventricle. More often, they are nodular and isolated. The widespread use of noninvasive techniques has contributed to the early detection of cardiac tumors. Echocardiography has proven to be very helpful in predicting the etiology of most intracavitary masses, computed tomography can evaluate the extracardiac extension of the tumor, and magnetic resonance imaging establishes the amount of myocardial involvement. Compression, obstruction, effusion, and bleeding with relative clinical picture may be the responsible mechanism for the symptoms, depending on the size, invasiveness, and location of the tumor. Cardiac hemangiomas may be radically resected with excellent surgical results. The natural story is unpredictable; hence, surgical intervention under cardiopulmonary bypass is mandatory, although the excision may be incomplete even in these rare benign tumors [19].

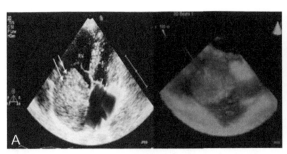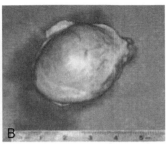

**FIG. 8.29**

The image shows a pheochromocytoma. (A) The 2D transthoracic and 3D transesophageal echocardiographic examinations of a 46-year-old woman presenting with palpitations, sweating, dyspnea, and a feeling of anxiety, as well as new hypertension, show a large mass in the right atrium. The mass originates from the junction of the superior vena cava and the right atrium. Laboratory data showed elevated neurohormones, and a pheochromocytoma was suspected. (B) Surgery consisted of a midline sternotomy, cardiopulmonary bypass, and complete resection of the tumor, which measured 3 × 4 cm in size, with free margins. The pathology results confirmed the diagnosis of a cardiac pheochromocytoma.

Pheochromocytomas comprise a type of catecholamine-producing paraganglioma derived from the chromaffin cells of the sympathetic nervous system. Most thoracic pheochromocytomas are located in the posterior mediastinum, and intrapericardial pheochromocytomas are rare. Around 60% of cardiac pheochromocytomas are located in the roof of the left atrium; the rest are located (in order of frequency) in the interauricular septum, the anterior surface of the heart, and the aortopulmonary window. Clinically, they manifest themselves as uncontrolled hypertension, severe headache, orthostatic hypotension, palpitations, sweating, and abdominal or chest pain. Transesophageal echocardiography is useful for determining the extension of the tumor and planning surgery [20].

**Table 8.30** Symptoms of pheochromocytoma.

| Symptoms of pheochromocytoma | |
| --- | --- |
| **More common** | **Less common** |
| Hypertension | Abdominal pain, nausea, vomiting, and diarrhea |
| Sweating | Pallor |
| Headache | Hallucinations |
| Anxiety and panic | Agitation |
| | Tremor |

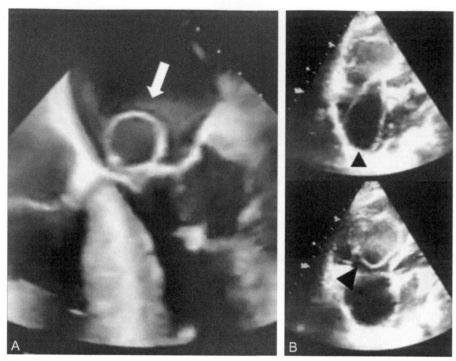

**FIG. 8.31**

The images demonstrate two cases of valvular blood cysts. (A) Transesophageal echocardiography shows a large cystic lesion attached to the atrial side of the mitral valve (Supplementary Video 8.5). (B) Transthoracic echocardiography shows a huge cystic lesion attached to the tricuspid valve. The cystic lesion oscillates between the right atrium and the right ventricle in the systole and the diastole, respectively.

**Table 8.32** Echocardiographic appearances of cardiac blood cysts.

| Echocardiographic appearances of cardiac blood cysts |
| --- |
| They are attached to the valve leaflet (most commonly, the mitral valve) |
| They are thin-walled cystic lesions |
| They have echolucent cores |
| They may be multilobed |
| They are usually not opacified by the use of the echo contrast; nonetheless, if channels are present, the contrast may show up in the cyst |
| They may cause valvular regurgitation and left ventricular outflow tract obstruction |

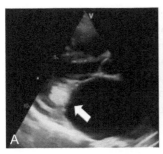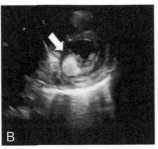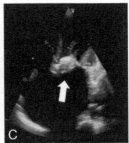

**FIG. 8.33**

The images illustrate calcium amorphous tumors. Transesophageal echocardiography in the parasternal long-axis (A), parasternal short-axis (B), and apical 4-chamber (C) views shows a large, echogenic, round, and mobile mass attached with a short pedicle on the ventricular surface of the mitral valve leaflet, indicative of a calcium amorphous tumor on the mitral valve (*white arrows*).

Intracardiac blood cysts are usually asymptomatic, small, and congenital. They are mainly seen during autopsies in fetuses and infants under the age of 6 months. The cysts regress spontaneously in most patients, and they are consequently rare in adults. Most commonly, blood cysts are asymptomatic in adults and often discovered incidentally during routine echocardiographic evaluations. Nevertheless, depending on which area of the heart is affected, blood cysts may result in a variety of clinical phenomena, including embolism, valvular dysfunction, and heart blocks. Therefore surgical resection should be considered in patients with symptoms or valvular dysfunction, and resection is also suggested to rule out malignancy (Supplementary Video 8.5 in the online version at https://doi.org/10.1016/B978-0-323-84906-7.00012-1).

Echocardiography is deemed the imaging modality of choice for the diagnosis. Cardiac blood cysts have typical ultrasound features, including an echolucent core and a thin wall with clean boundaries. Furthermore, contrast echocardiography can accurately demonstrate the attachment and absence of blood perfusion in the mass. Echocardiography can also demonstrate the effects of the blood cyst on cardiac function (e.g., the presence of mitral regurgitation, mitral valve stenosis, and outflow tract obstruction). It also helps differentiate a blood cyst from solid tumors such as fibroelastomas and myxomas, as well as vegetations [21,22].

Cardiac calcium amorphous tumors, which have been recently described as distinct pathological entities, are extremely rare, benign cardiac nonneoplasms. The most common symptoms of these masses are progressive dyspnea, chest pain, syncope, and symptoms related to embolism. Rarely, they may also present with cardiac arrhythmias such as ventricular tachycardia. Further, mobile calcium amorphous tumors have a higher chance of embolic events than immobile lesions. The size of calcium amorphous tumors was recently reported to range from several millimeters to 90 mm. Although they may occur in any chamber of the heart, calcium amorphous tumors are found most commonly in the left ventricle (31.25%) and the mitral valve (25%). Approximately, 12.5% of cases of calcium amorphous tumors originate from the right atrium. Surgical excision is mandatory because of the risk of complications or embolization and also for accurate diagnosis. The recurrence and fatal outcomes of cardiac calcium amorphous tumors have rarely been reported after surgical resection; consequently, long-term follow-ups with cardiac imaging studies, especially in patients with incomplete resection, are required [23,24].

## References

[1] Bruce CJ. Cardiac tumors: diagnosis and management. Heart 2011;97. https://doi.org/10.1136/hrt.2009.186320, 151e160.

[2] Colin GC, Gerber BL, Amzulescu M, et al. Cardiac myxoma: a contemporary multimodality imaging review. Int J Cardiovasc Imaging 2018. https://doi.org/10.1007/s10554-018-1396-z.

[3] Rourke F, Dean N, Mouradian MS, et al. Atrial myxoma as a cause of stroke: case report and discussion. CMAJ 2003;169(10).

[4] Bussani R, Castrichini M, Restivo L, et al. Cardiac tumors: diagnosis, prognosis, and treatment. Curr Cardiol Rep 2020;22:169. https://doi.org/10.1007/s11886-020-01420-z.

[5] Abels B, Pfeiffer S, Stix J, Schwab J. Multimodal imaging for the assessment of a cardiac mass—a case of primary cardiac sarcoma. J Radiol Case Rep 2017;11(11):11–9. https://doi.org/10.3941/jrcr.v11i11.3194.

[6] Avakian SD, Takada JY, Mansur ADP. Giant obstructive left atrial myxoma resembling mitral valve stenosis. Clinics (Sao Paulo) 2012;67(7):853–4. https://doi.org/10.6061/clinics/2012(07)25.

[7] Hsuan CF, Tseng WK, Yang CH, et al. Primary myxosarcoma of the right inferior pulmonary vein presenting clinically as benign left atrial myxoma with a concurrent right lower lung tumor. Circ J 2009;73:1547–9.

[8] Nina V, Silva N, Gaspar S, et al. Atypical size and location of a right atrial myxoma: a case report. J Med Case Reports 2012;6:26. https://doi.org/10.1186/1752-1947-6-26.

[9] Barik R. A biatrial myxoma with triple ripples. J Cardiovasc Echogr 2018;28(1):59–60. https://doi.org/10.4103/jcecho.jcecho_47_17.

[10] Park JS, Song JM, Shin E, et al. Cystic cardiac mass in the left atrium: hemorrhage in myxoma. Circulation 2011;123:e368–9. https://doi.org/10.1161/CIRCULATIONAHA.110.004655.

[11] Gribaa R, Slim M, Kortas C, et al. Right ventricular myxoma obstructing the right ventricular outflow tract: a case report. J Med Case Reports 2014;8:435. https://doi.org/10.1186/1752-1947-8-435.

[12] Birla S, Aggarwal S, Sharma A, Tandon N. Rare association of acromegaly with left atrial myxoma in Carney's complex due to novel PRKAR1A mutation. Endocrinol Diabetes Metab Case Rep 2014;2014:1–5. https://doi.org/10.1530/edm-14-0023.

[13] Tyebally S, Chen D, Sanjeev B, et al. Cardiac tumors: JACC CardioOncology state-of-the-art review. JACC CardioOncol 2020;2(2):293–311. https://doi.org/10.1016/j.jaccao.2020.05.009.

[14] Gomadam PS, Stacey RB, Johnsen AE, Kitzman DW, Kon ND, Upadhya B. Papillary fibroelastoma of the mitral valve chordae with systemic embolization. J Cardiol Cases 2014;10(4):125–8. https://doi.org/10.1016/j.jccase.2014.06.004.

[15] Srivatsa SV, Adhikari P, Chaudhry P, Srivatsa SS. Multimodality imaging of right-sided (tricuspid valve) papillary fibroelastoma: recognition of a surgically remediable disease. Case Rep Oncol 2013;6(3):485–9. https://doi.org/10.1159/000355419.

[16] Baker CA. Apical papillary fibroelastoma. J Diagn Med Sonogr 2006;22(6):382–6. https://doi.org/10.1177/8756479306293294.

[17] Sarkar S, Siddiqui WJ. Cardiac rhabdomyoma [Updated 2021 Jun 11]. In: StatPearls. Treasure Island, FL: StatPearls Publishing; 2021 Jan. [Internet]. Available from: https://www.ncbi.nlm.nih.gov/books/NBK560609.

[18] Mankad R, Herrmann J. Cardiac tumors: echo assessment. Echo Res Pract 2016;3(4): R65–77. https://doi.org/10.1530/ERP-16-0035.

[19] Manasse E, Nicolini F, Canziani R, et al. Left ventricular hemangioma. Eur J Cardiothorac Surg 1999;15(6):864–6. https://doi.org/10.1016/S1010-7940(99)00117-7.

[20] Cabo RA, Castedo E, Pastrana M, et al. Right atrial pheochromocytoma. Rev Esp Cardiol 2003;56(6):626–8.

[21] Park MII, Jung S, Youn HJ, et al. Blood cyst of subvalvular apparatus of the mitral valve in an adult. J Cardiovasc Ultrason 2012;20(3):146–9. https://doi.org/10.4250/jcu.2012.20.3.146.

[22] Beale RA, Russo R, Beale C, et al. Mitral valve blood cyst diagnosed with the use of multimodality imaging. CASE 2021;5(3):173–6. https://doi.org/10.1016/j.case.2021.01.004.

[23] Teshnizi MA, Ghorbanzadeh A, Zirak N, et al. Cardiac calcified amorphous tumor of the mitral valve presenting as transient ischemic attack. Hindawi, Case Rep Cardiol 2017. https://doi.org/10.1155/2017/2376096.

[24] Maleki M, Alizadehasl A, Haghjoo M. Practical cardiology. 2nd ed. Elsevier; 2021.

# Echocardiography in malignant cardiac tumors (diagnosis, approach, and follow-up)

**Azin Alizadehasl[a] and Niloufar Akbari Parsa[b]**

[a]Cardio-Oncology Research Center, Rajaie Cardiovascular Medical and Research Center, Iran University of Medical Sciences, Tehran, Iran [b]Echocardiography Department, Guilan University of Medical Sciences, Rasht, Iran

## Key points

- Most malignant cardiac tumors are metastatic, most commonly from lung and breast carcinomas, melanomas, soft tissue sarcomas, and renal carcinomas.
- Malignant primary cardiac tumors are rare and mostly consist of various sarcomas and lymphomas.
- Twenty-five percent of primary cardiac tumors are malignant.
- Echocardiography is a readily available, portable, low-cost imaging modality that gives the first clue as to the etiology of a cardiac mass. The characteristics of a mass such as location, mobility, attachment, and appearance can help determine whether a mass is benign or malignant.
- Magnetic resonance imaging offers incremental value owing to its larger field of view, superior tissue contrast, versatility in image planes, and unique ability to enable the discrimination of different tissue characteristics such as water and fat content, causing particular signal patterns with T1- and T2-weighted techniques (Table 9.1; Chart 9.2; Figs. 9.3 and 9.4).

Primary cardiac lymphomas are extremely rare in that they account for fewer than 2% of heart tumors. The most common pathological type is diffuse large B-cell lymphomas, followed by Burkitt lymphomas, T-cell lymphomas, small lymphocyte lymphomas, and plasmablastic lymphomas. The most frequent pathological types of secondary cardiac lymphoma are diffuse large B-cell lymphomas, T-lymphoblastic lymphomas, and Hodgkin lymphomas. Because most cardiac lymphomas are secondary, tumors outside the heart appear before cardiac tumors. Through the invasion of the mediastinum or the surrounding mass, the lymphatic circulation, or blood dissemination, the heart is involved and heart-related symptoms appear. Therefore most of the relevant cardiac symptoms are late or mild, indicating that they can be easily ignored [3].

**131**

**Table 9.1** Imaging features suggesting benign and malignant cardiac tumors [1].

| Imaging features suggesting benign and malignant cardiac tumors | | |
|---|---|---|
| **Features** | **Benign** | **Malignant** |
| Site/number | Small (<5cm), single lesion | Large (≥5cm), multiple lesions |
| Location | Left ≫ Right | Right ≫ Left |
| Morphology | Intracameral | Intramural |
| Attachment | Narrow stalk, pedunculated | Broad base |
| Borders | Smooth/well defined | Irregular |
| Invasion | None | Free wall and adjacent structures |
| Pericardial effusion | None | May be present |
| Calcification | Rare | Large foci in osteosarcomas |
| CT enhancement | Absent/minimal | Modest/intense |
| CMR T1W-TSE | Predominantly isointense | Predominantly isointense |
| CMR T2W-TSE | Predominantly hyperintense | Predominantly hyperintense or isointense |
| First-pass perfusion | May be present | Very frequent (70%) |
| Delayed enhancement | Usually present | Very frequent (80%) |

CMR, *cardiac magnetic resonance;* CT, *computed tomography;* T1W-TSE, *T1-weighted sequences turbo-spin-echo;* T2W-TSE, *T2-weighted sequences turbo-spin-echo.*

Cardiac lymphomas are easily missed or misdiagnosed, and medical personnel must increase their awareness of this malignancy. Echocardiography cannot be excluded from diagnostic examinations. In addition, the extensive application of positron emission tomography, which combines imaging and functional metabolism, effectively reveals the proliferation and metabolism of tumors throughout the body. It represents a more accurate method for the diagnosis and treatment of lymphomas with cardiac involvement (Fig. 9.5).

Although osteosarcomas are known to spread hematogenously, few imaging findings of cardiovascular involvement by osteosarcomas have been reported. Imaging findings of cardiovascular involvement by osteosarcomas can be subtle and are, thus, likely to be missed or misinterpreted, with potentially undesirable consequences. The incidence of cardiovascular metastases and the impact of its early recognition are not clear. Cardiovascular involvement usually happens early in the course of the disease within the systemic vein draining the primary tumor and in small pulmonary arterial branches, and in advanced cases within the veins draining the lung and extrapulmonary metastases. Extension into the left atrium is generally considered a feature of advanced osteosarcomas [4] (Figs. 9.6–9.8).

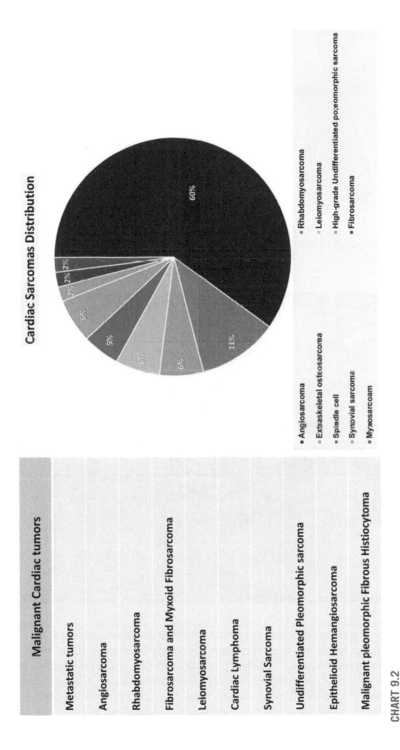

**Malignant Cardiac tumors**

Metastatic tumors

Angiosarcoma

Rhabdomyosarcoma

Fibrosarcoma and Myxoid Fibrosarcoma

Leiomyosarcoma

Cardiac Lymphoma

Synovial Sarcoma

Undifferentiated Pleomorphic sarcoma

Epithelioid Hemangiosarcoma

Malignant pleomorphic Fibrous Histiocytoma

**Cardiac Sarcomas Distribution**

60%

11%

6%

6%

5%

6%

2% 2% 2%

- Angiosarcoma
- Extraskeletal osteosarcoma
- Spindle cell
- Synovial sarcoma
- Myxosarcoam

- Rhabdomyosarcoma
- Leiomyosarcoma
- High-grade Undifferentiated pleomorphic sarcoma
- Fibrosarcoma

**CHART 9.2**

(Left) World Health Organization classification of malignant cardiac tumors. (Right) The image depicts the frequency distribution of cardiac sarcomas.

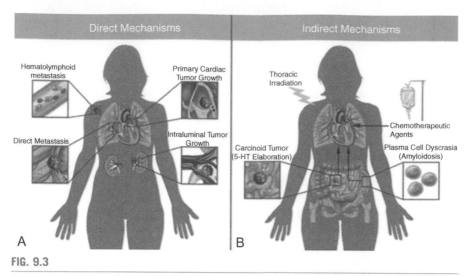

**FIG. 9.3**

The images illustrate the mechanisms of cardiac involvement in neoplasms [2].

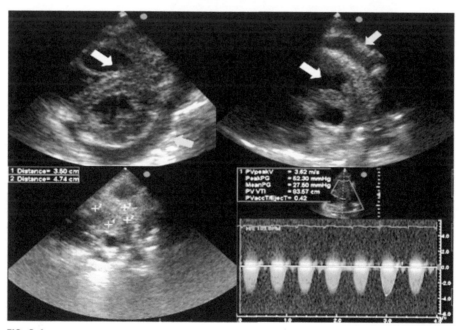

**FIG. 9.4**

The images demonstrate a lymphoma visualized by transthoracic echocardiography in a 24-year-old man with a history of a mediastinal lymphoma 2 years previously subjected to chemotherapy and radiotherapy. The patient presented with fatigue and exertional dyspnea (functional class II). The echocardiographic findings reveal a large, mural, echogenic mass in the right ventricular outflow tract *(white arrows)*, measuring about 3.5 cm × 4.7 cm in size. The mass results in a moderate obstruction (peak gradient =52 mmHg) and extends into the pulmonary artery branches. Additionally, a large heterogeneous pericardial effusion can be observed with the tumoral involvement of the pericardial cavity *(yellow arrows)*.

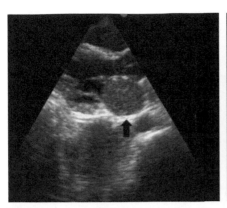
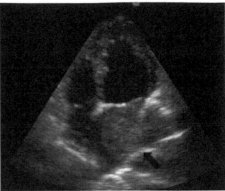

**FIG. 9.5**

The images illustrate cardiac metastases of an osteosarcoma. The transthoracic echocardiographic examination of a 61-year-old woman with a history of an osteosarcoma with lung metastases shows a large homogeneous left atrial mass (4.6 cm × 4 cm), which almost fills the atrium and originates from the left pulmonary veins and extends into the left atrium *(black arrows)*. The mass is the extension of the lung tumor from the pulmonary veins into the heart.

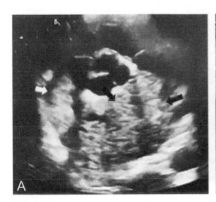
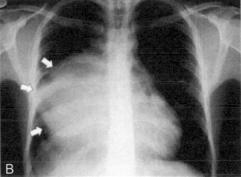

**FIG. 9.6**

The images show mediastinal germ cell tumors. The parasternal short-axis view shows that the right atrium is filled with a large heterogeneous mass (A, *white arrow*). The pulmonary trunk is infiltrated with a huge, heterogeneous mass that compresses the branches (A, *black arrows*), resulting in right ventricular dilatation and dysfunction. The chest X-ray shows the right-heart border silhouette (B, *white arrows*), suggestive of right-side enlargement with a mediastinal origin. Mediastinal germ cell neoplasms are rare and account for between 10% and 15% of all the mediastinal tumors. These tumors are usually asymptomatic and discovered incidentally during routine chest X-rays. Considering the close relationship between mediastinal germ cell tumors and the heart, echocardiography by an experienced cardiologist may be necessary for early detection [5].

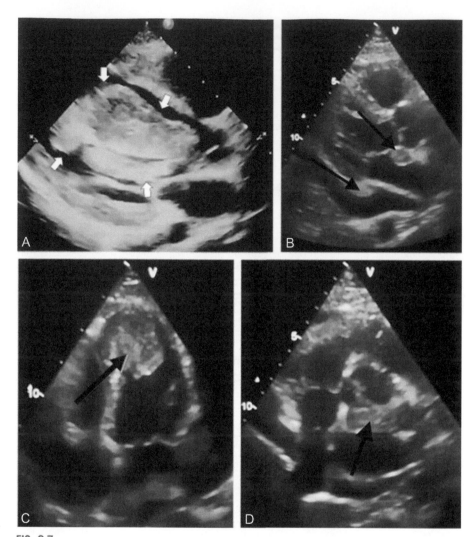

**FIG. 9.7**

The images depict metastatic melanomas involving the heart visualized by transthoracic echocardiography in 2 patients. A huge, semimobile, heterogeneous mass (A, *white arrows*) is seen attached to the mitral-annular intervalvular fibrosa, causing a life-threatening left ventricular outflow obstruction (Supplementary Video 9.S1 in the online version at https://doi.org/10.1016/B978-0-323-84906-7.00001-7). Multiple heterogeneous lesions can be seen with myocardial and pericardial invasions (B, C, and D, *black arrows*), suggestive of metastatic lesions. Malignant melanomas involve the heart frequently. However, they are diagnosed late in the course of the disease due to the absence of specific clinical signs and the low sensitivity of routine examinations. Complementary imaging modalities, including transesophageal echocardiography, cardiac magnetic resonance, and fluorodeoxyglucose-positron emission tomography, represent major advances in the assessment of metastatic melanomas [6].

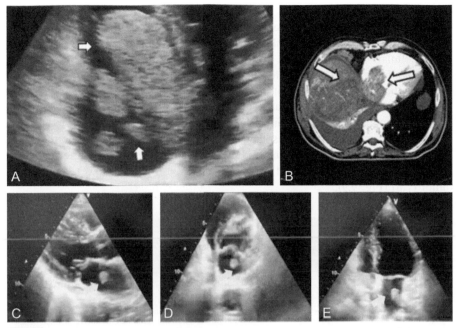

**FIG. 9.8**

The images illustrate 2 cases of cardiac metastases of hepatocellular carcinomas. (A and B) A large, multilobulated, semimobile, heterogeneous mass is seen in the right atrium (A, *white arrows*). The axial image in the computed tomography scan shows a large mass in the liver and its invasion to the right atrium (B, *white arrows*). The parasternal long-axis (C), parasternal short-axis (B), and apical 4-chamber (E) views of the transthoracic echocardiographic examination of a patient with a history of a hepatocellular carcinoma with metastases to the lung show a mobile mass with infiltration to the left atrium through a pulmonary vein.

Advanced hepatocellular carcinomas represent a disease with a poor prognosis and a median survival time of 4 to 7 months. Hepatocellular carcinoma metastases tend to spread through the intrahepatic blood vessels and the lymphatic system or direct infiltration. They frequently invade the vascular system at points such as the portal and hepatic veins. The extrahepatic metastases of hepatocellular carcinomas may reach around 18%, with the most common sites of involvement being the lungs, lymph nodes, adrenal glands, and bones. The intracardiac involvement of hepatocellular carcinomas rarely develops (2%), and the main mechanism of metastases into the cardiac cavity is the direct extension of the tumor to the heart via the hepatic vein and the inferior vena cava. The prognosis of hepatocellular carcinomas with intracardiac metastases is poor, with a median survival range of 1 to 4 months. The most common causes of death in patients with hepatocellular carcinomas with intracardiac involvement are heart failure and sudden death, which account for 25% of the patients. Most patients with right-sided metastases will have signs and symptoms of right-sided heart failure, or they could be totally asymptomatic. Irrespective of the symptoms, the presence of right-sided metastases renders the prognosis extremely poor. Other cardiac symptoms or findings such as dyspnea, lower extremity edema, dilatation of the jugular veins, and sudden death are generally seen in hepatocellular carcinomas with intracardiac involvement. Echocardiography is widely available, and it provides a simple, noninvasive technique for the initial evaluation of the cardiac involvement of any tumor. Echocardiography images both the myocardium and the cardiac chambers and can usually identify the presence of a mass in conjunction with its mobility and functional effects. Both computed tomography (CT) and magnetic resonance imaging (MRI) provide noninvasive, high-resolution images of the heart and the liver. MRI is generally preferred since, in addition to furnishing detailed anatomic images, it offers clues as to the type of tumor [7,8] (Fig. 9.9).

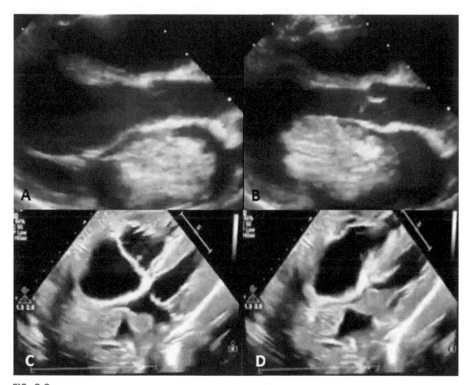

**FIG. 9.9**

The images demonstrate cardiac metastases of lung cancers in the transthoracic echocardiographic examinations of 2 patients. The upper panels show the cardiac metastases of lung squamous cell carcinomas. A large, multilobulated, heterogeneous mass is seen in the left atrium in the systole (A) with protrusion into the left ventricle in the diastole (B). The lower panels show another case of a lung tumor with cardiac metastases. A large, elongated hypermobile mass is seen in the systole (C) with protrusion into the left ventricle in the diastole (D).

Metastases comprise the most common cause of death from lung cancer. The most common sites of the metastases of lung cancer are the lymph nodes, liver, brain, bone, and adrenal glands in decreasing order of frequency. Cardiac metastases occur predominantly between the sixth and eighth decades of life, and there is no sex predisposition. The rate of the metastases of lung cancer to the heart varies with the histopathological subtype. Adenocarcinomas metastasize to the heart in 26% of cases, as opposed to squamous cell carcinomas in 23.4%, undifferentiated carcinomas in 21.2%, and bronchoalveolar carcinomas in 17.4% of cases. The most common site of cardiac metastases is the epicardium/pericardium. Myocardial involvement is less common. Endocardial, intracavitary, and valvular metastases are very rare. The right atrium is the most commonly affected chamber, and 80% of metastases occur to the right chambers. This is due to the filtering role of the pulmonary circulation and the slower flow in the right chambers. The mechanisms of cardiac metastases are lymphatic spread (most common), direct extension from the adjacent viscera, hematogenous spread, and transvenous extension [9] (Fig. 9.10).

In the majority (approximately 90%) of patients, cardiac metastases are silent and diagnosed only on autopsy. The clinical features are extremely variable and depend on the anatomic location and size of the tumor, as well as the invasion of the adjacent tissues. Clinical manifestations are caused by the direct obstruction of cardiac or valve function, interruption of the coronary flow (by obstruction or embolization), interference with the electrophysiology of contraction, and pericardial effusion. Intramural tumors cause arrhythmias and may cause obstruction in the right or left outflow tract or the compression of the cardiac chambers. Intracardiac tumors cause clinical features of right-sided (peripheral edema) or left-sided (orthopnea) heart failure. Echocardiography is the investigation of choice for the diagnosis. TEE confers better visualization of the atria and the great vessels than TTE, CT, MRI, and angiography. CT and MRI are also useful tools in imaging cardiac metastases in that they image the location, morphological features, extent, the presence of local invasion, and mediastinal or pulmonary involvement. They also offer some degree of histological characterization of metastases by identifying fat, calcification, fibrous tissue, melanin, hemorrhage, and cystic changes. The administration of contrast assists in differentiating between tumors and thrombi [9] (Fig. 9.11).

Cardiac metastases of primary prostate carcinomas are extremely rare. Metastases of prostate cancer, similar to those of other solid tumors, involve multiple steps, including angiogenesis, local migration, invasion, intravasation, circulation, and extravasation of tumor cells and then angiogenesis and colonization in the new site (Figs. 9.12 and 9.13).

The regional lymph nodes, liver, and lung are the most common sites of metastases from colorectal cancer, and cardiac metastases are extremely rare. In colorectal cancer, to our knowledge, only 9 reports have been published in the literature; however, the incidence of cardiac metastases is 1.4% to 7.2% in autopsy studies. Thus the true incidence of cardiac metastases from colorectal cancer might be higher than the cases reported so far. The differential diagnoses of cardiac myxomas and cardiac metastases from colorectal cancer might be difficult to determine by

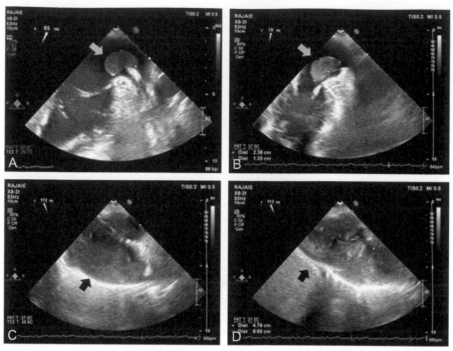

**FIG. 9.10**

The images illustrate cardiac metastases of lung cancer in the transesophageal echocardiographic examination of a 46-year-old man with a history of lung cancer. (A and B) A large (2.5 cm × 1.5 cm), homogeneous, mobile, solid, lobulated mass is seen in the left atrium. The mass originates from the left lower pulmonary vein, suggestive of a metastatic mass, although a large clot should be considered with less probability. (C and D) Additionally, there is a large (4.7 cm × 6.65 cm), heterogeneous mass posterior to the left atrium.

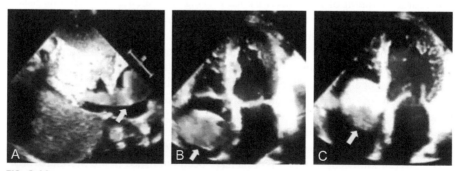

**FIG. 9.11**

The images demonstrate cardiac metastases of prostate cancer in the transthoracic echocardiographic examination of a man with a history of prostate cancer. (A) A large, elongated tumor thrombus in the inferior vena cava extends into the right atrium. (B) A large metastatic mass is visualized in the right atrium in the systole. (C) The mass protrudes into the right ventricle in the diastole (Supplementary Video 9.S2 in the online version at https://doi.org/10.1016/B978-0-323-84906-7.00001-7).

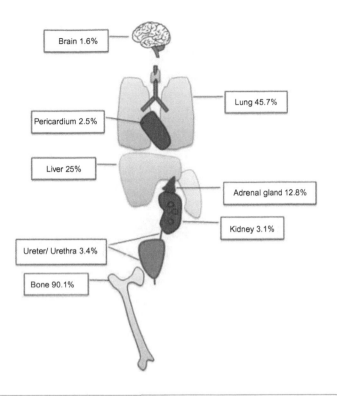

**FIG. 9.12**

The image depicts the distribution of the hematogenous metastases of prostate cancer [10].

echocardiography alone, and MRI is effective in the evaluation of secondary cardiac tumors because it can accurately define the pericardium, the myocardial walls, and the cardiac chambers, especially in cases with an infiltrative nature. Surgery as a treatment modality has not been investigated, but it could be especially effective in occurrences of obstructive and solitary lesions to ensure relief from symptoms and prolongation of life expectancy. With the improvement of diagnostic procedures and a prolonged life span, the incidence of cardiac metastases from colorectal cancer is likely to increase. Therefore the delineation of the role of surgical treatment in cardiac metastases from colorectal cancer requires further studies [11] (Fig. 9.14).

Sarcomas represent 65% of all malignant primary cardiac tumors. Because of their rarity, knowledge about this disease and possible therapeutic strategies are limited. Due to the silent progression and nonspecific symptoms caused essentially by mass location, cardiac sarcomas are usually diagnosed at advanced stages. Therefore the prognosis of primary cardiac sarcomas is very poor and worse than that of sarcomas in other anatomical districts. Clinical history focuses on previous extracardiac malignancies. Echocardiography can identify the mass and evaluate its mobility and hemodynamic impact. Cardiac magnetic resonance confers better soft tissue

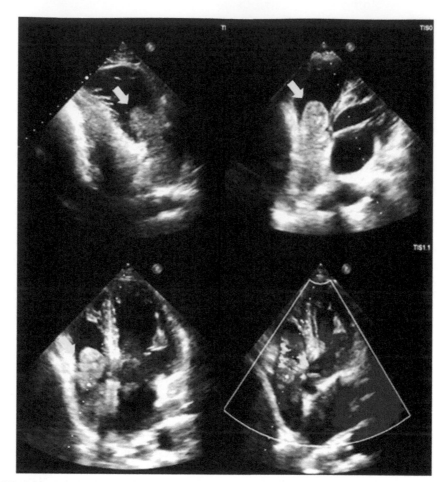

**FIG. 9.13**

The images show cardiac metastases of colon cancer in a 41-year-old man with a history of colon cancer presenting with dyspnea and palpitation. Transthoracic echocardiography shows a large, multilobulated, hypermobile mass that infiltrates into the right atrium from the inferior vena cava and protrudes into the right ventricle in the diastole (arrows) (Supplementary Video 9.S3 in the online version at https://doi.org/10.1016/B978-0-323-84906-7.00001-7).

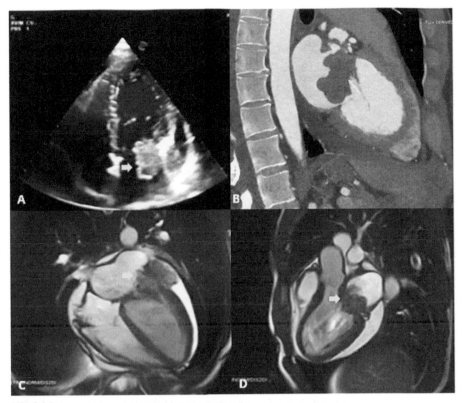

**FIG. 9.14**

The images illustrate a cardiac chondrosarcoma in a young man admitted to the emergency department due to worsening dyspnea. (A) Transthoracic echocardiography shows a large, nonhomogeneous left atrial mass (36 mm × 21 mm in diameter). The mass is adherent to the mitral ring and features irregular borders. (B) The cardiac computed tomography scan shows a large solid mass. The mass is adherent to the mitral ring and involves the ventricular cavity. (C) Cardiac magnetic resonance in the 4-chamber view shows an isointense cardiac mass infiltrating the myocardial wall and the pericardial space, with mild pericardial effusion. (D) Cardiac magnetic resonance in the 3-chamber view shows the cardiac mass. The surgical resection of the mass was incomplete, as was confirmed during surgery, due to parietal infiltration. Macroscopically, the tumor had a scirrhous consistency and a diameter of about 5 cm. The histologic examination showed a high-grade sarcoma with spindle cells and chondrosarcoma elements.

characterization, high resolution, and multiplane image acquisition. CT provides morphostructural information of the mass. Coronary artery imaging is the method of choice when cardiac magnetic resonance is contraindicated. Cardiac surgery aimed at radical resection is the cornerstone of the treatment, with chemotherapy used for neo- and adjuvant purposes. Radiation therapy, a still debated issue, is

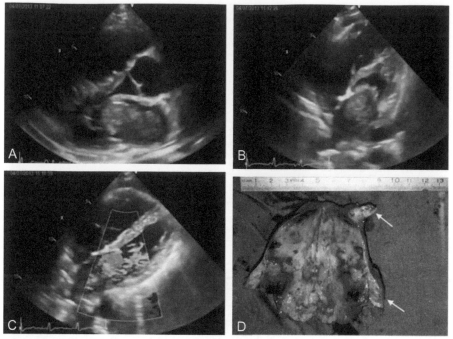

**FIG. 9.15**

The images illustrate a rhabdomyosarcoma in a 46-year-old woman admitted in a state of cardiogenic shock and pulmonary edema. (A and B) Transthoracic echocardiography shows a large, mobile mass in the left atrium. The mass protrudes into the left ventricle in the diastole and results in left ventricular inflow obstruction (C and D). The internal surface of the neoplasm (in cross-section) shows both necrotic and hemorrhagic areas. The *arrows* indicate the obstruction of the right pulmonary veins. The pathology results confirmed a rhabdomyosarcoma.

usually performed after surgery. Autotransplantation is a possible alternative approach, while conventional heart transplantation is to be reserved for patients in whom metastases have been excluded through a multidisciplinary evaluation [12] (Fig. 9.15).

Rhabdomyosarcomas account for almost 20% of all primary malignant neo-plasms of the heart and are the second most common primary cardiac sarcomas. These tumors usually arise from the ventricular or atrial walls but tend to occur in multiple sites within the heart and can cause obstruction at multiple levels. They grow rapidly and invade the pericardium early in their course, resulting in a poor prognosis.

Sarcomas, in general, grow rapidly and extensively and metastasize early. Complete resection is the most ideal option; still, metastatic disease and recurrence limit long-term survival even with complete excision. Adjuvant chemotherapy and radiation have been tried to improve the poor overall survival; no randomized trials have been undertaken, however. Radiation typically is used for metastatic disease [13] (Fig. 9.16).

Rhabdomyosarcomas make up almost 20% of primary cardiac sarcomas. These tumors usually arise from the ventricular walls and frequently interfere with valvular motion because of their intracavitary bulk. The involvement of the ventricular septum and ventricular walls, which often occurs, makes complete excision impossible. In adult patients, these tumors sometimes arise from the atrial walls and mimic atrioventricular valve stenosis. Rhabdomyosarcomas of the heart are very aggressive; and although survival of up to 5 years has been reported, the prognosis is very poor. Indeed, the patients usually survive less than 1 year, despite the excision of the primary tumor and subsequent radiation and chemotherapy.

TTE and TEE can diagnose the presence of the mass. Nonetheless, these imaging techniques rarely define the true nature of the mass, especially when it is located in the atria. In such cases, the tumor is usually given a presumptive diagnosis of a thrombus or a myxoma, and the patient is sent to surgery. Nuclear MRI can be useful in defining the nature of an intracardiac mass. Despite its poor midterm prognosis, surgery is indicated to remove the mass, thereby relieving acute symptoms and extending the life of the patient by perhaps a few months [14] (Fig. 9.17).

There are "red flags" regarding malignancy: a diameter exceeding 5 mm, right-heart localization, pericardial effusion, and the involvement of the right atrioventricular groove. Primary cardiac angiosarcomas are primarily endothelial cell tumors. About 90% of the tumors are in the right atrium as multicentric masses. The aggressive and permeating growth within the surrounding myocardial wall may result in the filling of the atrial chamber and the invasion of the vena cava and the tricuspid valve. The involvement of the left heart occurs in fewer than 5% of cases [15] (Fig. 9.18).

Leiomyosarcomas are known as mesenchymal tumors arising from smooth muscle cells. Cardiac leiomyosarcomas are usually located in the left atrium with the involvement of the pulmonary veins. The common presentations include dyspnea, pericardial effusion, chest pain, atrial arrhythmias, peripheral embolism, and heart failure. The prognosis is poor (mean survival ≈ 6 months) owing to the rapid growth, high rates of remote metastases, and postremoval recurrence [16] (Fig. 9.19).

The clinical presentation of cardiac synovial sarcomas is nonspecific, so the diagnosis is almost always at the advanced stage in most cases. Patients usually present with more than 1 symptom such as shortness of breath, dyspnea, chest pain, and weight loss. Patients with left-sided tumors present earlier than those with right-sided tumors due to the effects of the mass and the obstruction of the pulmonary veins. The mean age at presentation of cardiac synovial sarcomas is 32.5 years with a range from 13 to 66 years. All 3 treatment modalities of surgery, chemotherapy, and radiotherapy are given to patients, but surgery is the mainstay of treatment. Wide excision of the tumor is required for better outcomes, although it is anatomically difficult to

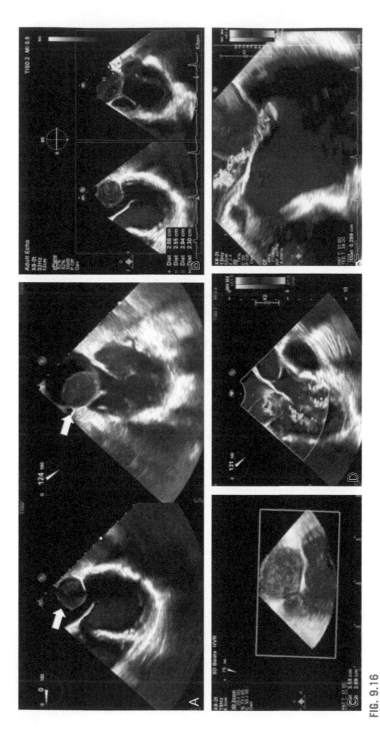

**FIG. 9.16**

The images show a rhabdomyosarcoma in the transesophageal echocardiographic examination of a 42-year-old woman with a history of left atrial rhabdomyosarcoma resection 3 years earlier presenting with atypical chest pain. (A) A round, large, fixed, homogeneous mass is attached to the posterolateral wall of the left atrium and the posterior mitral valve leaflet, suggestive of recurrence or a rhabdomyosarcoma. (B) The interrogation of the mass in 2 perpendicular views (the biplane mode) is presented herein. (C) The 3D image shows that the tumor is 2.7 cm × 3.6 cm in size. (D) A diastolic turbulent flow over the mitral valve due to functional obstruction by the tumor is visualized herein. (D) The mass has resulted in the malcoaptation of the mitral valve leaflets and moderate eccentric mitral regurgitation.

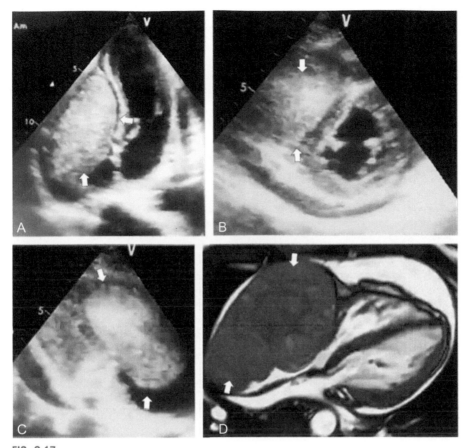

**FIG. 9.17**

The images demonstrate primary cardiac angiosarcomas in the transthoracic echocardiographic examination of a patient. There is a large, heterogeneous mass in the right atrium and the right ventricle (A, B, and C, *white arrows*) (Supplementary Video 9.S4 in the online version at https://doi.org/10.1016/B978-0-323-84906-7.00001-7). The mass breaches anatomical boundaries, making malignancy the first differential diagnosis.

obtain large, tumor-free margins in the heart. The prognosis of synovial sarcomas is poor, with most patients dying within 1 year. The most common cause of death is local recurrence. Because synovial sarcomas are rare, prognostic factors are hard to ascertain; nevertheless, younger age at diagnosis, the absence of chromosomal abnormalities, and the origination of the tumor from the pericardium seem to be favorable factors [17–19] (Fig. 9.20).

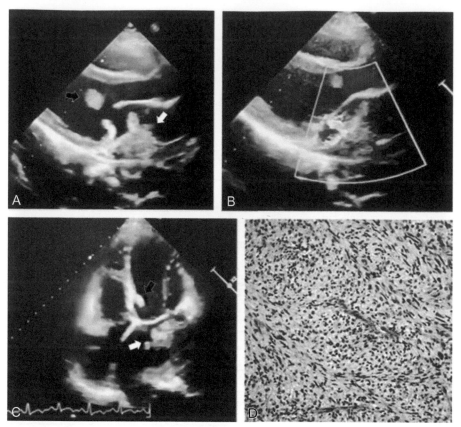

**FIG. 9.18**

The images illustrate a primary cardiac leiomyosarcoma in the transthoracic echocardiographic examination of a patient. A large, multilobulated, heterogeneous mass (A and C, *white arrows*) is seen. The mass extends from the pulmonary vein into the left atrium, resulting in interference with mitral valve coaptation and significant regurgitation (B). There is another hypermobile mass attached to the interventricular septum with a narrow stalk (A and C, *black arrows*).

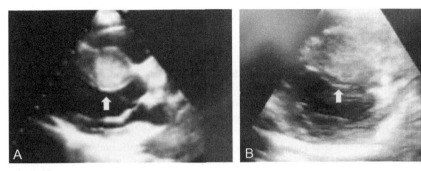

**FIG. 9.19**

The images present a synovial sarcoma. Transthoracic echocardiography shows a large, fixed mass in the interventricular septum *(arrows)*. The diagnosis is a synovial sarcoma.

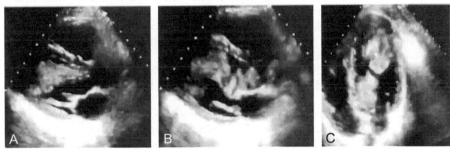

**FIG. 9.20**

The images demonstrate the relapse of a primary cardiac sarcoma. The transthoracic echocardiographic examination of a patient with a history of a primary cardiac sarcoma and surgical resection presenting with dyspnea shows a large, heterogeneous, hypermobile mass that extends from the left ventricular apex to the ascending aorta, suggestive of a relapsed left ventricular sarcoma. The patient underwent surgery again, and the pathology results confirmed the diagnosis.

## Appendix: Supplementary material

Supplementary material related to this chapter can be found on the accompanying CD or online at https://doi.org/10.1016/B978-0-323-84906-7.00001-7.

## References

[1] Andrei V, Scheggi V, Stefàno PL, et al. Primary cardiac sarcoma: a case report of a therapeutic challenge. Eur Heart J Case Rep 2020;4(6):1–6. https://doi.org/10.1093/ehjcr/ytaa404.

[2] Maleszewski JJ, Bois MC, Bois JP, et al. Neoplasia and the heart pathological review of effects with clinical and radiological correlation. J Am Coll Cardiol 2018;72(2):202–7.

[3] Zhao Y, Huang S, Ma C, et al. Clinical features of cardiac lymphoma: an analysis of 37 cases. J Int Med Res 2021;49. https://doi.org/10.1177/0300060521999558, 300060521999558.

[4] Yedururi S, Morani A, Gladish GW, et al. Cardiovascular involvement by osteosarcoma: an analysis of 20 patients. Pediatr Radiol 2016;46(1):21–33. https://doi.org/10.1007/s00247-015-3449-y.

[5] Karas SM, Parissis JT, Antoniades C, Loulias A. A rare case of large mediastinal germ cell tumor detected by echocardiography. Int J Cardiol 2005;101(1):159–61. https://doi.org/10.1016/j.ijcard.2004.01.044.

[6] Ramchand J, Wong GR, Yudi MB, Sylivris S. Cardiac metastatic melanoma. BMJ Case Rep 2016;2016:2–4. https://doi.org/10.1136/bcr-2016-215881.

[7] Senarslan O, Kantarci UH, Eyuboglu M, et al. Is it possible? Invasion of the heart with hepatocellular carcinoma in a short time. Int J Cardiovasc Acad 2016;2(3):124–6. https://doi.org/10.1016/j.ijcac.2016.06.002.

[8] Salehi M, Yee T, Alatevi E, et al. Clinically silent intracardiac metastasis with extremely poor prognosis in a patient with hepatocellular carcinoma. Case Rep Gastroenterol 2017;11(2):416–21. https://doi.org/10.1159/000477379.

[9] Prasad R, Karmakar S, Hussain A. Cardiac metastasis of lung cancer: case report and review of literature. J Assoc Chest Physicians 2016;4(2):84–6. https://doi.org/10.4103/2320-8775.183838.

[10] Pasoglou V, Michoux N, Tombal B, et al. Optimising TNM staging of patients with prostate cancer using WB-MRI. J Belg Soc Radiol 2016;100(1):101. https://doi.org/10.5334/jbr-btr.1209.

[11] Choi PW, Kim CN, Chang SH, et al. Cardiac metastasis from colorectal cancer: a case report. World J Gastroenterol 2009;15(21):2675–8. https://doi.org/10.3748/wjg.15.2675.

[12] Andrei V, Scheggi V, Stefàno PL, et al. Primary cardiac sarcoma: a case report of a therapeutic challenge. Eur Heart J Case Rep 2020;4(6):1–6. https://doi.org/10.1093/ehjcr/ytaa404.

[13] Mankad R, Herrmann J. Cardiac tumors: echo assessment. Echo Res Pract 2016;R65–77. https://doi.org/10.1530/ERP-16-0035.

[14] Castorino F, Masiello P, Quattrocchi E, et al. Primary cardiac rhabdomyosarcoma of the left atrium: an unusual presentation. Tex Heart Inst J 2000;27(2):206–8.

[15] Patel SD, Peterson A, Bartczak A, et al. Primary cardiac angiosarcoma—a review. Med Sci Monit 2014;20:103–9. https://doi.org/10.12659/MSM.889875.

[16] Andersen RE, Kristensen BW, Gill S. Cardiac leiomyosarcoma, a case report. Int J Clin Exp Pathol 2013;6(6):1197–9. https://pubmed.ncbi.nlm.nih.gov/23696944.

[17] Maleki M, Alizadehasl A, Haghjoo M. Practical cardiology. 2nd ed. Elsevier; 2021.

[18] Sharma A, Dixit S, Sharma M, et al. Primary synovial cell sarcoma of the heart: a rare case. Heart Views 2015;16(2):62–4. https://doi.org/10.4103/1995-705X.159223.

[19] Ziyaeifard M, Alizadehasl A, Aghdaii N, et al. The effect of combined conventional and modified ultrafiltration on mechanical ventilation and hemodynamic changes in congenital heart surgery. J Res Med Sci 2016;21:113. https://doi.org/10.4103/1735-1995.193504.

# Contrast echocardiography in cardiac masses

# 10

**Azin Alizadehasl[a], Shirin Habibi Khorasani[a], Niloufar Akbari Parsa[b], and Amir Abdi[c]**

*[a]Cardio-Oncology Research Center, Rajaie Cardiovascular Medical and Research Center, Iran University of Medical Sciences, Tehran, Iran [b]Echocardiography Department, Guilan University of Medical Sciences, Rasht, Iran [c]School of Medicine, Islamic Azad University Tehran Medical Branch, Tehran, Iran*

## Key points

- Newer echocardiographic techniques may provide incremental information to help characterize cardiac masses.
- Myocardial contrast echocardiography allows an improved definition of intracavity structures and an assessment of vascularity.
- The difference in the perfusion of cardiac masses may help distinguish between vascular tumors and nonvascular tumors or thrombi.
- Contrast agents improve the opacification of the cardiac cavities and the delineation of the endocardial borders in addition to helping perfusion evaluation.

Contrast echocardiography is based on the intravenous injection of microbubbles that act as blood flow tracers and increase ultrasound signals. Contrast agents enhance the opacification of the cardiac cavities and the delineation of the endocardial borders in addition to helping perfusion evaluation. Contrast echocardiography has recently been used to evaluate cardiac masses and shown to be valuable in the diagnosis of the different types of cardiac masses (Table 10.1).

Transthoracic echocardiography remains a versatile and globally the most common cardiac diagnostic imaging modality. Nonetheless, there is still a need to improve image resolution when acoustic windows are limited and endocardial definition suboptimal, which may result in potentially missed or incorrect diagnoses and consequential adverse outcomes. Microbubble ultrasound contrast is now regarded as an essential tool in the day-to-day practice of the clinical echocardiography laboratory to overcome some of these limitations. The contemporary approved and appropriate indications for the use of ultrasound contrast agents include left ventricular opacification and improvement of endocardial border detection [1]. Currently, the validity of this method for the differential diagnosis of cardiac masses is argued based on their vascular pattern analysis. Intracardiac masses can be a normal variant of cardiac structures such as false chordae, accessory papillary muscles, or prominent

**151**

**Table 10.1** Indications for contrast echocardiography [1].

| Indications for contrast echocardiography |
| --- |
| Left ventricular opacification during resting transthoracic echocardiography in difficult-to-image patients for<br><br>• improved left ventricular endocardial border definition (when ≥2 contiguous segments are not well visualized)<br>• improved accuracy and reproducibility of the quantitative left ventricular ejection fraction<br>• definitive diagnosis of left ventricular structural abnormalities, including apical thrombi, apical hypertrophic cardiomyopathy, left ventricular noncompaction, and complications of myocardial infarction (i.e., left ventricular aneurysms and pseudoaneurysms)<br>• left ventricular opacification during stress echocardiography (when ≥2 contiguous segments are not well visualized) to augment the sensitivity and accuracy of wall motion analysis for the detection of myocardial ischemia |

trabeculations or can be pathological such as thrombi, vegetations, and tumors. Any suspicious cardiac mass, when not evident on baseline images, can be confirmed or refuted after the injection of the intravenous contrast for a better delineation of the structures. As is the case with unenhanced echocardiography, off-axis images and longer loop acquisitions may be required to identify and characterize intracardiac thrombi or masses [2] with the general understanding that benign tumors have lower vascularization, thrombi are avascular, and malignant tumors are highly irrigated.

Despite advances in other imaging modalities, echocardiography remains the initial tool for diagnosis and risk stratification in patients predisposed to developing cardiac thrombi. The use of ultrasound-enhancing agents facilitates left ventricular thrombus detection by providing opacification within the cardiac chambers so that the filling defect of an intracardiac thrombus can be demonstrated. Ultrasound-enhancing agents can increase the sensitivity for the detection of left ventricular thrombi, improve the negative predictive value, and increase the certainty that a thrombus is truly absent when it is not visualized on echocardiography. It is recommended that nontraditional "off-axis" views be obtained in order to visualize the entire apex while imaging with ultrasound-enhancing agents. While delayed enhancement cardiac magnetic resonance (CMR) has the highest sensitivity and specificity for the detection of left ventricular thrombi, performing echocardiography with an ultrasound-enhancing agent is a more clinically feasible initial test. Nevertheless, CMR should be considered when echocardiography with ultrasound-enhancing agents fails to detect an intracardiac thrombus but clinical suspicion persists [2] (Figs. 10.2 and 10.3).

By differentiating malignant/highly vascular tumors from benign tumors and thrombi, echocardiographic contrast perfusion imaging may aid in the early identification and appropriate treatment of cardiac masses. A complete lack of enhancement, signaling thrombi, would be an indication for anticoagulation with a follow-up imaging study to evaluate resolution and could prevent unnecessary cardiac surgery. A further application is the detection and evaluation of malignant or highly vascular tumors or metastases within the myocardium that do not protrude into cardiac cavities. The objective hyperenhancement of an area of the myocardium may raise the suspicion of intramyocardial tumor infiltration [4,5] (Fig. 10.4).

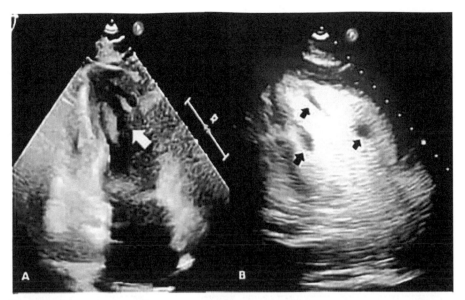

**FIG. 10.2**

The images depict contrast echocardiography in left ventricular clots. (A) Transthoracic echocardiography in a patient with breast cancer shows the normal size and function of the left ventricle with 2 hypermobile clots attached to the inner surface of the ventricle *(white arrow)*. (B) The contrast study reveals the third clot, not detected by transthoracic echocardiography *(black arrows)*.

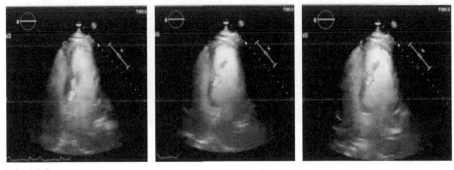

**FIG. 10.3**

The images illustrate a hypermobile left ventricular clot in contrast echocardiography. The use of the contrast agent in transthoracic echocardiography shows an elongated hypermobile mass at different time points in the cardiac cycle. The mass is attached to the inner surface of the left ventricular inferior wall, but it oscillates in the ventricle and carries the high risk of systemic embolization *(yellow arrows)* (Video 10.S1 in the online version at https://doi.org/10.1016/B978-0-323-84906-7.00002-9) [3].

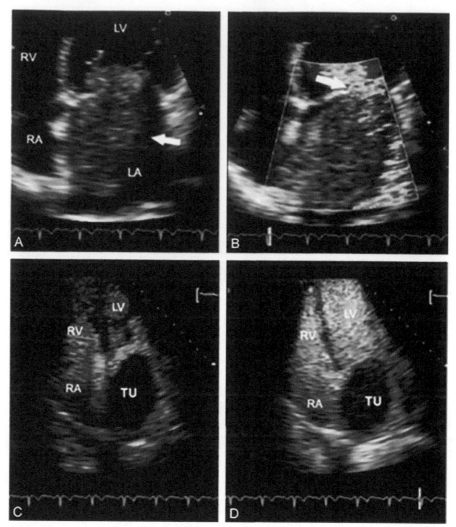

**FIG. 10.4**

The images demonstrate a left atrial myxoma. (A and B) Transthoracic echocardiography shows a large heterogeneous mass in the left atrium, resulting in the obstruction of the functional mitral valve inflow. (C) Contrast echocardiography exactly at the time of flash injection shows a large filling defect inside the atrium. Additionally, no contrast is observed immediately after the flash inside the mass. (D) After 5 s, the mass shows mild contrast filling, indicating low vascularization. The patient underwent surgical excision, and the pathology results confirmed the diagnosis of a myxoma [3].

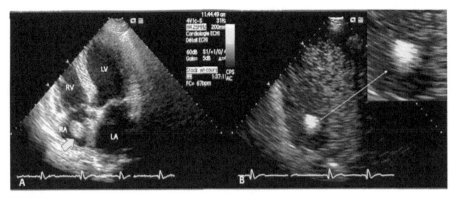

**FIG. 10.5**

The images depict a cardiac metastatic renal sarcoma. (A) The apical 4-chamber view of transthoracic echocardiography shows a round, well-defined mass in the right atrium *(yellow arrow)*. (B) Contrast injection shows the complete enhancement of the mass by the contrast agent and is indicative of the high vascularity of the mass and suggestive of the presence of a malignant tumor. The pathology results confirmed the diagnosis of a renal sarcoma.

Most malignant tumors have abnormal neovascularization with high blood supplies, which explains why these tumors present an enhancement of the mass by the contrast agent. Myxomas have poor blood supplies, with partial enhancement by the contrast agent. Finally, thrombi are avascular, with no enhancement. Thus, regardless of the experience of the physician, contrast echocardiography is highly reproducible and confers an accurate diagnosis with a simple and fast injection of the contrast agent, which permits heart opacification [6,7] (Fig. 10.5).

## Appendix: Supplementary material

Supplementary material related to this chapter can be found on the accompanying CD or online at https://doi.org/10.1016/B978-0-323-84906-7.00002-9.

## References

[1] Chong A, Haluska B, Wahi S. Clinical application and laboratory protocols for performing contrast echocardiography. Indian Heart J 2013;65:337–46. https://doi.org/10.1016/j.ihj.2013.04.002.

[2] Lindner JR, Porter TR, Park MM. American society of echocardiography guidelines and recommendations for contrast echocardiography: a summary for applications approved by the U.S. Food and Drug Administration. JASE; 2018.

[3] Ziyaeifard M, Alizadehasl A, Aghdaii N, et al. Heparinized and saline solutions in the maintenance of arterial and central venous catheters after cardiac surgery. Anesthesiol Pain Med 2015;5(4). https://doi.org/10.5812/aapm28056, e28056. 26478866.

[4] Uenishi EK, Caldas MA, Saroute ANR, et al. Contrast echocardiography for the evaluation of tumors and thrombi. Arq Bras Cardiol 2008;91(5):e56–60.

[5] Kirkpatrick JN, Wong T, Bednarz JE, et al. Differential diagnosis of cardiac masses using contrast echocardiographic perfusion imaging. JACC 2004;43(8):1412–9. https://doi.org/10.1016/j.jacc.2003.09.065.

[6] Maleki M, Alizadehasl A, Haghjoo M. Practical cardiology. 2nd ed. Elsevier; 2021.

[7] Mansencal N, Revault-d'Allonnes L, Pelage JP, et al. Usefulness of contrast echocardiography for assessment of intracardiac masses. Arch Cardiovasc Dis 2009;102:177–83. https://doi.org/10.1016/j.acvd.2008.12.007.

# CT in benign cardiac tumors (diagnosis, approach, and follow-up)

# 11

**Hamidreza Pouraliakbar and Kiara Rezaei-Kalantari**

*Department of Radiology, CardioOncology Research Center, Iran University of Medical Sciences, Rajaie Cardiovascular Medical and Research Center, Tehran, Iran*

## Key points

- CT has emerged as an important imaging modality in the evaluation of cardiac and paracardiac neoplasms. CT has several advantages including wide availability, rapid acquisition time, excellent isotropic spatial resolution, and multiplanar reconstruction capabilities.
- CT is a robust technique for assessment of the relationship of the mass to the myocardium, cardiac valves, pericardium, coronary arteries, great vessels including pulmonary and systemic, and adjacent tissues, such as lung and lymph nodes, in a way that no other imaging modality can often reach.
- Cardiac CT possesses a fairly good capability for tissue characterization through assessment of the lesion density (distinguishing calcium and fat components from soft tissue). Cardiac CT is the best modality for determining calcification.
- Myxomas are the most common and lipomas are the second primary cardiac tumor in adults.
- The most common primary cardiac tumors in pediatric are rhabdomyoma and fibroma.

## Tissue characterization

Primary benign cardiac neoplasms are more common than the primary malignant ones, most of them being myxomas. The CT features of the tumor that help distinguish benign from malignant neoplasms include location, size, margins, the presence of a feeding artery, calcification, or pericardial effusion [2] (Table 11.1).

## Technical issues

The scan protocol used can vary given the variety of clinical scenarios that may precede referral to CT.

Multimodal Imaging Atlas of Cardiac Masses. https://doi.org/10.1016/B978-0-323-84906-7.00017-0

**Table 11.1** CT characteristic features of various benign cardiac neoplasms.

| Tumor | Age | Sex | Chamber | Location | Morphology | Before contrast | After contrast | Functional |
|---|---|---|---|---|---|---|---|---|
| Myxoma | 30–60 y | M=F | LA | IAS, IC | Pedunculated, lobular | Heterogeneous, low density | Heterogeneous | Mobile, narrow stalk |
| Lipoma | Any | M=F | Any | IM, IC | Smooth, large, broad-based, lobular | Homogeneous, fat density | None | Maybe be mobile |
| Fibroelastoma | Middle, elderly | M=F | Valves | Valves | Small, smooth, pedunculated | Round, maybe difficult to see | Minimal | Usually mobile, narrow stalk |
| Hemangioma | Birth to middle age | F>M | Any | IC | Broad-based, lobular | Heterogeneous, fat areas, calcification | Heterogeneous, marked | Usually mobile |
| Paraganglioma | Young adults, 30s, 40s | F>M | Any (left atrium, coronary arteries, aortic root) | IC | Broad-based, circumscribed or infiltrative | Hypodense, no calcification | Intense enhancement | Usually mobile |
| Rhabdomyoma | Children | | Ventricles | IM | Broad-based, smooth | Hypo to isodense | None | Nonmobile |
| Fibroma | Infants, children, young adults | | Ventricles | IM | Broad-based, smooth, calcification | Hypodense, may be calcified | Minimal to none | Nonmobile |

F, female; IAS, interatrial septum; IC, intracavitary; IM, intramural; LA, left atrium; LV, left ventricle; M, male; RA, right atrium; RV, right ventricle.

Adapted from Rajiah P, Kanne JP, Kalahasti V, Schoenhagen P. Computed tomography of cardiac and pericardial masses. J Cardiovasc Comput Tomogr 2011;5(1):16–29 with permission.

If possible, clinical history and any available prior imaging (echocardiography, prior CT of the chest, or PET scan) should be reviewed before CT imaging. Our routine protocol for most examinations on patients sent with cardiac mass is to obtain three-phase imaging (gated nonenhanced, coronary CT angiography phase, and 20-second delay phase).

Prospective ECG triggering is the default mode due to lower radiation exposure, but retrospective ECG gating is recommended if ventricular functional estimation, mass mobility, and valvular motion need to be evaluated. We use retrospective gating with tube current modulation and iterative reconstruction to reduce radiation dose [1].

If available, dual energy or perfusion techniques are selectively used to gain additional information about the mass characteristics or usefully display that information to referring clinicians. If the scan is to be combined with imaging of the chest or abdomen and pelvis, we generally scan the whole chest on the delay phase outlined previously and can obtain abdominal and pelvic phase imaging with the same contrast bolus on the portal venous phase, 70 s after contrast injection [3].

For cardiac masses, it is advantageous to use a triphasic injection protocol that enables visualization of all the cardiac chambers and reduction of streak artifacts in the SVC and right atrium. This involves initial contrast injection at a flow rate of 5–7 mL/s to opacify the left heart, followed by either a contrast injection at a slower rate of 2–4 mL/s or injection of a mixture of contrast and saline (50: 50 or 60·40 ratio) at the same flow rate of 5–7 mL/s to opacify the right heart and finally by saline bolus injection to minimize streak artifact [3].

## Myxoma

Myxomas are the most common primary cardiac tumor in adults [4]. They are benign lesions characterized by myxoid tissue and spindle cells, often arising along the left side of the interatrial septum, sometimes with a stalk. They are more common in women than men, by a nearly 2:1 ratio.6.

CT typically demonstrates a low-attenuation (usually water values for Hounsfield units) lobular mass with or without a stalk, usually attached to the left side of the atrial septum (Figs. 11.2 and 11.3). Enhancement is typically absent or minimal. Calcification may be present in some cases [3].

Prospective ECG-gated cardiac CTA from a young male with syncope displays a huge mobile mass arising from the ventricular aspect of the mitral valve and protrudes into LVOT. A late image acquisition shows mild enhancement at some parts of the tumor.

Left upper extremity CT angiography reveals a filling defect at the distal part of the brachial artery. Due to critical limb ischemia, surgery was done for the patient, and metastatic myxoma was excised.

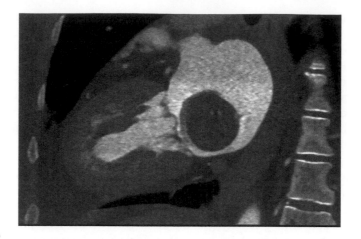

**FIG. 11.2**

Prospective ECG-gated cardiac CT scan. (A) A hypodense mass lesion with punctuate calcification, noncontrast cardiac CT. (B and C) Hypodense well-defined mass lesion, pedunculated from interatrial septum and fossa ovalis, without enhancement. The mass is mobile and protrudes through the mitral valve into the left ventricular cavity. Systolic phase (B), diastolic phase. MPR reconstruction of image (four chamber reconstruction). (D and E) Two chamber MPR reconstruction, systolic phase (D) and diastolic phase (E). (F and G) Volume rendering (VR) reconstruction, systolic phase (F), and diastolic phase(G).

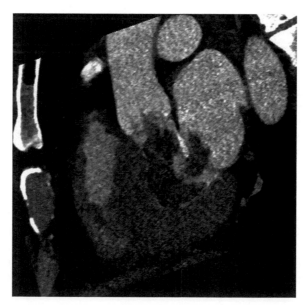

**FIG. 11.3**

Cardiac MYXOMA.

## Lipoma

Lipoma is the second most common primary benign cardiac neoplasm (8%–12%) and most commonly occurs in middle-aged and older adults. Half of the cardiac lipomas originate from the subendocardial layer, and the other half arise from the subepicardial or myocardial layers and grow into the pericardial sac. Endocardial lipomas are small with a broad base of attachment and usually occur in the left ventricle or along the septal wall or roof of the right atrium.

On CT, lipomas are well defined, homogeneous, nonenhancing masses with fat attenuation (Hounsfield units less than −50) located within the cardiac chamber (Fig. 11.4), the myocardium, or in the pericardium. Large tumors can cause cavitary obstruction, compressive effects, and cardiac dysrhythmias [2].

## Papillary fibroelastoma

Papillary fibroelastomas frequently have a classic appearance on imaging, arising from a stalk attached to a valvular surface. Larger papillary fibroelastomas typically demonstrate a classic "frond-like" appearance that has been likened to a sea anemone or broccoli floret. However, smaller lesions may not demonstrate this as clearly on some imaging modalities, especially if the spatial resolution is not sufficient. CT can provide an excellent characterization of many of these lesions owing to the high spatial resolution (Fig. 11.5) [3].

Papillary fibroelastomas are the most commonly diagnosed tumor of the heart valves [4]. They arise from the heart valves, with the aortic and mitral valves the most common sites of involvement. The differential diagnosis includes vegetation, thrombus, or myxoma. Vegetations typically destroy leaflets and cause functional abnormalities with systemic signs and symptoms, whereas fibroelastomas usually spare the free edges of the valve leaflets [2].

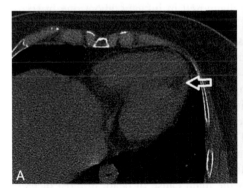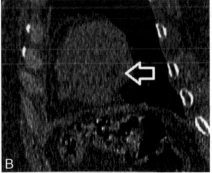

**FIG. 11.4**

Cardiac lipoma. Echogenic mass lesion detected in middle-aged women in echocardiography. Cardiac CT without intravenous contrast media displays a low-density mass in the LV cavity and densitometry of −100 HU.

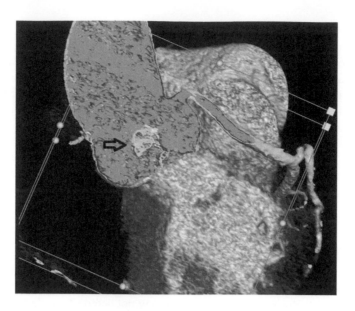

**FIG. 11.5**

Cardiac CT angiography with sequential ECG-gated acquisition, MPR (A and B), and VRT reconstruction (C and D). Coronal and three-chamber oblique CT image (A and B) of a 50-year-old woman with a fibroelastoma (*arrow*) shows a hypodense well-defined round mass with a frond-like surface, with a stalk arising from the left cusp of the aortic valve.

## Fibroma

Cardiac fibromas are the second most common benign cardiac tumor in children after rhabdomyoma [5]. While it is typically diagnosed in infancy, about one in six of lesions occur in adolescents and adults [6]. The mean age of affected patients is 13 years, with an age range of 0–60 years [7,8]. More than half of tumors arise from the left ventricle, followed by right ventricle and interventricular septum (27.5% and 17%, respectively) [9].

The tumor becomes larger accordingly in diameter until the somatic cardiac growth ceases. However, the overall lesion mass decreases relative to cardiac mass. Unlike rhabdomyoma, fibromas never resolve completely [5].

Septal involvement—with the risk of conduction system invasion—and age less than 17 years old at the time of diagnosis are associated with a poorer prognosis [5]. If symptomatic, often present with heart failure and arrhythmias, mostly ventricular tachycardia [10], which is considered as the main cause of death in most of these patients. Embolic sequelae are not a feature of cardiac fibromas.

The most frequent abnormality in chest X-ray is cardiomegaly or a contour bulge. CT usually shows a bulging almost well-defined oval-shape tumor within the ventricular wall. They are always single and range in size from 2 to 10 cm. Dystrophic

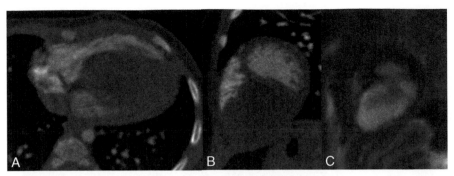

**FIG. 11.6**

Cardiac fibroma in an 11-year-old infant. (A and B) A large well-circumscribed mass involving inferior RV and RV insertion point. (C) Corresponding late-gad sequence reveals the characteristic almost homogenous avid enhancement of the lesion.

calcification is seen in about 25% of cases; and when present, its mural location is considered as a prominent finding to suggest the diagnosis [6]. Due to its fibrotic nature, it shows no discernible enhancement in early contrast-enhanced CT unless delayed (7–10 min) image is acquired which demonstrates the characteristic distinct homogenous enhancing lesion (Fig. 11.6).

## Hemangioma

Cardiac hemangioma (CH) is a rare tumor of the heart which comprises less than 10% of benign primary cardiac tumors [11].

Although he reported that the range of age at diagnosis comprises the fetal period to 9th decade of life [12,13], most patients are detected in their 40s with no significant gender preponderance [11].

It is usually an asymptomatic well-marked lesion that can arise from either layer (endo to pericardium) or chamber and valve of the heart [14]. The mean diameter of encountered lesions was about 4.5 cm [11]. And, there was no chamber predilection [11,15]. Usually, cardiac fibroma is solitary and the only one in the visceral body.

CT is capable of helping for almost exact lesion location and sometimes tissue characterization. Lesion often shows varying degrees of hypodensity compared to the myocardium. Phleboliths or nodular calcifications although uncommon but are suggestive [16]. The high vascularity of CH is also of great diagnostic value resulting in a characteristic early avid uniform enhancement of the smaller (<3 cm) and heterogeneous, eccentric, and progressive for the larger ones till the point that becomes homogenous on delayed (7–10 min) images (Fig. 11.7).

The surgical indication for CH remains controversial. But, most CH, especially the septum-related ones, should undergo surgical excision if possible [11].

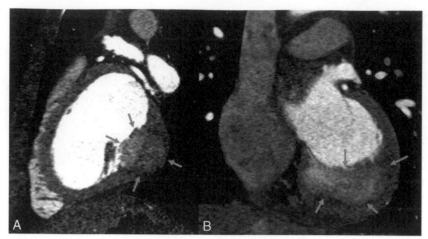

**FIG. 11.7**

Cardiac hemangioma in a 14-year-old boy. *Small arrows* in sagittal (A) and coronal (B) views of a ECG-gated cardiac CT demonstrate the basal inferior location of the mass. Note the remarkable enhancement of the lesion in early arterial phase.

## Rhabdomyoma

Rhabdomyomas are the most common primary cardiac tumors in infants and children. They are typically detected during gestational ultrasound exam or newborn's health checks in the ventricular myocardium. Most (nearly 90%) are multiple and often are associated with tuberous sclerosis [9].

They are well circumscribed sometimes lobulated tumors of varying diameters with the average of 3–4 cm but may measure up to 10 cm, especially in sporadic cases [6].

The majority stand asymptomatic and spontaneously regress till the age of 4 years without the need for surgical removal [9]. Symptom, if happens, is mostly due to outflow tract obstruction or less frequently arrhythmia [17].

Microscopically, they are hamartomas, composed of altered myocytes that are enlarged, highly vacuolated, and laden with glycogen [18].

On cardiac CT imaging, they typically appear as smooth and likely multiple masses with attenuation similar to myocardium while showing no considerable enhancement with contrast material [19]. Absence of calcification and cystic degeneration are features that help differentiation from other benign tumors like fibromas [6] (Fig. 11.8).

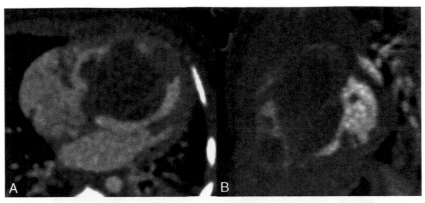

**FIG. 11.8**

Multiple rhabdomyomas in a newborn. (A) A large well-defined slightly hypo to isodense septal mass that is lobulated in some parts. (B) Sagittal view demonstrates another smaller round mass at right ventricular cardiac angle.

## Paraganglioma

Paragangliomas arise from intrinsic cardiac paraganglia, which are commonly located in the atria (L > R), along atrioventricular grooves, and near the root of the aorta and pulmonary artery. They often arise in the setting of predisposing genetic mutations.

On imaging, they appear as well-defined, extremely vascular lesions that infiltrate adjacent tissues, and more commonly project into the pericardial space than intraluminally. They are rare in ventricular walls. Surgeons comment that these tumors are difficult to separate out from adjacent normal tissue and have to be "cut" out rather than shelled out. Because of this, and their highly vascular nature, CT imaging is helpful to define the anatomy and blood supply of these lesions (Fig. 11.9) to aid surgical planning [3].

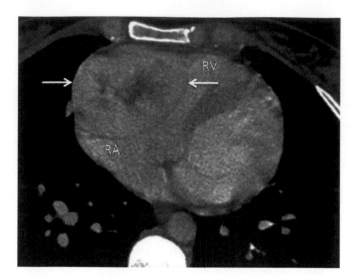

**FIG. 11.9**

Contrast-enhanced computed tomography of the chest demonstrating a well-defined hyperenhancing mass (*arrows*) with a thin hypoenhancing rim, and a central area of stellate hypoenhancement, in the right atrioventricular groove, indenting the RA and right ventricle outflow tract.

## References

[1] Schoepf UJ. CT of the heart. Humana Press; 2019.

[2] Rajiah P, et al. Computed tomography of cardiac and pericardiac masses. J Cardiovasc Comput Tomogr 2011;5(1):16–29.

[3] Young PM, et al. Computed tomography imaging of cardiac masses. Radiol Clin 2019; 57(1):75–84.

[4] Lam KY, Dickens P, Chan A. Tumors of the heart. A 20-year experience with a review of 12,485 consecutive autopsies. Arch Pathol Lab Med 1993;117(10):1027–31.

[5] Torimitsu S, et al. Literature survey on epidemiology and pathology of cardiac fibroma. Eur J Med Res 2012;17(1):5.

[6] Grebenc ML, et al. Primary cardiac and pericardial neoplasms: radiologic-pathologic correlation. Radiographics 2000;20(4):1073–103.

[7] Burke AP, et al. Cardiac fibroma: clinicopathologic correlates and surgical treatment. J Thorac Cardiovasc Surg 1994;108(5):862–70.

[8] Pittman S, et al. Cardiac fibroma: an uncommon cause of a fixed defect on myocardial perfusion imaging. Clin Nucl Med 2018;43(2):e56–8.

[9] Motwani M, et al. MR imaging of cardiac tumors and masses: a review of methods and clinical applications. Radiology 2013;268(1):26–43.

[10] Miyake CY, et al. Cardiac tumors and associated arrhythmias in pediatric patients, with observations on surgical therapy for ventricular tachycardia. J Am Coll Cardiol 2011; 58(18):1903–9.

[11] Li W, et al. Cardiac hemangioma: a comprehensive analysis of 200 cases. Ann Thorac Surg 2015;99(6):2246–52.

[12] Sharma J, Hirata Y, Mosca RS. Surgical repair in neonatal life of cardiac haemangiomas diagnosed prenatally. Cardiol Young 2009;19(4):403–6.

[13] Dod HS, et al. Two-and three-dimensional transthoracic and transesophageal echocardiographic findings in epithelioid hemangioma involving the mitral valve. Echocardiography 2008;25(4):443–5.

[14] Reynen K. Frequency of primary tumors of the heart. Am J Cardiol 1996;77(1):107.

[15] Hrabak-Paar M, et al. Hemangioma of the interatrial septum: CT and MRI features. Cardiovasc Intervent Radiol 2011;34(2):90–3.

[16] Bai Y, Zhao G, Tan Y. CT and MRI manifestations of mediastinal cavernous hemangioma and a review of the literature. World J Surg Oncol 2019;17(1):205.

[17] Sparrow PJ, et al. MR imaging of cardiac tumors. Radiographics 2005;25(5):1255–76.

[18] Mc Allister Jr HA. Primary tumors and cysts of the heart and pericardium. Curr Probl Cardiol 1979;4(2):1–51.

[19] Kassop D, et al. Cardiac masses on cardiac CT: a review. Curr Cardiovasc Imaging Rep 2014;7(8):9281.

# CT in malignant cardiac tumors (diagnosis, approach, follow-up)

# 12

**Hamidreza Pouraliakbar**

*Department of Radiology, CardioOncology Research Center, Iran University of Medical Sciences, Rajaie Cardiovascular Medical and Research Center, Tehran, Iran*

## Key points

- Cardiac CT has several advantages including wide availability, rapid acquisition time, excellent isotropic spatial resolution, and multiplanar reconstruction capabilities.
- CT is a robust technique for assessment of the relationship of the mass to the myocardium, cardiac valves, pericardium, coronary arteries, great vessels including pulmonary and systemic, and adjacent tissues, such as lung and lymph nodes, in a way that no other imaging modality can often reach.
- Metastasis to the heart is more common than a primary malignant tumor.
- Metastasis may involve the heart and pericardium by one of four pathways: retrograde lymphatic extension, hematogenous spread, direct contiguous extension, or transvenous extension. The predominant route is a retrograde lymphatic extension.
- The most common primary malignant cardiac mass is sarcoma and angiosarcoma is the most common.
- The right atrium is the most common cardiac chamber involved by a primary malignant tumor.

CT has emerged as an important imaging modality in the evaluation of cardiac and paracardiac masses. CT has several advantages including wide availability and rapid acquisition time, excellent isotropic spatial resolution, and multiplanar reconstruction capabilities. CT demonstrates excellent, three-dimensional rendering of the masses, which is essential for surgical planning. The wide field of view of CT enables visualization of paracardiac and other extracardiac structures, which is essential for staging malignancies.

Malignant masses are often more challenging to specifically diagnose, but the differential diagnosis can often be narrowed, and more importantly, the examination may document the extent of the lesion and presence or absence of additional (extracardiac) metastatic lesions, perform preoperative coronary evaluation, and be used to help plan biopsy or resection.

Multimodal Imaging Atlas of Cardiac Masses. https://doi.org/10.1016/B978-0-323-84906-7.00029-7

Cardiac computed tomography (CT) is particularly helpful in establishing the presence of thrombus versus enhancing tissue, and the pattern of enhancement in perfused masses may lead to insights that a mass is hypervascular, has a dominant fibrous component, or demonstrates features typical of a vascular malformation.

Newer techniques, such as CT perfusion and dual energy CT, may be useful in characterizing tissue and enhancement characteristics [1].

## Tissue characterization

Metastases to the heart and pericardium are much more common than primary cardiac tumors and are generally associated with a poor prognosis. A primary malignant tumor is less common than a primary benign tumor, with most of them being sarcomas. Imaging features of tumors in CT that help distinguish benign from malignant neoplasms include location, size, margins, the presence of a feeding artery, calcification, or pericardial effusion (Table 12.1) [3].

## Technical issues

See Chapter 11.

**Table 12.1** CT features that distinguish benign and malignant neoplasms.

| Feature | Benign | Malignant |
|---|---|---|
| Location | More on left side | More in right atrium |
| Size | Small | Large, may fill chamber |
| Margin | Smooth, well defined | Lobulated, ill defined, invasive, infiltrative |
| Invasion | None | Myocardium, pericardium, extracardiac |
| Attachment | Pedicle may be seen | Broad based |
| Feeding Vessels | Absent | May be present |
| Calcification | Rare, except for small foci in fibroma, myxoma | Large foci in osteosarcoma |
| Pericardial Effusion | Not seen | Suspicious for malignancy |
| Metastasis | None | May be present |

*Rajiah P, Kanne JP, Kalahasti V, Schoenhagen P. Computed tomography of cardiac and pericardiac masses. J Cardiovasc Comput Tomogr 2011;5:16–29.*

# Primary malignant cardiac tumors
## Sarcoma

Sarcoma is the most common primary cardiac malignancy, accounting for one-third of cases [2].

Angiosarcoma is the most common type of sarcoma [3,4].

### Angiosarcoma

These tumors usually arise from the right atrium or pericardium but may also arise from the pulmonary artery. Up to 25% of these tumors are partly intracavitary and can cause valvular obstruction, right-sided heart failure, and pericardial tamponade with hemorrhagic fluid. Two main morphologic types have been described in angiosarcoma. The first is a well-defined mass protruding into a cardiac chamber; the second is a diffusely infiltrative mass extending along the pericardium [5].

On CT imaging (Fig. 12.2), a low-attenuation intracavitary mass, which may be irregular or nodular and usually arising from the right atrial free wall with areas of necrosis, may be seen [4,6]. Tumor infiltration of the myocardium, compression of the cardiac chambers, direct extension into the pericardium with features of pericardial thickening or effusions, and involvement of the great vessels are other features discernible on CT imaging.

On post-contrast enhancement acquisition, the tumors show a heterogeneous enhancement pattern [5]. Multiple lesions occur in 60% of patients, and pulmonary metastases are present in 66%–89% [3].

### Undifferentiated sarcoma

On CT, these tumors appear as large, irregular, low-attenuation intracavitary lesions [7]. Tumor infiltration of the myocardium may appear as thickening and irregularity. The tumor may also manifest as a hemorrhagic mass replacing the pericardium, similar to angiosarcoma. Several reports have demonstrated a tendency to involve the valves [8,9].

### Rhabdomyosarcoma

This tumor is the most common cardiac malignancy in infants and children. There is a slight male predilection, but because there is no predilection for any cardiac chamber.

Rhabdomyosarcomas may arise anywhere in the myocardium and are more likely than other sarcomas to involve or arise from cardiac valves [10].

They are often multiple and may invade the pericardium [10].

In contrast to angiosarcomas, rhabdomyosarcomas tend to always involve the myocardium, and when they involve the pericardium, the appearance is that of nodular masses rather than sheetlike thickening of the pericardium [10]. CT imaging may demonstrate a smooth or irregular low-attenuation mass in a cardiac chamber. CT is also useful in identifying extracardiac extension of the tumor (Fig. 12.3) [5].

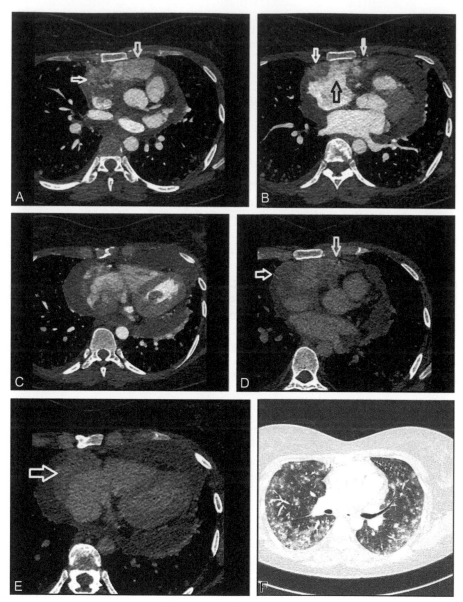

**FIG. 12.2**

Prospective ECG gated cardiac CT angiography shows infiltrating tumor in the middle-aged woman with a chief complaint of malaise, fever, and dyspnea who evaluates for COVID-19 pneumonia. The tumor arising from the right atrium (RA) (*white arrow*) shows early enhancement in the early acquisition phase (A–C). These images show a defect in the wall of RA (*black arrow*) and sealed IV contrast in pericardial space (*yellow arrow*). The mass displays heterogeneous enhancement at the late acquisition phase (D, E). Large pericardial effusion is noted (E). Multiple pulmonary ground-glass nodules in both lungs suggest metastasis (F).

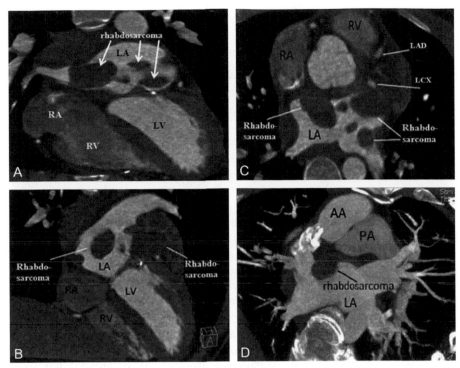

**FIG. 12.3**

Several soft tissue masses in the left atrium (LA) were demonstrated by computed tomography 60 days after the operation, which suggested tumor recurrence.
(A) Computed tomographic 4-chamber view showed three masses in the left atrium.
(B) Computed tomographic 2-chamber view indicated two tumors in the left atrium.
(C) Computed tomographic short-axis view showed several masses in the left atrium.
(D) Computed tomographic reconstructed image showed the rhabdomyosarcoma in the left atrium close to the anterior wall. *AA*, ascending aorta; *LAD*, left anterior descending coronary artery; *LCX*, left circumflex artery; *LV*, left ventricle; *PA*, pulmonary artery; *RA*, right atrium; *RV*, right ventricle.

### Osteosarcoma

Osteosarcomas that are metastatic to the heart tend to occur in the right atrium. By contrast, primary cardiac osteosarcomas (Fig. 12.4) tend to occur in the left atrium, and their obstructive nature results in signs and symptoms of congestive heart failure. CT imaging demonstrates dense calcifications within a low-attenuation mass [11]. Because these tumors are most commonly observed in the left atrium, they may be confused with atrial myxomas, especially in the early stages, when calcifications may be absent. Distinguishing features on imaging that are more suggestive of an osteogenic sarcoma include a broad base, an aggressive growth pattern such as

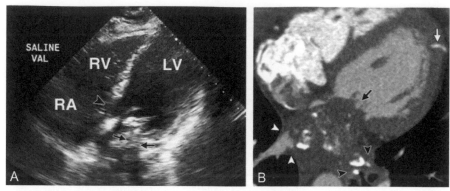

**FIG. 12.4**

Four-chamber reconstruction from retrospectively gated cardiac CT angiography demonstrates a 6 × 5.6-cm mass with internal calcifications that fills a large portion of the left atrium and extends to the mitral valve (*black arrow*). The mass has invaded the left inferior pulmonary vein (*black arrowheads*) and left superior pulmonary vein (not shown). The mass also obstructs the ostium of the right inferior pulmonary vein (*white arrowheads*). A linear area of calcification in the left ventricular wall (*white arrow*) was suggestive of a metastatic lesion.

extension into the pulmonary veins, invasion of the atrial septum, or infiltrative growth along the epicardium [12]. It has been contended that primary cardiac osteosarcoma should be in the differential diagnosis of all atypical left atrial myxomas [5].

### *Leiomyosarcoma*

Leiomyosarcomas (Fig. 12.5) are malignant tumors with smooth muscle differentiation. They may arise from smooth muscle bundles lining the subendocardium, but many cardiac leiomyosarcomas may arise from the smooth muscle of the pulmonary veins and arteries, and then spread into the heart [6]. Cardiac leiomyosarcomas constitute 8% to 9% of all cardiac sarcomas, they have a predilection for the left atrium and manifest commonly with congestive heart failure signs and symptoms.

On CT, they usually appear as lobulated, irregular, low-attenuation masses in the left atrium, most commonly arising from the posterior wall, a feature that distinguishes them from left atrial myxomas. Additional imaging findings include a tendency to invade the pulmonary veins and mitral valve, the former with the appearance of a low-attenuation filling defect [5].

### Primary lymphoma

Primary cardiac lymphomas preferentially involve the right cardiac chambers and the pericardium. At CT, lymphomas commonly appear as an infiltrating epicardial or myocardial mass that is often isoattenuating to hypoattenuating relative to the

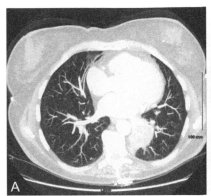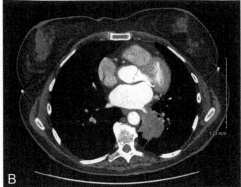

**FIG. 12.5**

(A) Transverse section of chest computed tomography in lung window showing a large left lower lobe mass. (B) Transverse section of chest computed tomography in a mediastinal window demonstrating the close involvement of the mass with the inferior pulmonary veins.

myocardium. Heterogeneous enhancement after administration of intravenous contrast material is routinely demonstrated. A curious feature of cardiac lymphoma is the tendency of the tumor to extend along the epicardial surfaces of the heart, primarily encasing adjacent structures including coronary arteries and the aortic root (Fig. 12.6). Frequently, it also follows along the right atrioventricular groove and involves the base of the heart.

Left atrial and ventricular infiltration has been described but is far less common [12–16]. Note that structures including the cardiac valves, ventricles, and aortic root tend to be spared from tumor encroachment [12].

Pericardial thickening or effusion is not an uncommon feature and in certain cases may be the only imaging finding. Pericardial effusions can be large and in severe cases may result in tamponade [17].

Metastatic lung carcinoma is the most common tumor that is similar in appearance to cardiac lymphoma. Cardiac sarcomas can be difficult to discern from lymphomas. Accounting for approximately 40% of cases, angiosarcoma is the most common form of cardiac sarcoma; research suggests a slight male predominance. Angiosarcomas usually involve the right side of the heart and may also manifest with pericardial effusion.

Angiosarcomas are typically far more aggressive than lymphomas, involve larger areas of the heart, and even penetrate the valves and great vessels—an atypical finding in cardiac lymphoma. Central necrosis is another common feature of angiosarcoma and is less likely seen with lymphoma. In addition, angiosarcomas tend to show prominent enhancement after contrast material administration at both CT and MR imaging, whereas lymphoma typically does not have such strong enhancement patterns [17].

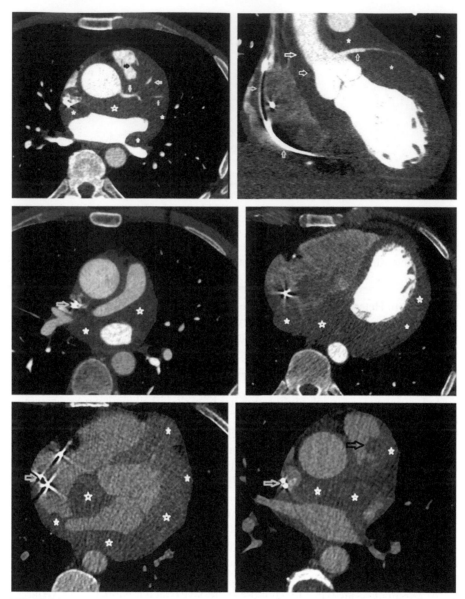

**FIG. 12.6**

Prospective ECG-gated contrast-enhanced cardiac CT image displays primary cardiac B-cell lymphoma in a young male patient. Early acquisition phase images (A–D) reveal extensive infiltration of tumor (*) along the epicardial surface with infiltration into the myocardium to involve the lateral wall of the left ventricle, interatrial septum, and atrial wall. The tumor shows encasement of coronary arteries (*yellow arrow*), ascending aorta (*white arrow*), and pulmonary arteries with invasion into the main pulmonary artery (*black arrow*). In the late acquisition phase images, the mass shows homogenous enhancement (E, F).Pericardial effusion is seen. Implanted leads of the intracardiac device in RV and RA cavities (*green arrow*).

# Secondary malignant cardiac tumors
## Metastases
### Introduction
Metastases to the heart and pericardium are much more common than primary cardiac tumors and are generally associated with a poor prognosis.

### Pathways of spread
A tumor may involve the heart and pericardium by one of four pathways: retrograde lymphatic extension (Fig. 12.7), hematogenous spread (Figs. 12.8 and 12.9), direct contiguous extension (Fig. 12.10), or transvenous extension (Figs. 12.11–12.13). The predominant route is retrograde spread through lymphatic channels in the mediastinum to the heart, producing small tumor implants on the epicardial surface of the heart. The visceral pericardium contains most of the lymphatic channels that drain the pericardial space [18].

Other tumors, such as melanoma, usually spread hematogenously and often produce tumor implants in the myocardium. Hematogenous metastases to the myocardium and epicardium occur via the coronary arteries or, less commonly, by implantation of cancer fragments carried through the vena cava. Therefore hematogenous metastases in the heart and pericardium are usually accompanied by evidence

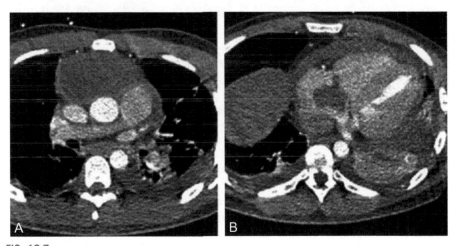

**FIG. 12.7**

Cardiac CT with IV contrast reveals a large anterior mediastinal germ cell tumor (A) that involves the pericardium. The metastatic tumor is seen in the RA cavity (B).

*Courtesy from Dr. Saeed Mirsadraee, Consultant Cardiothoracic Radiologist, Royal Brompton, and Harefield Hospitals, London, England.*

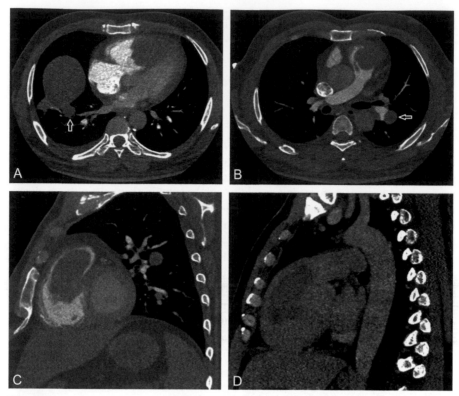

**FIG. 12.8**

Metastasis of thyroid cancer. Multiplanar reconstruction images of multislice CT with IV contrast from middle-aged patient displays hypodense mass lesion in the RV cavity and RVOT in the axial and sagittal reformatted images in the early perfusion phase (A–C). Two round tumors are seen in the lungs (*arrow*). A delayed phase image shows enhancing tumor in the RV cavity (D). The patient had a history of papillary thyroid carcinoma and metastasis to the heart and lungs.

of hematogenous metastases in other organs. In particular, pulmonary metastases are usually present [18].

Direct extension of tumors into the heart and pericardium typically occurs in patients with large bronchogenic carcinomas (Fig. 12.14) but may also occur in patients with esophageal carcinoma, breast carcinoma that erodes through the chest wall, or mediastinal lymphoma. In these cases, it can be difficult to determine whether the cardiac involvement is the result of lymphatic obstruction or direct invasion.

The transvenous route of tumor spread relies on the extension of tumor thrombus into the right atrium via the superior or inferior vena cava (see Fig. 12.11) or extension into the left atrium via the pulmonary veins (see Fig. 12.13).

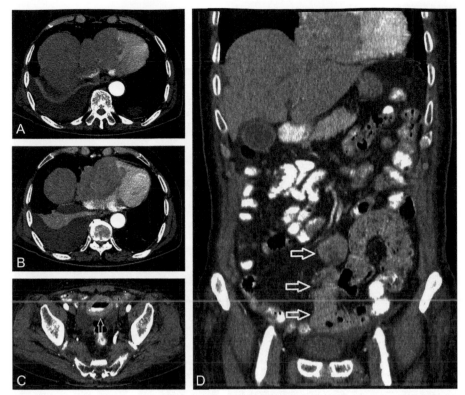

**FIG. 12.9**

Adenocarcinoma of the small bowel and large cardiac metastasis. Cardiac CT angiography (A, B) reveals an infiltrative enhancing mass in RA, RV, and extension through the wall of the right atrium. Mass encased the aortic root. Abdominal and pelvic CT (C, D) with contrast displays circumferential tumor (*white arrow*) of small bowel with mesenteric extension.

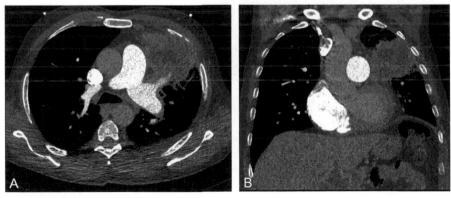

**FIG. 12.10**

Bronchogenic tumor. Multiplanar reconstruction of pulmonary CT angiography displays infiltrative bronchogenic carcinoma with invasion into the pericardium and left upper lobe pulmonary artery. A hypodense area is seen in the tumor due to necrosis. The left hemidiaphragm shows upward displacement due to paralysis. The tumor invades the chest wall and reveals rib erosion.

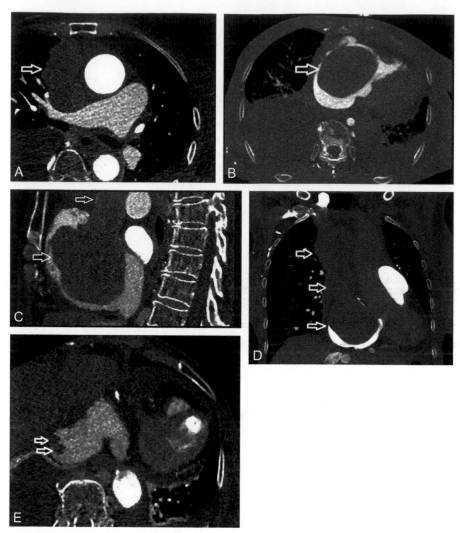

**FIG. 12.11**

High pitch prospective ECG gated computed tomography with IV contrast and MPR reconstruction from a 55-year-old woman with dyspnea and RA mass in echocardiography. Infiltrative bronchogenic carcinoma tumor (*white arrow*) at the medial side of the superior lobe of the right lung (A) is detected which invades to mediastinum and SVC and extended along the SVC into RA (C, D). The tumor fills a large space of RA and protrudes toward the tricuspid valve (B). Satellite tumoral lesions in RA (E).

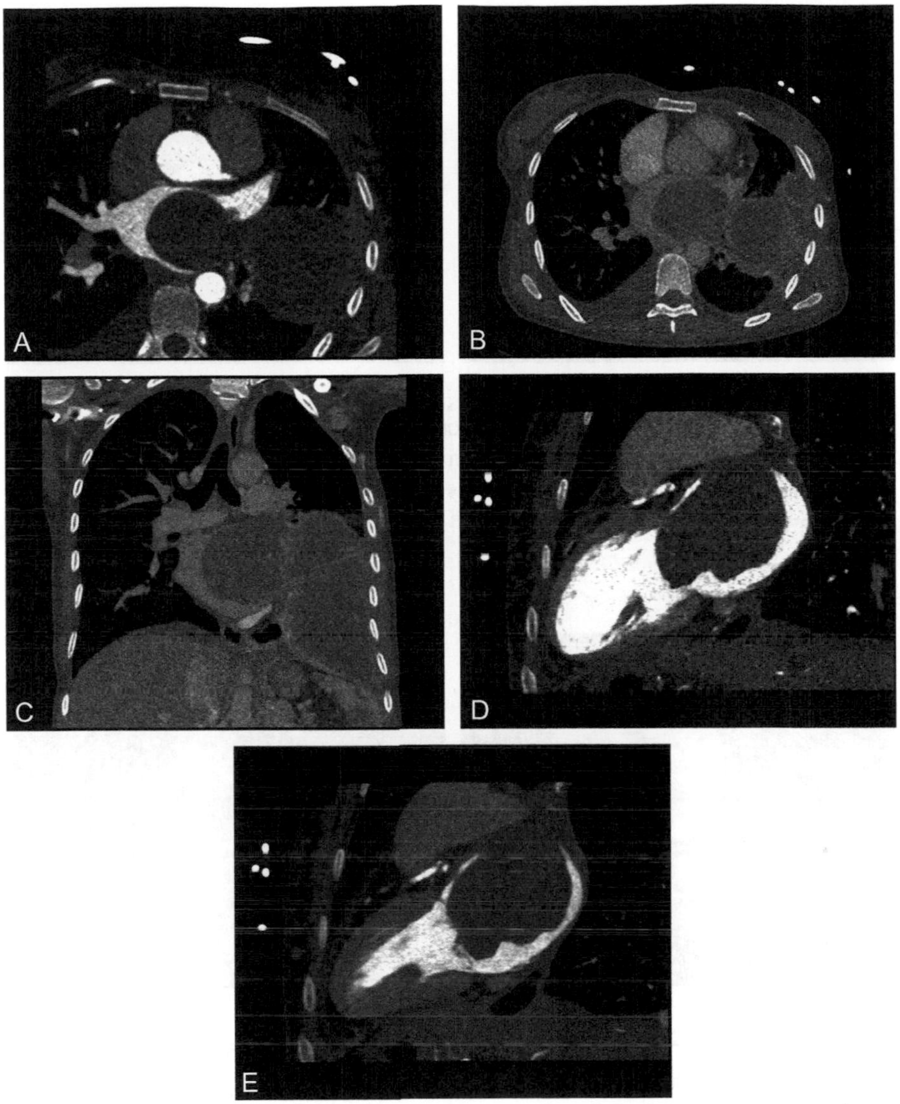

**FIG. 12.12**

The patient had a history of excision of left breast mass and pathology report of phyllodes tumor. The patient had a history of dyspnea and send to the radiology department due to a tumoral lesion in LA which was found in the transthoracic echocardiography. Multiphase MDCT was done for her. The large hypodense pleural-based tumor is detected from the left lung into the LA via the pulmonary vein due to recurrent phyllodes tumor. Prospective ECG-gating MDCT, arterial phase (A). Prospective ECG-gating high pitch MDCT, delayed phase (B, C), peripheral enhancement, and central necrosis of tumor. Left atrial (LA) tumor protruded through the mitral valve into LV during the diastolic phase (D) and return into LA during the systolic phase (E).

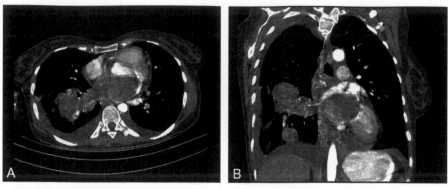

**FIG. 12.13**

Metastatic osteosarcoma. Chest CT with IV contrast reveals a huge hypodense mass lesion (*white arrow*) that invades the right inferior pulmonary vein (PV) and extends along with the PV to the left atrium. Large tumor identifies in the LA cavity (*yellow arrow*). Another round hypodense mass represents metastasis in the lower lobe of the right lung.

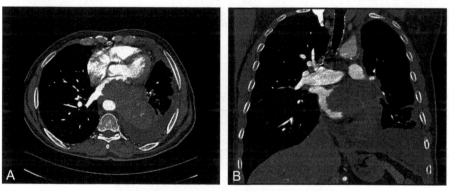

**FIG. 12.14**

Bronchogenic tumor. Thorax multislice CT with IV contrast reveals infiltrative bronchogenic carcinoma from the left lung and direct invasion into the left atrium. Descending aorta encases by tumor and left pleural effusion.

This mechanism provides the means for the spread of tumors from the kidney or liver (IVC) and some lung cancers (superior vena cava, pulmonary veins). The transvenous route of tumor extension is most common in patients with renal cell carcinoma; in these patients, tumor thrombus may spread into the right atrium via the IVC [18].

# References

[1] Young PM, Foley TA, Araoz PA, Williamson EE. Computed tomography imaging of cardiac masses. Radiol Clin North Am 2019;57(1):75–84.

[2] McAllister Jr HA, Fenoglio Jr JJ. Tumors of the cardiovascular system. In: Atlas of tumor pathology, 2nd Series, Fascicle 15. Washington, DC: Armed Forces Institute of Pathology; 1978.

[3] Rajiah P, Kanne JP, Kalahasti V, Schoenhagen P. Computed tomography of cardiac and pericardiac masses. J Cardiovasc Comput Tomogr 2011;5:16–29.

[4] Matheis G, Beyersdorf F. Primary cardiac angiosarcoma. A case report. Cardiology 1995;86(1):83–5.

[5] Anavekar NS, Bonnichsen CR. Computed tomography of cardiac pseudotumors and neoplasms. Radiol Clin North Am 2010;48:799–816.

[6] Shin MS, Kirklin JK, Cain JB, et al. Primary angiosarcoma of the heart: CT characteristics. AJR Am J Roentgenol 1987;148(2):267–8.

[7] Baumgartner RA, Das SK, Shea M, et al. The role of echocardiography and CT in the diagnosis of cardiac tumors. Int J Card Imaging 1988;3(1):57–60.

[8] Itoh K, Matsumura T, Egawa Y, et al. Primary mitral valve sarcoma in infancy. Pediatr Cardiol 1998;19(2):174–7.

[9] Ludomirsky A, Vargo TA, Murphy DJ, et al. Intracardiac undifferentiated sarcoma in infancy. J Am Coll Cardiol 1985;6(6):1362–4.

[10] Raaf HN, Raaf JH. Sarcomas related to the heart and vasculature. Semin Surg Oncol 1994;10(5):374–82.

[11] Chaloupka JC, Fishman EK, Siegelman SS. Use of CT in the evaluation of primary cardiac tumors. Cardiovasc Intervent Radiol 1986;9(3):132–5.

[12] Araoz PA, Eklund HE, Welch TJ, et al. CT and MR imaging of primary cardiac malignancies. Radiographics 1999;19(6):1421–34.

[13] Lam KY, Dickens P, Chan ACL. Tumors of the heart: a 20-year experience with a review of 12,485 consecutive autopsies. Arch Pathol Lab Med 1993;117:1027–31.

[14] Dorsay TA, Ho VB, Rovira MJ, Armstrong MA, Brissette MD. Primary cardiac lymphoma: CT and MR findings. J Comput Assist Tomogr 1993;17(6):978–81.

[15] Khuddus MA, Schmalfuss CM, Aranda JM, Pauly DF. Magnetic resonance imaging of primary cardiac lymphoma. Clin Cardiol 2007;30(3):144–5.

[16] Ryu SJ, Choi BW, Choe KO. CT and MR findings of primary cardiac lymphoma: report upon 2 cases and review. Yonsei Med J 2001;42(4):451–6.

[17] Jeudy J, Kirsch J, et al. From the radiologic pathology archives: cardiac lymphoma: radiologic-pathologic correlation. Radiographics 2012;32:1369–80.

[18] Chiles C, Woodard PK, Gutierrez FR, Link KM. Metastatic involvement of the heart and pericardium: CT and MR imaging. Radiographics 2001;21:439–49.

# CMR in benign cardiac tumors (diagnosis, approach, and follow-up)

# 13

## Hamidreza Pouraliakbar and Kiara Rezaei-Kalantari

*Department of Radiology, CardioOncology Research Center, Iran University of Medical Sciences, Rajaie Cardiovascular Medical and Research Center, Tehran, Iran*

## Key points

- Cardiac magnetic resonance (CMR) is a robust technique in the evaluation of cardiac mass.
- The advantage of CMR includes the large field of view, superior tissue contrast, multiplanar reconstruction, and unique ability to discriminate tissue characteristics.
- CMR core protocol for assessment of cardiac mass includes cine SSFP, T1-W, T2-W, first pass perfusion, postcontrast T1-W, and late gadolinium enhancement (LGE) sequences.
- Strong early contrast enhancement on postcontrast T1-weighted images is more suggestive of a malignant, highly vascular lesion, although mild contrast enhancement is still seen in 40%–50% of benign tumors.
- Secondary cardiac tumors (metastasis) are more common than primary benign cardiac masses.
- Myxoma is the most common primary benign cardiac mass.
- Lipoma is the second most common primary cardiac tumor.
- The most common primary benign cardiac tumors in pediatric patients are rhabdomyoma and fibroma.
- The left atrium is the most common chamber is involved by primary benign cardiac mass.

## CMR protocols for cardiac and paracardiac masses, including thrombous

A core protocol for the MR imaging assessment of cardiac masses and tumors mention, follow. However, cardiac masses vary widely and therefore any standardized protocol needs to be tailored to the specific mass lesion.

Multimodal Imaging Atlas of Cardiac Masses. https://doi.org/10.1016/B978-0-323-84906-7.00025-X

1. LV structure and function
2. T1w FSE—slices through the mass and surrounding structures (number of slices depends on size of the mass)
3. T2w FSE with fat suppression (optional—without fat suppression)—through the mass and surrounding structures as earlier
4. First-pass perfusion module with slices through mass
5. Repeat T1w FSE with fat suppression (early after GBCA)
6. Optional—Repeat selected bSSFP cine images postcontrast
7. LGE
   a. Images with the TI set to null thrombus (approximately 500–550 ms at 1.5 T, 850–900 ms at 3 T) will help differentiate thrombus from the tumor as well as delineate thrombus surrounding or associated with tumors
   b. Serial imaging can help distinguish hypoperfused tumor necrotic core from thrombus [1]

## Tissue characteristics

In MR imaging, the relative signal intensity from a particular tissue depends principally on its proton density and the T1 and T2 relaxation times. Different tissues have different T1 and T2 relaxation times owing to different internal biochemical environments surrounding protons. By weighting images to emphasize on either T1- or T2-based contrast, MR imaging can exploit differences in signal intensity to discriminate between different tissue types (Table 1). Neoplastic cells tend to be larger than normal cells, contain more free intracellular water, and are usually associated with surrounding inflammatory reactions and increased interstitial fluid. Because water molecules are small and move so rapidly for an efficient relaxation, the higher free

**Table 13.1** MR imaging tissue characteristics of benign cardiac masses.

| Cardiac mass | T1-weighted[a] | T2-weighted[a] | After contrast administration |
|---|---|---|---|
| Myxoma | Isointense | High | Heterogeneous |
| Lipoma | High | High | No enhancement |
| Fibroma | Isointense | Low | hyperenhancement |
| Rhabdomyoma | Isointense | Iso to high intense | No or minimal |
| Fibroelastoma | Isointense | High | No enhancement |
| Paraganglioma | Hypo to Isointense | High | Strong enhancement |
| Hemangioma | Isointense | High | Hyperenhancement |

The table reveals typical characterization of mentioned tumors. Sometimes tumors demonstrate the atypical feature.
[a]T1- and T2-weighted imaging signal intensity is given relative to myocardium.

water content of the malignant tissue, as well as other changes in tissue composition, leads to prolonged T1/T2 relaxation times and thus an inherent contrast between tumors and normal tissue [1,2]. In addition, tumors containing fibrotic or lipomatous material show characteristic signal intensity patterns on MR images (Table 1) [3].

*T1-weighted imaging.* Targeted black-blood T1-weighted FSE images (e.g., pulse sequence parameters at our department: 1000/40; flip angle, 90°; section thickness, 6–8 mm, no gap; matrix, 512*512) in the optimal imaging planes defined earlier are acquired to cover the entire mass, with and without a fat saturation prepulse. Acquisition of T1-weighted images can be repeated after the intravenous injection of gadolinium-based contrast agent for further tissue characterization. Strong early contrast enhancement on postcontrast T1-weighted images is more suggestive of a malignant, highly vascular lesion, although mild contrast enhancement is still seen in 40%–50% of benign tumors. Differential enhancement due to variation in tumor vascularity and altered capillary permeability allows some discrimination between the various tumor types as will be discussed in their individual section later [3].

*T2-weighted imaging.* Prior to the administration of contrast material, T2-weighted images should be acquired in the same imaging planes as T1-weighted images. These T2-weighted FSE images are acquired with breath hold, preferably triple inversion recovery with blood and fat suppression (e.g., pulse sequence parameters at our department: 2000/100; flip angle, 90°; inversion time, 160 msec; section thickness, 6–8 mm, no gap; matrix, 192*192), and can be used to detect regions of edema or liquefactive necrosis in the mass, which demonstrate high signal intensity, or regions of coagulative necrosis, which have low signal intensity [4,5]. The presence of hemorrhage or thrombus also affects T2-weighted signal intensity depending on their chronicity.

## First-pass perfusion and delayed enhancement imaging

After infusion of gadolinium chelate, first-pass rest perfusion imaging (based on a T1-weighted gradient echo sequence) of the tumor followed by 10–15 min delayed enhancement imaging (based on a T1-weighted inversion recovery sequence) assess lesion vascularity. Considerable first-pass enhancement is a typical feature for highly vascular tumors such as hemangioma or angiosarcoma. The presence of late phase gadolinium enhancement (LGE) implies delayed contrast washout from the lesion, usually as the result of extracellular space expansion or necrosis [4]. LGE can be seen with both benign and malignant lesions. Benign tumors like fibroma usually display uniform LGE whereas tumors with a more heterogeneous composition like myxoma or angiosarcoma (containing a mixture of tumor tissue, necrosis, and foci of hemorrhage) usually show patchy areas of LGE.

## Myxoma

Myxomas are the most common type of primary cardiac tumor (50%) and usually occur in the fourth to seventh decade of life. They are typically solitary, vary in size from 1 to 15 cm, and have a predilection for the interatrial septum near the fossa ovalis. Approximately 75% occur in the left atrium, 20% in the right atrium, and 5% concomitantly in both sides, either involving the atrium, ventricle, or mitral valve. They are generally well defined, smooth, lobular or oval, and often pedunculated. On MR images, they appear isointense on T1-weighted images and have higher signal intensity on T2-weighted images owing to the high extracellular water content (Figs. 13.2–13.4). Regions of acute hemorrhage within myxomas appear hypointense on both T1- and T2-weighted images, while the older ones appear hyperintense as the hemoglobin becomes deoxidized to methemoglobin [6–9]. Cine imaging is very useful in the workup of myxomas as they are highly mobile, occasionally prolapsing through the mitral valve causing an obstruction. With SSFP cine techniques, myxomas appear hyperintense relative to the myocardium but hypointense relative to the blood pool (Movie [online]).

Internally, myxomas may contain cysts, regions of necrosis, fibrosis, hemorrhage, and calcification, which lead to a typically heterogeneous appearance after contrast enhancement [3].

Many myxomas have a layer of surface thrombus, with low signal intensity on LGE images [10]. The majority occur sporadically but approximately 7% constitute part of an autosomal dominant syndrome known as Carney complex, comprising skin lentigines, endocrine tumors, fibroadenomas, and melanotic schwannomas [11]. They can be asymptomatic if they are small, but most patients present with symptoms due to mass effect (e.g., inflow/outflow obstruction), embolization, or constitutional symptoms (owing to the release of IL-6) [3].

## Lipoma

Lipoma is the second most common primary benign cardiac neoplasm (8%–12%) and most commonly occurs in middle-aged and older adults [12].

The two most common fat-containing lesions in the heart are cardiac lipomas and lipomatous hypertrophy of the interatrial septum.

True cardiac lipomas are encapsulated, contain neoplastic fat cells, and occur at a young age. Lipomas constitute 8%–12% of primary cardiac tumors. Half of the lipomas arise from the subendocardial layer and are relatively small (Fig. 13.5), whereas the other half are from either subepicardial or mid-myocardial layers (Fig. 13.6) [13]. Lipomas usually have a homogeneous signal on cardiac MR images (Table 1). They have the same signal intensity as fat tissue—that is, high intensity on T1 and lower intensity on T2-weighted FSE images. An invaluable sequence if this type of tumor is suspected is pre- and post-fat-saturated T1-weighted FSE sequences, in which signal dropout is identified in the mass on the fat saturation sequence, confirming a fat-containing lesion [14].

Lipomatous hypertrophy of the interatrial septum is often found in older and overweight patients. Unlike true lipomas, they are not capsulated and contain lipoblasts and mature fat cells. The bilobed, dumbbell-shaped fatty mass must be greater than 20 mm in thickness and characteristically spares the fossa ovalis [15].

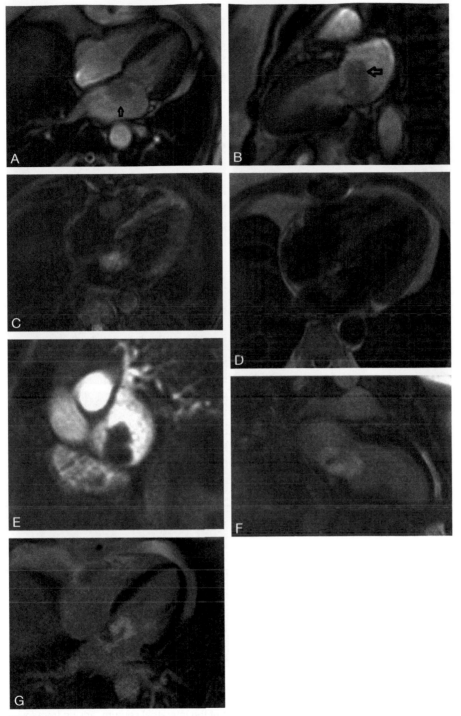

**FIG. 13.2**

Cardiac myxoma. In 4-chamber and longitudinal 2-chamber cine SSFP sequences (A and B), the mass shows heterogeneous low signal intensity and is well defined. The tumor is pedunculate, mobile, and adheres to the interatrial wall, arising from fossa ovalis. In STIR images the tumor is strongly hyperintense (C) whereas in T1-weighted image it is isointense to the myocardium. In short-axis oblique view early perfusion sequence, no evidence of early enhancement (D). Four chamber and longitudinal 2-chamber post gadolinium IR image reveal hyperenhancement of tumor (E and F).

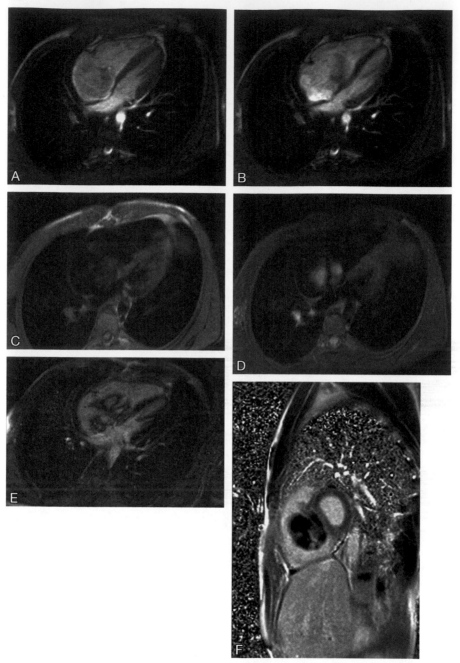

**FIG. 13.3**

Right atrium myxoma. Cardiac magnetic resonance images demonstrate a large pedunculated mobile myxoma from the RA side of the interatrial septum, arising from fossa ovalis. In the four-chamber Cine SSFP sequence in the systole (A) and diastole (B) phase, the lesion reveals high signal intensity heterogeneous mass in the RA cavity. The tumor protrudes through the tricuspid valve into RV in the diastolic phase. In the four-chamber T1-W sequence (C) and STIR sequence (D) image, the mass shows hyposignal intensity and high signal intensity in the RA cavity, respectively. In the four-chamber (E) and short-axis (F) late gadolinium enhancement (LGE) images, the tumor displays heterogeneous enhancement.

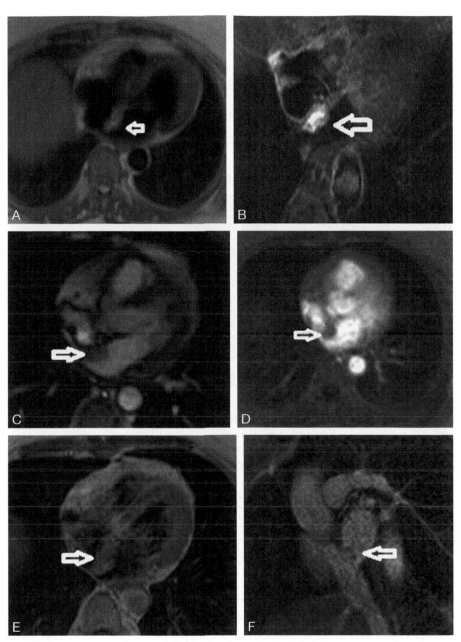

**FIG. 13.4**

Sessile myxoma of the left atrium. Iso signal T1-w mass (A) in LA arising from IAS adjacent to fossa ovalis and high T2 signal in STIR sequence (B). The tumor shows Iso signal in four-chamber cine SSFP sequence (C) and without enhancement in early perfusion sequence (D). Mass displays enhancement in postcontrast T1–W sequence (E) and in late gadolinium enhancement (LGE) sequence.

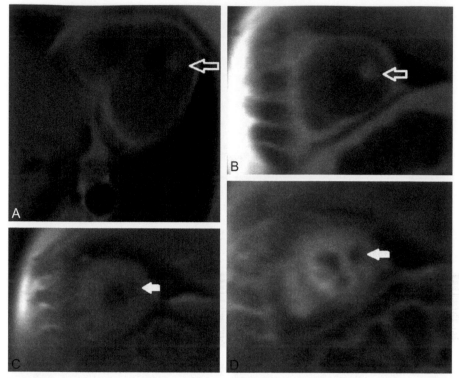

**FIG. 13.5**

Cardiac Lipoma. Round well-defined tumor in the apical lateral segment of LV cavity *(arrow)*. High signal mass in T1-W sequence axial (A) and short-axis (B) view, hyposignal mass in fat suppression sequence (C), and hyposignal mass in early perfusion sequence (D). The mass shows no late gadolinium enhancement (not shown).

In lipomatous hypertrophy, a bilobed atrial septum thickening with a signal intensity comparable to subcutaneous fat on T1- and T2-weighted images can be visualized.

## Papillary fibroelastoma

Papillary fibroelastomas are small (usually, 1.5 cm), benign endocardial papillomas that predominantly affect the cardiac valves (90%), accounting for 75% of all valvular neoplasms. In surgical series, they account for approximately 10% of primary cardiac tumors, but their prevalence in the general population is uncertain as they are often asymptomatic and discovered incidentally (Table 1). Because of their small size and high mobility, they are usually best diagnosed with echocardiography, and MR imaging is rarely additive except in atypical cases. Typical MR imaging features are of a small, highly mobile homogeneous valvular mass (usually attached to

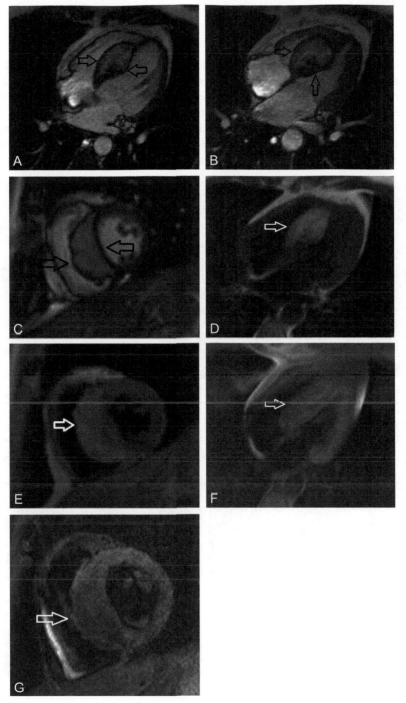

**FIG. 13.6**

Interventricular septum lipoma. Intramural sigmoid shape, well-defined, and capsulated tumor *(arrow)* in the interventricular septum. Hypersignal tumor in axial view cine SSFP sequence, diastole (A), and systole (B). Hypersignal mass in axial and short-axis views T1-W sequence (C and D). Hyposignal tumor in axial view T1-W fat saturation sequence (E). Hyposignal mass in short-axis view, short tau inversion recovery (STIR) sequence.

the downstream side with a small pedicle); hypointense signal intensity and surrounding turbulent flow on cine images; and isointense T1 and hyperintense T2 signal intensity patterns (Fig. 13.7). Movie [online]) [16,17] (Table 1). The main differentials include vegetations and thrombus.

Vegetations are usually present in the clinical context of suspected infected endocarditis and cause destruction of valvular leaflets, whereas fibroelastomas are rarely associated with an impact on the valve function.

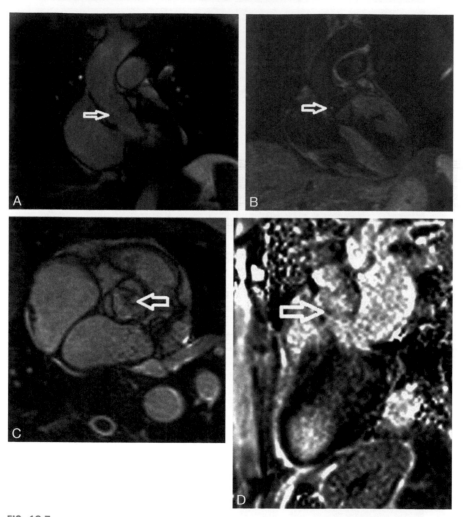

**FIG. 13.7**

Aortic valve fibroelastoma. Tiny mass *(arrows)* is displayed on the ventricular side of the right aortic valve leaflet in a patient with a history of TIA. The mass is iso to low signal in coronal oblique cine SSFP sequence (A), high signal intensity in coronal oblique STIR sequence (B), low signal intensity in high-resolution cross-section of aortic valve cine SSFP sequence (C), and without enhancement in the late gadolinium enhancement sequence.

Surgical excision is only recommended in symptomatic patients or in those with larger (>1 cm), highly mobile, left-sided tumors [3].

## Fibroma

Cardiac fibromas are the second most common benign cardiac tumor in children (after rhabdomyoma) [18] but it is the most commonly resected pediatric cardiac tumor. It typically presents in infancy, but approximately 15% of cardiac fibromas occur in adolescents and adults [19]. The mean age at diagnosis is 13 years, with an age range of 0–60 years [13,20]. It sometimes carries associations with genetic conditions; for example, up to 14% of patients with nevoid basal cell carcinoma syndrome (NBCCS), also called Gorlin syndrome, can have cardiac fibromas [15,21].

The most common site is the left ventricle (approximately 57% of the cases), followed by right ventricle (27.5%) and interventricular septum (17%). Those associated with polyposis syndromes (e.g., familial adenomatous polyposis or Gardner syndrome) occur more commonly in the atria [3].

Unlike rhabdomyoma, fibromas never resolve completely [18]. In fact, although not accordingly, tumor increases in size until the somatic cardiac growth ceases.

MRI demonstrate a mural mass that are usually round, well-circumscribed tumors located within the ventricular myocardium, bulging internally or externally or even obliterating the chamber lumen. They are always single and range in size from 2 to 10 cm (Fig. 13.8) [19]. The tumor appears as an isointense to hyperintense mass

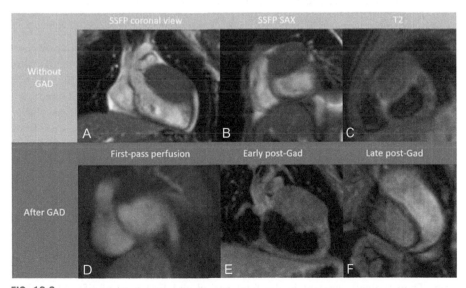

**FIG. 13.8**

Cardiac fibroma. (A and B) A one-year-old infant with a well-defined isosignal cardiac mass involving the anteroseptal and anterior left ventricular wall. (C) Characteristic T2 hypointensity of the lesion. (D–F) After Gad injection, there is no first-pass, minimal early and brisk homogeneous late enhancement of the tumor, respectively.

on T1-weighted and characteristically hypointense on T2-weighted sequences [19]. Owing to its nature, there is often little or no enhancement during the first-pass perfusion or early phase images after contrast injection while progressive intense enhancement of the poorly vascularized fibrotic tissues on delayed images (7–10 min)—due to slow and persistent contrast diffusion into large extracellular space component—which make it of utmost diagnostic importance.

## Hemangioma

Cardiac hemangioma (CH) is a rare primary tumor of the heart which comprises about 2.8% of all and 5%–10% of benign primary cardiac tumors [22]. The reported range of age when detected comprises the 20th gestational week to 86 years [23,24] but most manifest in the 40's decade with no significant gender preponderance [22]. The lesion diameter ranges from 0.5 to 14 cm [25,26], but the average size is about 4.5 cm [22].

It is typically a well-circumscribed tumor and can originate either in the pericardium, myocardium, or endocardium [27]. It can involve all cardiac chambers and valves with no chamber predilection [22,28]. Cardiac hemangiomas are usually asymptomatic until hemodynamic, conduction system, or coronary flow alterations happen.

Usually, the lesion is solitary and the heart is the only place of involvement. There are only few reports of multiplicity [25,29] and accompanied hemangiomas in other location, including liver [30,31], lung [32], and pleura [33]. However, histopathologic features of CH are identical to those of hemangiomas elsewhere in the body and more than 50% of cardiac hemangiomas are of cavernous type [22].

While echocardiographic features of hemangioma although suggestive but are nonspecific in most instances [22], MRI is more capable of assessment of extension, tissue characterization, and involvement to surrounding structures. Typically, CH shows intermediate T1 and homogeneously high T2 signal intensity compared with myocardium, respectively, owing to slow internal blood flow. The high vascularity of CH is noteworthy leading to a characteristic early filling of contrast during first-pass sequence. For larger lesions fast eccentric puddling of contrast material via feeder arter(ies) on delayed images is a typical pattern of enhancement. This "fast in and slow out" enhancement pattern [34], in addition to high signal intensity on T2-weighted images [28], is characteristic for diagnosis (Fig. 13.9).

## Rhabdomyoma

Rhabdomyomas are the most common primary cardiac tumors in infants and children. They typically present in the fetal period and first year of life. More than 50% of cardiac rhabdomyomas are associated with tuberous sclerosis [3]. They originate within the myocardium, typically in the ventricles and unlike fibromas, they are

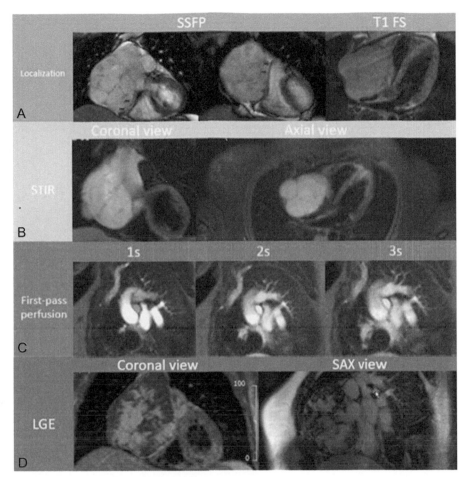

**FIG. 13.9**

Cardiac Hemangioma. A 35-year-old female, complaining of palpitation from 3months before. Echocardiography suggested a mediastinal mass. (A) SSFP and T1 fat-sat sequences revealed the location of the lesion. Red arrows depict the pericardial origin of the mass. (B) The bright homogeneous T2 hyperintensity of the mass. (C) First-pass perfusion demonstrates the rapid early fill-in and slow outward propagation of contrast material. (D) Slow progressive enhancement of the cavernous spaces. *SSFP*, steady-state free precession; *STIR*, short-tau inversion recovery; *LGE*, late gadolinium enhancement; *S*, second.

multiple in up to 90% of cases [1]. Tumors may measure up to 10cm, especially in sporadic cases, but it averages 3–4cm [19].

On cardiac MR imaging, they typically appear as well-defined occasionally lobulated tumors isointense similar to that of the adjacent normal myocardium on T1-weighted images and intermediate to hyperintense, unlike fibromas, on T2-weighted

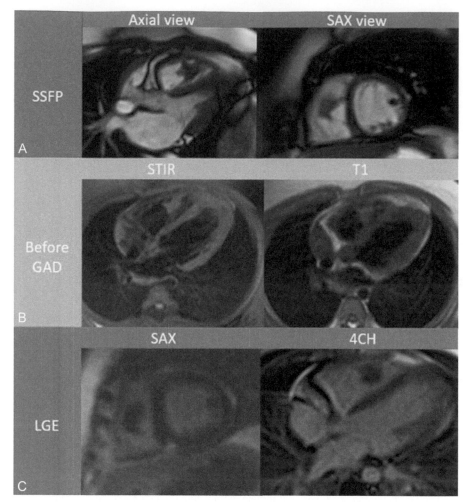

**FIG. 13.10**

Cardiac rhabdomyoma. (A) 2-year-old boy referred for an incidental endocavitary RV mass. (B) The lesion shows iso to intermediate signal on T1 and STIR sequences. (C) No evident or minimal enhancement of the lesion even in late gad sequences.

images while showing minimal or no enhancement with gadolinium-based contrast material (Fig. 13.10) [14,35,36]. Lack of calcification or internal cystic component are features that assist in discrimination from other benign tumors like fibromas [19].

The majority stand asymptomatic and spontaneously regress till the age of 4 years without the need for surgical removal [3].

## Paraganglioma

Cardiac paragangliomas are extremely rare neoplasms that arise from intrinsic cardiac paraganglial (chromaffin) cells, which are normally predominantly located within the atria. Most lesions have been reported in adult patients with an age range of 18–85 years (mean age, 40 years).

MR imaging typically demonstrates a mass that is hypointense on T1-weighted and very hyperintense on T2-weighted images. The intrapericardial location of the mass and its relationship to the cardiovascular structures is usually clearly demonstrated (Fig. 13.11) [37].

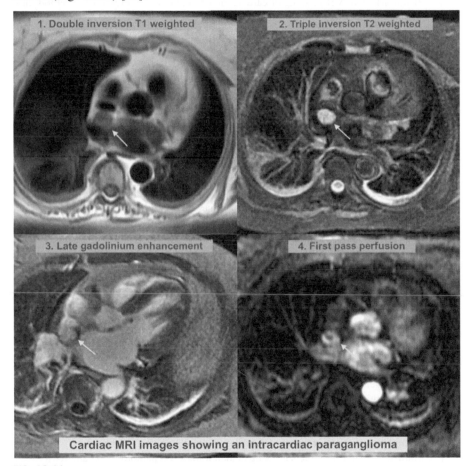

**FIG. 13.11**

Cardiac paraganglioma. Cardiac MRI shows a mass, hypointense to myocardium on T1-weighted (1), and hyperintense on T2-weighted images (2). First-pass perfusion (4) reveals rapid uptake of contrast in the lesion after administration, whereas late gadolinium enhancement (3) displays avid enhancement with contrast with a central stellate scar.

These tumors usually strongly enhance on first-pass perfusion and LGE imaging. Not infrequently, the central portion remains hypoenhanced likely representing central necrosis or liquefaction.

## References

[1] Sparrow PJ, et al. MR imaging of cardiac tumors. Radiographics 2005;25(5):1255–76.

[2] Mitchell DG, et al. The biophysical basis of tissue contrast in extracranial MR imaging. Am J Roentgenol 1987;149(4):831–7.

[3] Motwani M, et al. MR imaging of cardiac tumors and masses: a review of methods and clinical applications. Radiology 2013;268(1):26–43.

[4] Kramer CM, et al. Standardized cardiovascular magnetic resonance imaging (CMR) protocols: 2020 update. J Cardiovasc Magn Reson 2020;22(1):17.

[5] Simonetti OP, et al. "Black blood" T2-weighted inversion-recovery MR imaging of the heart. Radiology 1996;199(1):49–57.

[6] de Roos A, et al. Calcified right atrial myxoma demonstrated by magnetic resonance imaging. Chest 1989;95(2):478–9.

[7] Masui T, et al. Cardiac myxoma: identification of intratumoral hemorrhage and calcification on MR images. AJR. Am J Roentgenol 1995;164(4):850–2.

[8] Matsuoka H, et al. Morphologic and histologic characterization of cardiac myxomas by magnetic resonance imaging. Angiology 1996;47(7):693–8.

[9] Luna A, et al. Evaluation of cardiac tumors with magnetic resonance imaging. Eur Radiol 2005;15(7):1446–55.

[10] Basso C, et al. Surgical pathology of primary cardiac and pericardial tumors. Eur J Cardiothorac Surg 1997;12(5):730–8.

[11] Carney JA, et al. The complex of myxomas, spotty pigmentation, and endocrine overactivity. Medicine 1985;64(4):270–83.

[12] Tyebally S, et al. Cardiac tumors: JACC CardioOncology state-of-the-art review. JACC CardioOncol 2020;2(2):293–311.

[13] Pittman S, et al. Cardiac fibroma: an uncommon cause of a fixed defect on myocardial perfusion imaging. Clin Nucl Med 2018;43(2):e56–8.

[14] O'Donnell DH, et al. Cardiac tumors: optimal cardiac MR sequences and spectrum of imaging appearances. Am J Roentgenol 2009;193(2):377–87.

[15] Vidaillet Jr. HJ. Cardiac tumors associated with hereditary syndromes. Am J Cardiol 1988;61(15):1355.

[16] Wintersperger B, et al. Tumors of the cardiac valves: imaging findings in magnetic resonance imaging, electron beam computed tomography, and echocardiography. Eur Radiol 2000;10(3):443–9.

[17] Klarich KW, et al. Papillary fibroelastoma: echocardiographic characteristics for diagnosis and pathologic correlation. J Am Coll Cardiol 1997;30(3):784–90.

[18] Torimitsu S, et al. Literature survey on epidemiology and pathology of cardiac fibroma. Eur J Med Res 2012;17(1):5.

[19] Grebenc ML, et al. Primary cardiac and pericardial neoplasms: radiologic-pathologic correlation. Radiographics 2000;20(4):1073–103.

[20] Burke AP, et al. Cardiac fibroma: clinicopathologic correlates and surgical treatment. J Thorac Cardiovasc Surg 1994;108(5):862–70.

[21] Ritter AL, et al. Cardiac fibroma with ventricular tachycardia: an unusual clinical presentation of nevoid basal cell carcinoma syndrome. Mol Syndromol 2018;9(4):219–23.

[22] Li W, et al. Cardiac hemangioma: a comprehensive analysis of 200 cases. Ann Thorac Surg 2015;99(6):2246–52.

[23] Sharma J, Hirata Y, Mosca RS. Surgical repair in neonatal life of cardiac haemangiomas diagnosed prenatally. Cardiol Young 2009;19(4).

[24] Dod HS, et al. Two-and three-dimensional transthoracic and transesophageal echocardiographic findings in epithelioid hemangioma involving the mitral valve. Echocardiography 2008;25(4):443–5.

[25] Tadros NB, et al. Arteriovenous and capillary hemangiomas of the interventricular septum. Ann Thorac Surg 1988;46(2):236–8.

[26] Weir I, Mills P, Lewis T. A case of left atrial haemangioma: echocardiographic, surgical, and morphological features. Heart 1987;58(6):665–8.

[27] Reynen K. Frequency of primary tumors of the heart. Am J Cardiol 1996;77(1):107.

[28] Hrabak-Paar M, et al. Hemangioma of the interatrial septum: CT and MRI features. Cardiovasc Intervent Radiol 2011;34(2):90–3.

[29] Acikel S, et al. Multisided cardiac hemangiomas mimicking biatrial thrombus: atypically located cardiac hemangiomas of left atrial appendage and right atrium. J Am Soc Echocardiogr 2009;22(4):434.e7–9.

[30] Abad C, et al. Cardiac hemangioma with papillary endothelial hyperplasia: report of a resected case and review of the literature. Ann Thorac Surg 1990;49(2):305–8.

[31] Kan C-D, Yae C, Yang Y. Left ventricular haemangioma with papillary endothelial hyperplasia and liver involvement. Heart 2004;90(8):e49.

[32] Yang L, et al. Cardiac cavernous hemangioma and multiple pulmonary cavernous hemangiomas. Ann Thorac Surg 2014;97(2):687–9.

[33] Wender C, Acker Jr. JE. Constrictive pericarditis associated with hemangioma of the pericardium. Am Heart J 1966;72(2):255–8.

[34] Bai Y, Zhao G, Tan Y. CT and MRI manifestations of mediastinal cavernous hemangioma and a review of the literature. World J Surg Oncol 2019;17(1):205.

[35] Kiaffas MG, Powell AJ, Geva T. Magnetic resonance imaging evaluation of cardiac tumor characteristics in infants and children. Am J Cardiol 2002;89(10):1229–33.

[36] Fieno DS, et al. Cardiovascular magnetic resonance of primary tumors of the heart: a review. J Cardiovasc Magn Reson 2006;8(6):839–53.

[37] Grebenc ML, et al. Primary cardiac and pericardial neoplasms: radiologic-pathologic correlation. Radiographics 2000;20(4):1073–103.

# CMR for malignant cardiac tumors: Diagnosis, approach, and follow-up

**Shahrad Shadman[a], Charles Benton[a], Neha Gupta[b], Marcus Carlsson[a,c,d,f], and Ana Barac[c,e,f]**

[a]NHLBI, National Institutes of Health, Bethesda, MD, United States [b]Cleveland Clinic Foundation, Cleveland, OH, United States [c]Clinical Physiology Laboratory, NHLBI, National Institutes of Health, Bethesda, MD, United States [d]Lund University, Lund, Sweden [e]Cardio-Oncology Program, MedStar Washington Hospital Center, Washington, DC, United States [f]Georgetown University, Washington, DC, United States

## Key points

- Cardiac magnetic resonance (CMR) is the gold standard noninvasive imaging modality to assess tissue characteristics in vivo which gives it a unique advantage in discriminating benign cardiac masses from malignant tumors. CMR also provides visualization of tumor invasion, hemodynamic effects, and location relative to surrounding cardiac and extracardiac structures. These features make CMR an essential tool for diagnosis and management of cardiac tumors.

- The following sequences form part of a comprehensive CMR exam: cine imaging (e.g. balanced steady state free precession (bSSFP)), T1/T2-weighted black-blood (BB) images, T1/T2 mapping, first-pass perfusion, and delayed enhancement imaging. The characteristics of the tumor are often described as hyper/iso/hypo-intense, meaning higher, equal to, or lower signal intensity compared to normal myocardium. For instance, the extensive vascular networks associated with malignant tumors often present as hyperintense on first-pass perfusion and on late gadolinium enhancement (LGE) images. The high volume of intracellular free water content in malignant tumors and the frequently observed surrounding edema may lead to longer T1 and T2 relaxation times. At the same time, necrosis and hemorrhage within the tumor often result in heterogeneous signal on T1W and T2W BB images. The newer T1 and T2 mapping techniques provide quantitative T1 and T2 values, instead of the relative grayscale obtained through T1W and T2W BB imaging, providing an opportunity to further advance the diagnosis of malignant cardiac tumors.

- CMR limitations include absolute and relative contraindications for imaging in patients with devices that are not MR compatible (e.g., noncompatible pacemakers, internal defibrillators, mechanical circulatory support devices, etc.).

Breath-holds are often used in clinical protocols and patients that cannot hold their breath often have decreased image quality. Similarly, the need for ECG gating makes CMR a challenge in patients with irregular heart rhythm as it can lead to acquisition artifacts and poor image quality.

## Abbreviations

| | |
|---|---|
| **2CH** | 2-chamber |
| **4CH** | 4-chamber |
| **BB** | black blood |
| **bSSFP** | balanced steady-state free precession |
| **CMR** | cardiovascular magnetic resonance imaging |
| **CNS** | central nervous system |
| **CT** | computed tomography |
| **FPP** | first-pass perfusion |
| **FS** | fat saturation |
| **FSE** | fast spin echo |
| **LGE** | late gadolinium enhancement |
| **LV** | left ventricle |
| **RV** | right ventricle |
| **SAX** | short-axis |
| **SSFP** | steady-state free precession |
| **T1W** | T1 weighted |
| **T2W** | T2 weighted |
| **TEE** | transesophageal echocardiography |
| **TTE** | transthoracic echocardiography |

## Introduction

Cardiac masses entail a heterogeneous group of disorders that can be broadly divided into benign and malignant tumors. Malignant cardiac tumors are exceedingly rare (compared to benign masses) and often present with significant diagnostic and therapeutic challenges. Cardiac magnetic resonance (CMR) imaging has emerged as a key noninvasive technique in their evaluation, primarily due to the superior tissue characterization without ionizing radiation exposure. Moreover, CMR provides visualization of cardiac tumor extension/invasion, relationship with surrounding cardiac and extracardiac structures, and the evaluation of hemodynamic effects. Malignant tumors can be further divided into primary and secondary cardiac malignancies (Table 14.1). Among malignant primary cardiac tumors, the most common are sarcomas which account for about 75% of the cases, while primary cardiac lymphomas, mesotheliomas, neuroendocrine tumors, and others account for the remainder 25% of cases (Table 14.1) [8]. Secondary tumors can invade the heart by direct extension (e.g. pleural mesothelioma), intracavitary spread (e.g. renal cell carcinoma via

**Table 14.1** Malignant cardiac tumors—clinical, morphologic, and histopathologic characteristics and management.

| Primary cardiac tumors | Morphologic characteristics | Histopathologic characteristics | Treatment considerations and prognosis |
|---|---|---|---|
| **Cardiac sarcomas** | | | |
| Angiosarcoma | Invasive, sessile, and lobular [1] | Present with myocardial infiltration, often highly vascularized with pleomorphism, mitotic figures, and areas of necrosis [1] | When possible, surgical resection is recommended and is often considered to treat hemodynamic consequences and reduce tumor burden. Systemic chemotherapy and less often radiation therapy may be considered |
| Undifferentiated sarcoma | Large, irregular, intracavitary mass [1] | Typical spindle and polygonal cells, filled with eosinophilic cytoplasm [1] | Poor prognosis with aggressive course |
| Osteosarcoma | Invasive, sessile, lobular [2] | Spindle cell lesions with malignant fibrous histiocytoma, microscopic foci areas of osteosarcoma, and chondrosarcoma in the spindle regions [2] | |
| Leiomyosarcoma | Invasive, sessile, lobular [2] | Blunt nuclei with bundles of spindled cells, areas of necrosis, mitotic cells with epithelioid regions [2] | |
| Synovial cell sarcoma | Protruded mass with irregular, gelatinous appearance [3] | Monophasic: Only contains spindle cells, no epithelial cells [3] Biphasic: contains both epithelial and spindle cells [3] | |
| Intimal sarcoma | Invasive, arising from large blood vessels and heart [4] | Spindle and pleomorphic cells with myxoid area [4] | |
| Fibrous histiocytoma sarcoma (pleomorphic and undifferentiated high grade) | Invasive, knoblike lesion [5] | – *Storiform-pleomorphic type:* Pleomorphic cells with spoke wheel-like structure [5] – *Giant tumor cell type:* giant cells with a strong eosinophilic cytoplasm and irregular nuclei [5] | |

Continued

**Table 14.1** Malignant cardiac tumors—clinical, morphologic, and histopathologic characteristics and management—Cont'd

| Primary cardiac tumors | Morphologic characteristics | Histopathologic characteristics | Treatment considerations and prognosis |
|---|---|---|---|
| | | – *Inflammatory type:* Large number of foamy yellow tumor cells mixed with a large number of inflammatory cells [5]<br>– *Myxoid type:* Round or star-shaped, in a loose mucus matrix [5] | |
| Rhabdomyosarcoma | Invasive, lobular [2] | Embryonal type with rhabdomyoblasts containing abundant glycogen and expressing desmin, myoglobin, and myogenin [2] | |
| Primary cardiac lymphoma | Lobular, multiple lesions [2] | Commonly diffuse large B-cell lymphoma. Other variations include Burkitt lymphoma, T-cell lymphoma, and low-grade B-cell lymphoma [2] | Chemotherapy and immunotherapy, no role for surgery [2] |
| Pericardial mesothelioma | Pericardial effusion and a tumor encasing the heart [2] | Combination of epithelial or sarcomatous lesions, and/or biphasic [2] | Highly aggressive with poor prognosis Palliative management [2] |
| Secondary cardiac tumors | Smooth surface, often multiple lesions [2] | Varies depending on the primary disease | Cardiac involvement confers a similar prognosis to stage IV cancer [2] Management directed toward primary disease [2] |
| Metastatic melanoma | Smooth surface, often multiple lesions [6] | Malignant epithelioid cells with prominent nucleoli and frequent mitoses [2] | Systemic therapy with targeted therapy per clinical guidelines [7] |

inferior vena cava or lung carcinoma via pulmonary veins), and hematogenous or lymphatic, metastatic spread. The reports about the prevalence of cardiac metastases vary widely, from 2% to up to 18%; however, these estimates are largely based on autopsies and may not reflect the cases seen in cardiac imaging centers [9].

In this chapter we describe current clinical indications for CMR and detailed CMR imaging protocol recommended for the comprehensive assessment and management of cardiac tumors. We then provide examples of applied CMR imaging and specific CMR findings with primary and secondary cardiac tumors.

## Role of CMR imaging in establishing the diagnosis

The initial identification and evaluation of a cardiac mass most often starts with the readily available transthoracic echocardiogram (TTE). Echocardiographic findings, in turn, frequently represent an indication for CMR to (a) confirm abnormal cardiac mass (vs normal anatomical structure as described in Table 14.2) and (b) further differentiate between benign, malignant, and nontumorous masses (e.g. thrombus). CMR imaging protocols can be employed to evaluate hemodynamics, morphology, pericardial invasion, size, location, homogeneity, and signal characteristics of cardiac masses, and thus aid in differentiation between benign and malignant tumors [11,12]. Features concerning for malignancy include large tumor size, involvement of the pericardium and the right heart, tissue heterogeneity, and high extracellular volume (ECV) determined by T1 mapping before and after gadolinium contrast infusion. A position paper published in 2020 by the Society of Cardiovascular Magnetic Resonance (SCMR) outlines clinical indications for the use of CMR in the evaluation and management of cardiac masses [10]. Beyond diagnosis and differentiation of malignant masses, CMR is recommended for guidance of surgical therapy, assessment of treatment effect, as well as posttreatment surveillance (Table 14.3) [10].

**Table 14.2** Normal heart structures that may be misinterpreted as cardiac tumors [10].

| Anatomical structure | Comments |
|---|---|
| Crista terminalis | Seen as a protuberance in the right atrium, may be perceived as angiosarcoma or primary cardiac lymphoma |
| Eustachian valve | Frequently observed in the right atrium |
| "Coumadin ridge" | Lies in the left atrium, in between the left atrial appendage and the left superior pulmonary vein |
| Chiari network | Occasionally seen in the right atrium near the entry site of inferior vena cava and coronary sinus |
| Moderator band | Seen in the right ventricle |
| False tendons of LV | Seen in the left ventricle |

**Table 14.3** Society of cardiovascular magnetic resonance (SCMR) recommendations for CMR use in evaluation and management of cardiac tumors [10].

| CMR indications | Level of evidence |
|---|---|
| I. Suspected cardiac mass | I |
| II. Differentiation between benign, malignant, and nontumorous masses | I |
| III. Guide surgery and/or biopsy if this is deemed appropriate | I |
| IV. Follow-up of benign cardiac tumors that do not require urgent intervention for changes over time | I |
| V. Evaluation of tumor resection/debulking, monitoring recurrence after surgery, and regression or progression after chemotherapy or radiotherapy | I |
| VI. Extracardiac extension of cardiac tumors or cardiac extension of tumors originating from surrounding structures | I |
| VII. Impact of cardiac masses on hemodynamics | I |

Most clinically indicated CMR images are obtained on 1.5T field strength magnets, though in recent years 3T imaging has been making a significant advance in quality and availability. The signal intensity of a neoplastic lesion is dependent on the tissue morphology and CMR parameters employed to obtain the images. Fig. 14.4 illustrates a CMR protocol recommended for the evaluation of cardiac masses [13]. Axial plane images with T1-weighted (T1W) and T2-weighted (T2W) sequences are used for native tissue characterization and are the first step in CMR evaluation. In recent years, the evolution of CMR parametric mapping has provided us with the ability to quantify myocardial tissue alterations based on T1, T2, and T2*(star) relaxation times and extracellular volume (ECV) measurements [14]. In turn, these values can be used in conjunction with qualitative T1W and T2W images in differentiating between cardiac tumors. For instance, a hypointense mass on T1W (or low T1 on T1 mapping) may represent a calcified tumor, meanwhile, hyperintensity on T1W images (high T1 on T1 mapping) can be seen in masses with high-fat content (e.g. lipomas and liposarcomas), hemorrhagic or highly vascularized tumors (e.g. angiosarcoma and hemangioma), as well as in melanomas (Table 14.5). On T2W images, highly vascularized tumors such as angiosarcoma present with hyperintense signal (high T2 on T2 mapping), in contrast to fibrous tumors which are hypointense (low T2 on T2 mapping). Importantly, the most common benign primary tumor, cardiac myxoma, also presents as bright/hyperintense on T2W and with high values on T2 mapping and in instances may present a diagnostic challenge (Fig. 18.8).

In contrast to qualitative assessment on T1W and T2W images, mapping permits quantification and may allow visualization of the disease process related to intra- and

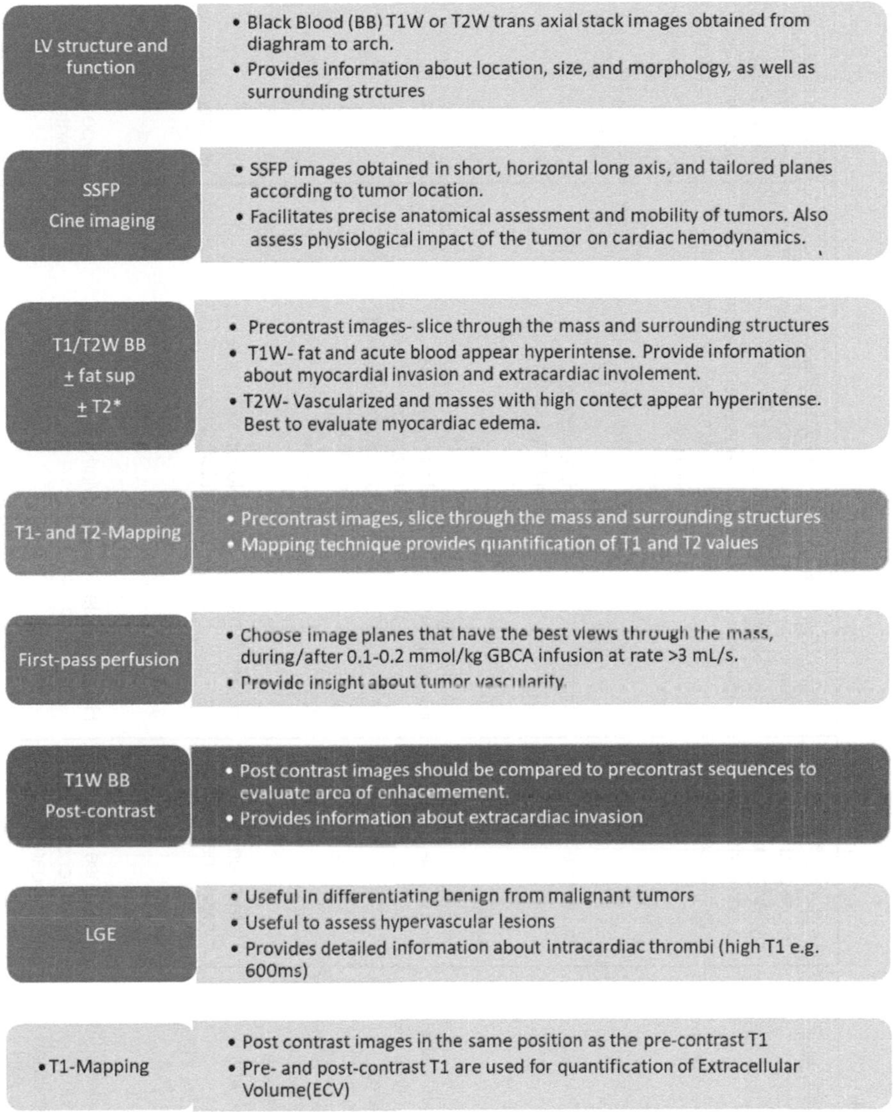

| | |
|---|---|
| **LV structure and function** | • Black Blood (BB) T1W or T2W trans axial stack images obtained from diaghram to arch.<br>• Provides information about location, size, and morphology, as well as surrounding strctures |
| **SSFP Cine imaging** | • SSFP images obtained in short, horizontal long axis, and tailored planes according to tumor location.<br>• Facilitates precise anatomical assessment and mobility of tumors. Also assess physiological impact of the tumor on cardiac hemodynamics. |
| **T1/T2W BB ± fat sup ± T2\*** | • Precontrast images- slice through the mass and surrounding structures<br>• T1W- fat and acute blood appear hyperintense. Provide information about myocardial invasion and extracardiac involement.<br>• T2W- Vascularized and masses with high contect appear hyperintense. Best to evaluate myocardiac edema. |
| **T1- and T2-Mapping** | • Precontrast images, slice through the mass and surrounding structures<br>• Mapping technique provides quantification of T1 and T2 values |
| **First-pass perfusion** | • Choose image planes that have the best views through the mass, during/after 0.1-0.2 mmol/kg GBCA infusion at rate >3 mL/s.<br>• Provide insight about tumor vascularity. |
| **T1W BB Post-contrast** | • Post contrast images should be compared to precontrast sequences to evaluate area of enhacemement.<br>• Provides information about extracardiac invasion |
| **LGE** | • Useful in differentiating benign from malignant tumors<br>• Useful to assess hypervascular lesions<br>• Provides detailed information about intracardiac thrombi (high T1 e.g. 600ms) |
| **• T1-Mapping** | • Post contrast images in the same position as the pre-contrast T1<br>• Pre- and post-contrast T1 are used for quantification of Extracellular Volume(ECV) |

**FIG. 14.4**

CMR imaging techniques—a comprehensive protocol for evaluation of cardiac masses. Abbreviations: *LV*, left ventricle; *BB*, black blood; *SSFP*, steady-state free precession; *FSE*, fast pin echo; *fat sup*, fat suppression; *bSSFP*, balanced steady-state free precession; *LGE*, late gadolinium enhancement.

**Table 14.5** CMR characteristics of malignant cardiac tumors.

| Tumor | Preferential location | T1W | T2W | LGE | Cine images |
|---|---|---|---|---|---|
| **Primary cardiac sarcomas** | | | | | |
| Angiosarcoma | Right atrium | Heterogeneous hypo- and hyperintensity due to hemorrhage and necrosis | Heterogeneous hyperintense, "cauliflower" appearance | Heterogeneous enhancement pattern with marked surface enhancement ("sunray appearance") and central necrosis | Fixed on the wall with a broad base, does not move with the heart Impaired right atrium and ventricular motion |
| Undifferentiated sarcoma | Left atrium | Isointense | Slightly hyperintense | Heterogeneous enhancement | Hypo- or isointense |
| Rhabdomyosarcoma | Frequently involves the valves Commonly not confined to one chamber | Isointense | Hyperintense | Homogeneous enhancement with areas of low central intensity due to necrosis | Isointense |
| Osteosarcoma | Left atrium | Heterogeneously hypointense | Hyperintense | Nonspecific due to calcification | Hypo- or isointense |
| Leiomyosarcoma | Posterior left atrium, pulmonary vein and mitral valve | Isointense or hypointense to myocardium | Hyperintense | Markedly enhanced | Hypo-or isointense |

**Table 14.5** CMR characteristics of malignant cardiac tumors—Cont'd

| Tumor | Preferential location | T1W | T2W | LGE | Cine images |
|---|---|---|---|---|---|
| Primary cardiac lymphoma | Right atrium (often involves more than one chamber) | Isointense ↕ | Heterogeneously hyperintense ← | Heterogeneous enhancement, with area of low enhancement in the center of the lesion ← | Isointense, large soft tissue mass ↕ |
| Pericardial mesothelioma | Pericardial space | Homogeneously isointense ↕ | Heterogeneously hyperintense with areas of necrosis ←← | Markedly heterogeneous enhancement ←←← | Hypointense nodule → |
| Metastatic melanoma | Right heart | Hyperintense ←← | Hyperintense ←← | Heterogeneous enhancement ←← | Nodular hyperintense appearance in the myocardium |
| Other metastatic involvement | Pericardium | Hypointense ⇉ | Hyperintense ←← | Heterogeneous enhancement ←← | Varies depending on the primary source |

extracellular disturbances. Though current clinical evidence is scarce, mapping techniques can be used to characterize masses, pericardial effusion, and fatty lesions within the heart. For example, vascularized tumors with high water content have long T1 and T2 relaxation times, while they have low T1 values postcontrast update due to significant gadolinium contrast uptake [14]. Although significant advances have been made in parametric mapping techniques, future research and validation are needed before routine clinical application for diagnoses of cardiac tumors. When describing T1W and T2W imaging with hyperintense or hypointense findings for various tumors, this information can also be obtained using T1 and T2 mapping.

Steady-state free precession (SSFP) technique is a valuable sequence to assess the relationship between the tumor with the myocardium, pericardium, blood pool, valves, and adjacent tissues. Assessment of tumor movement with respect to normal cardiac structure during cardiac cycle provides information on tumor attachment and whether tumor growth is invasive. Additionally, the hemodynamic effects on cardiac pumping and valvular function can be evaluated by cine SSFP images. Also, phase contrast flow imaging can be used to quantify hemodynamic effects with, e.g. increases in flow velocity if the tumor is affecting ejection or filling of blood.

Beyond native tissue characteristics, gadolinium contrast infusion can be employed to discern cardiac masses from normal cardiac structure through first-pass perfusion and late gadolinium enhancement (LGE). First-pass perfusion is conducted with dynamic imaging during infusion of contrast and is an important method to identify tumor vascularity and presence of necrosis. Masses such as hemangioma and to a lesser degree angiosarcoma tend to show early enhancement after contrast infusion and are easily distinguishable from other lesions [15]. As malignant tumors frequently cause tissue necrosis by obliteration of capillary beds, first-pass perfusion images may exhibit dark central areas (necrosis) with hyperenhancement of the surrounding tissue, an important diagnostic measure to differentiate benign from malignant tumors. Late gadolinium enhancement (LGE) sequences are obtained 10 min postcontrast administration. Benign cardiac masses more often present as markedly homogeneous enhancing lesions (with the exception of myxoma), while malignant tumors present heterogeneous contrast enhancement due to extensive vascularity and necrosis. To discriminate normal myocardium from neoplastic masses, the inversion time is set to null normal cardiomyocytes as the exact inversion time varies depending upon patient physiology, timing postcontrast administration, and type of sequence.

## Primary malignant tumors
### Cardiac sarcomas

Cardiac sarcomas are the most common primary malignant tumor of the heart and together represent more than two-thirds of all malignant primary tumors [2]. Cardiac sarcomas occur mainly in adulthood, usually between the third and fifth decades of life, and are often asymptomatic until advanced with dismal prognostic results [2]. Many subtypes have been described based on histological characteristics (e.g., angiosarcoma, rhabdomyosarcoma, fibrosarcoma, leiomyosarcoma, liposarcoma, synovial sarcoma, intimal sarcoma, myxofibrosarcoma, and undifferentiated pleomorphic sarcomas) which largely share imaging appearances (Table 14.1). Angiosarcomas are the most common subtype in adulthood, accounting for approximately 40% of all cardiac sarcomas, while rhabdomyosarcomas are the most common in the pediatric population [16].

### Angiosarcoma

Angiosarcomas commonly present in the right atrium, manifesting with symptoms of right-heart failure, hemorrhagic pericardial effusions, and metastatic invasion [2]. Histologically, angiosarcomas present with widespread infiltrative anaplastic cells derived from blood vessels, often highly vascularized with pleomorphic mitotic figures and areas of extensive hemorrhage and necrosis [2] (Table 14.1). These tissue characteristics may be seen on CMR imaging as heterogeneous T1W and T2W signal intensity, in part due to tissue necrosis and hemorrhage. On LGE images heterogeneous enhancement may be seen as a result of central necrosis (hypointense) and fibrotic margins (hyperintense) (Fig. 14.6).

### Rhabdomyosarcoma

Rhabdomyosarcomas are malignant tumors of striated muscle and are the most common pediatric cardiac malignancy [2]. Unlike other cardiac sarcomas, these tumors arise from the myocardium and frequently affect multiple sites within the heart, frequently involving the valves. Often times they grow to be >10 cm in diameter, and as described in Table 14.1, they are made up of rhabdomyoblasts containing glycogen and expressing desmin, myoglobin, and myogenin [2]. CMR findings of this tumor typically include isointensity on T1W and hyperintensity on T2W images, with diffuse enhancement after contrast administration. Depending on the extent of central necrosis and the volume of necrotic tissue, regions of hypointensity may be present at the center of the mass.

### Leiomyosarcoma

Primary cardiac leiomyosarcomas are the second most common type of cardiac sarcomas in adult patients, accounting for 8% to 9% of all cardiac sarcomas [2]. They are known to mimic myxomas and have a predilection for the posterior left atrium, pulmonary vein, and mitral valve. Leiomyosarcoma often presents as a sessile mass on SSFP cine images with a gelatinous base [2]. They arise from smooth muscle and as mentioned before, they have the propensity to involve the valves (Table 14.1). Leiomyosarcoma, as opposed to angiosarcomas, is characterized by slow and asymptomatic growth. Due to the oligosymptomatic course, they are usually diagnosed in advanced stages. CMR imaging descriptions are scarce due to the rarity of the condition, but it is commonly described

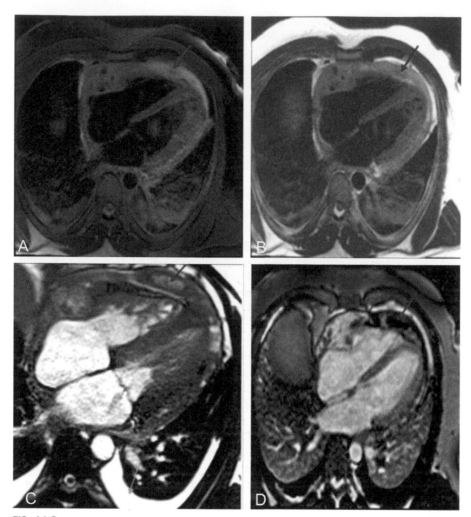

**FIG. 14.6**

Primary pericardial angiosarcoma. A previously healthy 40-year old man presented with fever, chills, and exertional dyspnea. He was found to have pericardial effusion with tamponade, requiring urgent pericardiocentesis. CMR images post pericardiocentesis are shown: 4CH BB T2W images, with FS (A) and without FS (B), show a circumferential, complex mass around the pericardium *(red arrow)*. The mass is located anterior to the RV with evidence of RV impingement, with extension to the RV groove. The mass appears heterogeneously hyperintense on 4CH Cine image (C) during diastole, in addition to bilateral pleural effusion (C—*blue arrow*). After administration of contrast, the mass depicted heterogeneous areas of hyper and hypointensity on 4CH LGE sequence (D), making the diagnosis of the angiosarcoma more plausible. Abbreviations: *4CH*, four chamber; *BB*, black blood; *T2W*, T2-weighted; *FS*, fat saturation; *RV*, right ventricle; *LGE*, late gadolinium enhancement.

as isointense or hypointense on T1W images, and hyperintense on T2W images [2]. Diffuse enhancement is frequently observed after administration of gadolinium contrast.

### Osteosarcoma

Primary cardiac osteosarcomas are extremely rare, making up 3% to 9% of primary cardiac sarcomas [2]. As opposed to metastatic osteosarcomas that frequently involve the right atrium, primary cardiac osteosarcomas predominantly involve the left atrium which makes it easy to be mistaken for myxomas. However, presence of dense calcification, wide-based attachment, and location away from fossa ovalis with frequent invasive behavior can be helpful in differentiation. They may have osteo-, chondro-, or fibro-blastic substances with atypical spindle or ovoid cells [2]. This tumor is best seen on computed tomography (CT) as low attenuated masses with dense calcifications will not be seen on CMR. (For details of CT imaging in malignant masses, we direct the reader to Chapter 12.) On CMR imaging, osteosarcomas tend to be heterogeneously hypointense on T1W and hyperintense on T2W images [2].

## Primary cardiac lymphoma

Primary cardiac lymphomas are rare tumors and when found, they most often fall in the category of aggressive large B cell lymphoma, a subtype of non-Hodgkin lymphoma (NHL). It is much more common for extracardiac NHL to metastasize to the heart, and approximately 25% of all patients with disseminated disease have evidence of heart involvement [17]. Primary cardiac lymphomas are more frequently seen in immunocompromised individuals and are strictly confined to the heart and/or pericardium [17]. They have the tendency to involve the right side of the heart, in particular the right atrium, and frequently involve multiple structures [2]. The pericardium is involved in approximately about one-third of reported cases and superior vena cava involvement is seen in up to 25% of all cases [17]. Microscopically, they consist of malignant lymphoid cells with firm nodules of homogeneously appearing tissue, without apparent hemorrhage or necrosis [17]. On CMR imaging, primary cardiac lymphomas are commonly hypointense on T1W and hyperintense on T2W (Fig. 14.7). On first-pass-perfusion, lymphomas often rapidly enhance while the appearance on LGE sequences may vary from homogeneous to heterogeneous enhancement. Postcontrast images also help delineate presence of pericardial nodularity, inflammation, and enhancement. Primary cardiac lymphomas may have adjacent thrombi that are seen as absence of enhancement on LGE sequences (Fig. 14.8).

## Primary pericardial mesothelioma

Pericardial mesothelioma is a highly aggressive malignancy of the pericardium, frequently associated with pericardial effusion and invasion of the underlying myocardium. Causal relationship between primary pericardial mesothelioma and asbestos

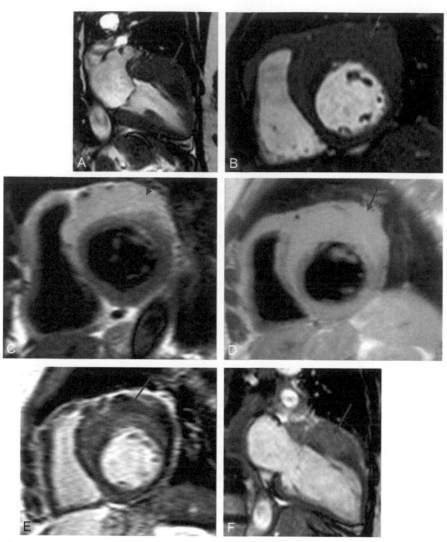

**FIG. 14.7**

Primary Cardiac Lymphoma—A 67-year-old woman with initial presentation of fatigue, weight loss, and pericardial effusion. CMR following pericardiocentesis showed a mass within the pericardium, adjacent to the anterolateral, anterior, septum, superior portion of the right ventricle and right ventricular outflow tract. The mass appeared isointense on SSFP cine images, in 2CH LV (A) and SAX projections (B). On SAX BB sequences with FS (C) and without FS (D), the mass appeared hyperintense *(arrows)*. Postgadolinium infusion, there was diffuse patchy hyperenhancement seen in the abnormal tumor mass affecting different myocardial territories including lateral wall, anterior wall, septum, as shown in SAX (E) and 2CH LV (F) projections *(arrows)*. Abbreviations: *SSFP*, steady-state free precession; *2CH*, two chamber; *LV*, left ventricle; *SAX*, short axis; *FS*, fat saturation; *RCA*, right coronary artery.

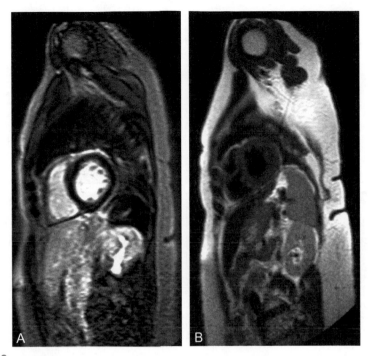

**FIG. 14.8**

Primary cardiac lymphoma post treatment—the patient described in Fig. 14.7 completed six cycles of dose-adjusted EPOCH and rituximab treatment. First chemotherapy was given in the CCU secondary to the concerns of possible arrhythmias with large tumor mass in the anterior wall. After completion of chemotherapy, CMR showed mildly thickened basal anterior wall and anterior septum possibly due to residual fibrotic changes (A and B). Abbreviations: *EPOCH*, etoposide, doxorubicin, vincristine, prednisone, and cyclophosphamide; *CCU*, cardiac care unit.

exposure has not been confirmed [1]. By definition, pericardial mesothelioma is distinguished from pleural mesothelioma by a lack of pleural involvement and with most of the disease being confined to the pericardial space. Despite being the most common primary malignancy of the pericardium, it is an exceedingly rare finding and it accounts for only <2% of all mesotheliomas [1]. It may present as pericardial effusion, atypical symptoms, or remain silent until hemodynamic symptoms of obstruction occur. On CMR imaging, pericardial mesotheliomas are often isointense on T1W images and heterogeneously hyperintense on T2W images, in part due to areas of necrosis. On LGE sequences, pericardial mesothelioma is most often seen as a hyperintense lesion which may help with delineating normal pericardium from tumor invasion (Fig. 14.9).

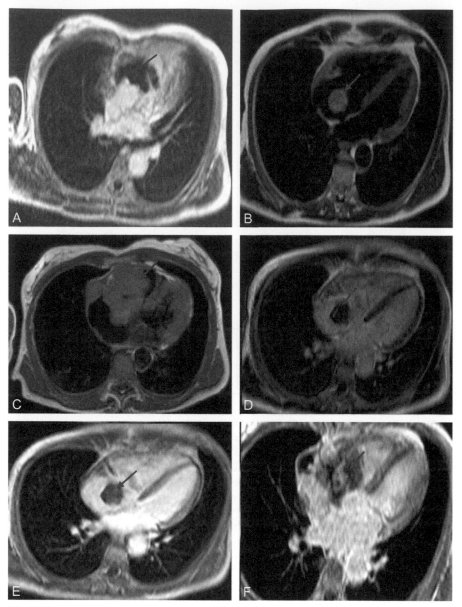

**FIG. 14.9**

Primary pericardial mesothelioma—A 56-year-old woman presented with a 6-month history of exertional chest pain and dyspnea and was found to have a mass in RA on echocardiography. On further evaluation, CMR confirmed a large mass occupying most of the RV and RVOT, involving the tricuspid valve, the RA, and extending into the AV groove surrounding the RCA. The mass appeared isointense on T1-bright blood axial localizer images (A) and hyperintense on 4CH BB T2W images (B and C). Shortly after infusion of gadolinium contrast, the mass did not enhance on FPP images (D); however, on LGE images contrast was seen within the mass in a heterogeneous pattern (E and F). Abbreviations: *LA*, left atrium; *RV*, right ventricle; *RVOT*, right ventricular outflow tract; *RA*, right atrium; *AV*, atrio-ventricular; *RCA*, right coronary artery; *T1W*, T1-weighted; *4CH*, four chamber; *BB*, black blood; *T2W*, T2-wighted; *FPP*, first-pass perfusion; *LGE*, late gadolinium enhancement.

## Secondary cardiac tumors

Metastasis to the heart and pericardium, also known as secondary cardiac tumors, is reported to be 20 to 40 times more common than primary cardiac tumors [18]. These data, however, are based on autopsies, and real clinical incidence remains difficult to ascertain. Distant invasion may occur directly from the mediastinum via large vessels, and/or through the lymphatic system. As previously shown by Bussani et al., the postmortem examination of 18,751 in-patients has demonstrated that the tumors with highest propensity to metastasize to heart or pericardium are pleural mesothelioma (48.4%), melanoma (27.8%), lung adenocarcinoma (21%), undifferentiated carcinomas (19.5%), lung squamous cell carcinoma (18.2%), breast carcinoma (15.5%), ovarian carcinoma (10.3%), lymphoproliferative neoplasms (9.4%), bronchioloalveolar carcinoma (9.8%), gastric carcinomas (8%), and renal carcinomas (7.3%) [19].

CMR with gadolinium administration is particularly important to detect the extent of myocardial tumor invasion and to recognize small, but significant, subset of patients with isolated lesions who should be considered for surgical resection. Metastatic lesions of the heart appear mostly hypointense on T1W and hyperintense on T2W (Fig. 14.10 and Table 14.5) [2]. A noteworthy exception is metastatic melanoma, which due to paramagnetic T1-shortening effects of melanin appears hyperintense on both T1W and T2W images (Table 14.5 and Fig. 14.11) [2]. Similar to other secondary cardiac masses, the postgadolinium images of metastatic melanoma also demonstrate enhancement.

## Differential diagnosis

Cardiac myxoma is the most common primary cardiac tumor. It falls into the category of benign tumors, described in Chapter 13 and is included here to highlight diagnostic challenges that may occur in the setting of less frequent locations and/or distal embolization. Importantly, CMR imaging characteristics may overlap with malignant masses including hyperintense appearance on T2W images and LGE enhancement (Fig. 14.12). Roughly 16% of all myxomas embolize systemically, and of those up to 45% may demonstrate neurologic symptoms secondary to embolic cerebral infarctions [20].

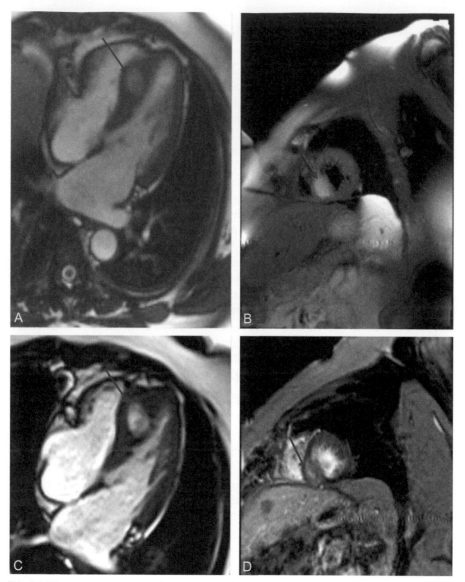

**FIG. 14.10**

Carcinoid heart metastasis—A 70-year-old woman with a well-differentiated carcinoid tumor of the small bowel with metastasis to the liver was incidentally found to have a cardiac mass on PET imaging. Further evaluation with CMR confirmed the presence of an oval-shaped well-circumscribed cardiac mass encased within the mid inferoseptal interventricular septum with no communication to the left or right ventricle. The mass appeared hyperintense on 4CH SSFP images (panel A, *red arrow*). The hyperintensity did not suppress on BB sequences with FS in SAX projection (panel B, *red arrow*). After gadolinium contrast infusion, the mass appeared hyperintense with predominantly homogenous intensity on LGE images, in 4CH (panel C, *red arrow*) and SAX (panel D, *red arrow*) projections. Abbreviations: *PET*, positron emission tomography; *4CH*, four chamber; *SSFP*, steady-state free precession; *BB*, black blood; *FS*, fat saturation; *SAX*, short axis; *LGE*, late gadolinium enhancement.

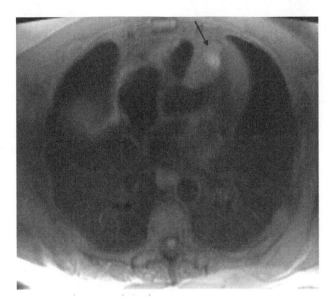

**FIG. 14.11**

Metastatic melanoma of the heart—while most secondary cardiac tumors appear
hypointense on T1-weighted (T1W) images, metastatic melanoma is a notable exception
reflecting as a hyperintense lesion. As shown by the arrow, the high concentration of melanin
results in a T1-shortening effect, making the tumor appear as a bright lesion on T1W.

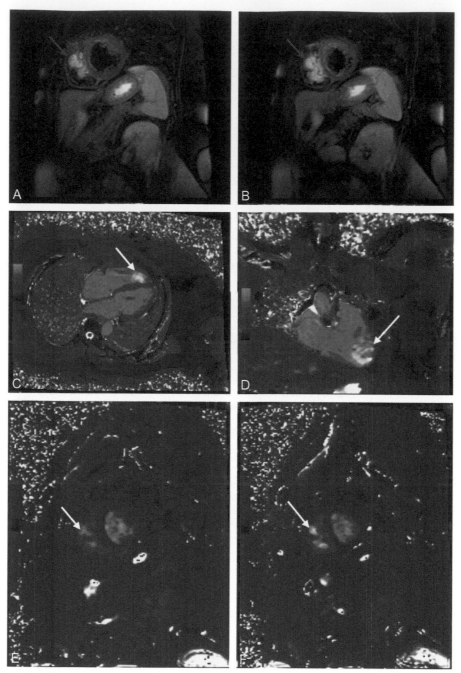

**FIG. 14.12**

Recurrent cardiac myxoma—a 61-year-old woman with history of large, left atrial cardiac myxoma, status postsurgical resection, was found to have new right ventricular (RV) mass on CMR imaging 8 months later. The mass was hyperintense on T2W BB images with FS in SAX projection (A and B). This mass had high T1 values on T1-mapping (C and D) in 4CH projection and high on T2-mapping (E and F) in SAX projection. RV biopsy, obtained via right heart catheterization, confirmed recurrent myxoma. Germline genetic testing was negative for Carney complex. Abbreviations: *T2W*, T2-weighted; *BB*, black blood; *FS*, fat saturation; *SAX*, short axis; *4CH*, four chamber.

# References

[1] Bussani R, et al. Cardiac tumors: diagnosis, prognosis, and treatment. Curr Cardiol Rep 2020;15343170. 22 [169, s.l.].

[2] Tyebally S, et al. Cardiac tumors—JACC cardiooncology state-of-the-art review. JACC Cardio Oncol 2020;2666-0873. 2 [2, s.l.].

[3] Varma T, Adegboyega P. Primary cardiac synovial sarcoma. Arch Pathol Lab Med 2012;1543-2165. 136 [4, s.l.].

[4] Neuville A, et al. Intimal sarcoma is the most frequent primary cardiac sarcoma. Am J Surg Pathol 2014;1532-0979. 38 [4, s.l.].

[5] Hirano Y. Editorial: primary cardiac malignant fibrous histiocytoma is a rare case of cardiac tumor. J Cardiol Cases 2015;18785409. 12 [5, s.l.].

[6] Allen BC, et al. Metastatic melanoma to the heart. Curr Probl Diagn Radiol 2012;15356302. 41 [5, s.l.].

[7] Swetter SM, et al. NCCN guidelines® insights: melanoma: cutaneous. J Natl Compr Canc Netw 2021;19(4):364–76.

[8] Ramlawi B, et al. Surgical treatment of primary cardiac sarcomas. Ann Thorac Surg 2016;2304-1021. 101:698–702 [2, s.l.].

[9] Bussani R, et al. Cardiac metastases. J Clin Pathol 2007;1472-4146. 60 [1, s.l.].

[10] Leiner T, Bogaert J, Friedrich MG, et al. SCMR position paper(2020) on clinical indications for cardiovascular magnetic resonance. J Cardiovasc Magn Reson 2020;1097-6647. 22 [76, s.l.].

[11] Sparrow PJ, et al. RSNA education exhibits. Radiographics 2005;27(2):1255–76. https://doi.org/10.1148/rg.272065049. https://pubs.rsna.org/doi/10.1148/rg.255045721. [Online] 1 September 2005. [Cited 17 October 2021].

[12] Fussen S, et al. Cardiovascular magnetic resosnance imaging for diagnsois and clincial management of suspected cardiac masses and tumours. Eur Heart J 2011;32:12.

[13] Kramer CM, Barkhausen J, Bucciarelli-Ducci C, et al. Standardized cardiovascular magnetic resonance imaging(CMR) protocols: 2020 update. J Cardiovasc Magn Reson 2020;1097-6647. 22 [17, s.l.].

[14] Messroghli DR, Moon JC, Ferreira VM, et al. Clinical recommendations for cardiovascular magnetic resonance mapping of T1, T2, T2* and extracellular volume: a consensus statement by the Society for Cardiovascular Magnetic Resonance (SCMR) endorsed by the European Association for Cardiovascular Imaging. J Cardiovasc Magn Reson 2017;1097-6647. 19 [75, s.l.].

[15] Motwani M, et al. MR imaging of cardiac tumors and masses: a review of methods and clinical applications. Radiology 2013;1527-1315. 268 [1, s.l.].

[16] Chen Y, Li Y, Zhang N, Shang J, Li X, Liu J, Xu L, Liu D, Sun Z, Wen Z. Clinical and imaging features of primary cardiac angiosarcoma. Diagnostics 2020;10:776.

[17] Jeudy J, Burke AP, Frazier AA. Cardiac lymphoma. Radiol Clin N Am 2016;0033-8389. 54 [4, s.l.].

[18] Sparrow PJ, Kurian JB, Jones TR, Sivananthan MU. MR imaging of cardiac tumors. Radiographics 2005;1527-1323. 25 [5, s.l.].

[19] Bussani R, De-Giorgio F, Abbate A, Silvestri F. Cardiac metastases. J Clin Pathol 2007;1472-4146. 60 [s.l.].

[20] Lee VH, Connolly HM, Brown RD. Central nervous system manifestations of cardiac myxoma. JAMA Neurol 2007;2168-6157. 64 [8, s.l.].

## Further reading

Pacheco-Velázquez SC, et al. Heart myxoma develops oncogenic and metastatic phenotype. J Cancer Res Clin Oncol 2019;1432-1335. 145 [5, s.l.].

# PET in benign cardiac tumors: Diagnosis, approach, and follow up

# 15

**Hadi Malek and Nahid Yaghoobi**

*Rajaie Cardiovascular Medical and Research Center, Iran University of Medical Sciences, Tehran, Iran*

## Key points

- Positron emission tomography (PET) measures two annihilation photons of an emitted positron from a radionuclide-labeled tracer with a specific biochemical distribution, resulting in molecular imaging of biological nature. Moreover, reduction in patient radiation dose could be achieved as the positron emitter radionuclides are usually short lived. However, in spite of functional imaging on a biochemical level, PET alone suffers from lack of anatomical details. In order to overcome this disadvantage, hybrid scanners were introduced in which computed tomography (CT) or magnetic resonance (MR) images are registered with the PET images.
- Currently, $^{18}$F-Fluorodexoglucose ($^{18}$F-FDG) is the most frequently used radiotracer for PET imaging. $^{18}$F-FDG is transported into the intracellular space by facilitated transport similar to glucose. However, contrary to glucose, $^{18}$F-FDG does not undergo further metabolism after phosphorylation. Thereby, this process allows mapping and measuring of the glucose metabolic activity. Despite the fact that elevated $^{18}$F-FDG uptake could be observed in a variety of inflammatory or benign lesions, it remains as the cornerstone in the workup of many cancers [1]. $^{18}$F-FDG PET/CT imaging enjoys the potential of noninvasive preoperative determination of cardiac malignancies and detection of metastatic lesions originated from primary malignant cardiac tumors in a single study [2].
- Benign neoplastic cardiac masses are usually of no to low FDG avidity; therefore, PET/CT imaging can play an important role in discrimination of malignant from benign neoplastic cardiac masses. Be that as it may, particular attention should be paid to normal variations and potential causes of false positive findings for cardiac masses and malignancies in interpretation (Boxes 15.1, 15.5, and 15.12).

Multimodal Imaging Atlas of Cardiac Masses. https://doi.org/10.1016/B978-0-323-84906-7.00026-1

## Box 15.1 Normal variations.

### Biodistribution of $^{18}$F-FDG

$^{18}$F-FDG accumulation is observed in different body organs, including brain, heart, urinary system, gastrointestinal tract, liver, spleen, and bone marrow. Myocardial uptake follows glucose metabolism, which is defined by myocardial perfusion and function along with available substrate. As a result of elevated plasma glucose and insulin levels, $^{18}$F-FDG myocardial uptake is increased after meal. Conversely, fasting state leads to decreased oxidative glucose metabolism while myocardial energy is supplied by fatty acids [3]. Focal or diffuse myocardial uptake might occur after standard period of fasting for oncologic studies [4]. Therefore, more prolonged fasting as well as consuming low carbohydrate diet is mandatory in order to decrease the normal cardiac background activity.

| Ventricular uptake | Atrial uptake |
|---|---|
| Various left ventricular (LV) $^{18}$F-FDG uptake patterns have been observed, including diffuse uptake throughout the LV myocardial walls, regional uptake in the lateral and posterior walls, and accumulation of radiotracer in the papillary muscles, which could sometimes be misinterpreted as thrombus or neoplasm when it occurs in the posterior muscle and in a globular pattern, or in base of the LV and posterolateral region, particularly in patients with a previous history of radiation therapy in an adjacent field to the heart (Figs. 15.2 and 15.3) [5]. On the other hand, increased uptake in the right ventricle (RV) has been reported to be correlated with RV dysfunction in patients with pulmonary hypertension [6]. | The atrial uptake is uncommon but increased uptake in the right atrium is usually associated with cardiac disease, particularly atrial fibrillation, and is a source of false positive finding in cancer assessment [7]. Moreover, $^{18}$F-FDG uptake in the crista terminalis is variable but increased uptake might occur in this structure, mimicking cardiac mass or thrombosis [5]. Right auricle is also a rare site of increased uptake with potential of misinterpretation as a pathologic mediastinal lymph node [6] (Fig. 15.4). |

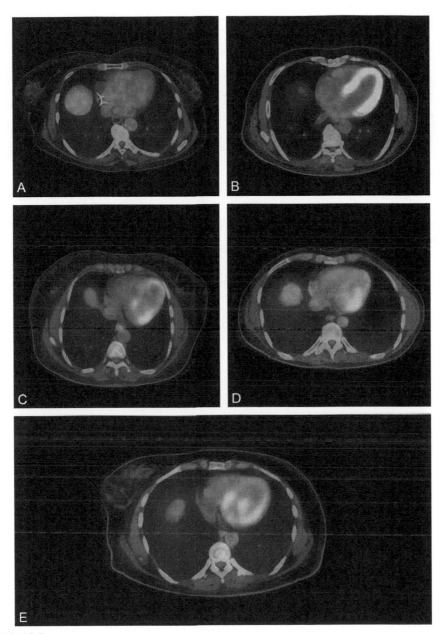

**FIG. 15.2**

Various patterns of left ventricular uptake in $^{18}$F-FDG PET/CT. Normal variation of left ventricular (LV) $^{18}$F-FDG uptake in fused axial PET/CT images. Absence of LV uptake (A); diffuse LV uptake (B); physiologic uptake in the base of the LV (basal ring uptake) (C); physiologic uptake in the posterior wall of the LV (D); and physiologic uptake in the lateral wall as well as base of the LV (E).

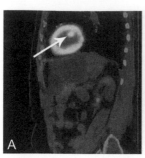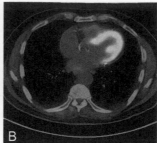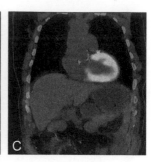

**FIG. 15.3**

Papillary muscle activity in $^{18}$F-FDG PET/CT. $^{18}$F-FDG uptake in papillary muscle as a focal area of radiotracer accumulation on fused PET/CT images in sagittal (A), axial (B), and coronal (C) planes. Particular attention should be paid in order to not mistake papillary muscle and/or chordae tendineae physiologic uptake as a cardiac mass.

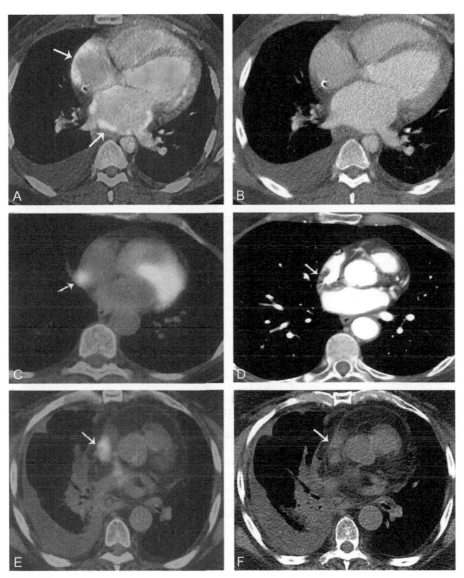

**FIG. 15.4**

Various patterns of atrial uptake in $^{18}$F-FDG PET/CT. *Upper row*: Diffuse biatrial uptake secondary to atrial fibrillation in a patient with a past medical history of lymphoma; *Middle row*: Increased uptake of $^{18}$F-FDG, corresponding to the crista terminalis in a patient with recurrent nonsmall cell lung carcinoma; *Lower row*: Increased radiotracer uptake in the right atrial appendage in a patient with the past medical history of nonsmall cell lung carcinoma and radiation therapy. Fused axial PET/CT images are shown on the left side and CT images of the same level are shown on the right side. Normal variations of physiologic uptake should be always considered in differential diagnosis with pathologic uptake, including thrombosis or cardiac masses.

*Adapted from Cuellar SLB, Palacio D, Benveniste MF, Carter BW, Gladish G. Pitfalls and misinterpretations of cardiac findings on PET/CT imaging: a careful look at the heart in oncology patients. Curr Prob Diagn Radiol. 2019;48(2):172–183; with permission.*

## Box 15.5 Diagnostic pitfalls.

*Different entities with the characteristics of increased accumulation of $^{18}F$-FDG are known, leading to inaccurate diagnosis of a FDG-avid cardiac lesion. Therefore, the interpreting physician should be aware of potential causes of false positive findings for cardiac masses and malignancies.*

| Entity | Description |
|---|---|
| *Lipomatous hypertrophy of interatrial septum* | Lipomatous hypertrophy of interatrial septum (LHIS) is a relatively uncommon finding which is characterized by fat deposition in the interatrial septum. Despite the fact that this entity represents a histologic benign process, adverse sequels of supraventricular arrhythmias, syncope, and sudden cardiac death have been reported. Since this fatty infiltration can appear as a fat-containing mass-like lesion with $^{18}$F-FDG avidity, other neoplastic processes, including myxoma, rhabdomyoma, rhabdomyosarcoma, and liposarcoma can be mimicked (Fig. 15.6) [8]. |
| *Epipericardial fat necrosis* | Epipericardial fat necrosis represents a benign entity of unknown etiology. The presenting symptom is usually pleuritic chest pain in a previously healthy subject. The CT component of PET/CT imaging allows characterization of the lesion as the presence of encapsulated pericardial fat density along with dense strands and/or thickening of the adjacent pericardium. The inflammatory infiltration of necrotic fat can explain the cause of $^{18}$F-FDG accumulation in this lesion (Fig. 15.7) [9]. |
| *Idiopathic hypertrophic cardiomyopathy* | Glucose metabolism increases in hypertrophic myocardium as a result of decreased expression of beta-oxidation enzymes. Idiopathic hypertrophic cardiomyopathy (HCM) is a genetic disease in which $^{18}$F-FDG uptake increases in the hypertrophic myocardium. The $^{18}$F-FDG uptake could be even more prominent in obstructive HCM [10]. HCM may present as a segmental FDG-avid mass-like lesion, which could be inseparable from cardiac metastasis in $^{18}$F-FDG PET/CT imaging unless additional cardiac imaging is performed (Fig. 15.8) [5]. |
| *Postradiation changes* | Radiation therapy as a fundamental measure of multimodality therapy for some of the malignancies can lead to pericardial or myocardial injury. Both radiation-induced myocarditis and acute as well as chronic pericarditis have been introduced. In both situations, postradiation $^{18}$F-FDG uptake may be falsely interpreted as malignant pericardial or myocardial involvement. Correlation with the radiation ports and CT component of PET/CT images as well as quantitative analysis by means of standardized uptake value (SUV) helps in differentiation of postradiation changes from malignant process (Fig. 15.9) [5]. |

| Box 15.5 Diagnostic pitfalls—Cont'd | |
|---|---|
| *Cardiac sarcoidosis* | Cardiac sarcoidosis is characterized pathophysiologically by accumulation of noncaseating granulomas in pericardium, myocardium, or endocardium of any of cardiac chambers, increasing the risk of morbidity and mortality in the process of the disease. Cardiac involvement can manifest as arrhythmias, heart failure, or sudden cardiac death. Despite the fact that active inflammatory process may pose diagnostic challenges in oncologic patients, the pattern of radiotracer uptake and the presence of hilar and mediastinal adenopathy or pulmonary involvement may help in differentiation between the two entities (Fig. 15.10) [11,12]. |
| *Infective endocarditis* | Infective endocarditis is a serious and potentially life-threatening condition. This condition can be visualized as a hypermetabolic focus in $^{18}$F-FDG PET/CT imaging, which should be differentiated from a hypermetabolic cardiac mass (Fig. 15.11) [13]. |

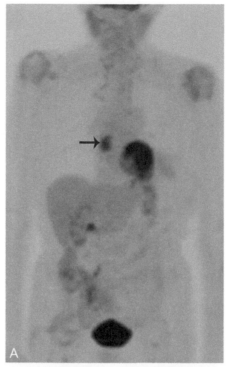

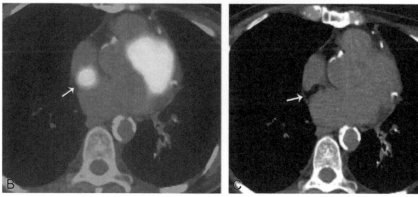

**FIG. 15.6**

Lipomatous hypertrophy of interatrial septum. $^{18}$F-FDG uptake in mass-like lesion in the interatrial septum with a relatively intense activity, representing lipomatous hypertrophy of interatrial septum. Maximum intensity projection (MIP) image (A), fused axial PET/CT image (B), and the corresponding slice of the CT component of PET/CT study (C). Particular attention should be paid in order to not mistake this histologically benign process with other fat-containing neoplastic lesions.

*Adapted from Cuellar SLB, Palacio D, Benveniste MF, Carter BW, Gladish G. Pitfalls and misinterpretations of cardiac findings on PET/CT imaging: a careful look at the heart in oncology patients. Curr Prob Diagn Radiol. 2019;48(2):172–183; with permission.*

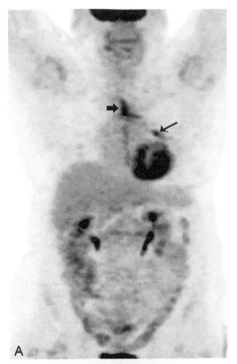

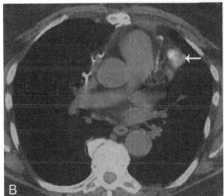

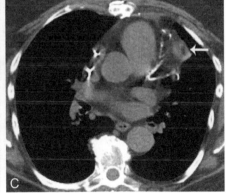

**FIG. 15.7**

Epipericardial fat necrosis. $^{18}$F-FDG accumulation and increased fat density along the anterior pericardium in a woman with the past medical history of lymphoma. Maximum intensity projection (MIP) image (A), fused axial PET/CT image (B), and the corresponding slice of the CT component of the study (C).

*Adapted from Cuellar SLB, Palacio D, Benveniste MF, Carter BW, Gladish G. Pitfalls and misinterpretations of cardiac findings on PET/CT imaging: a careful look at the heart in oncology patients. Curr Prob Diagn Radiol. 2019;48(2):172–183; with permission.*

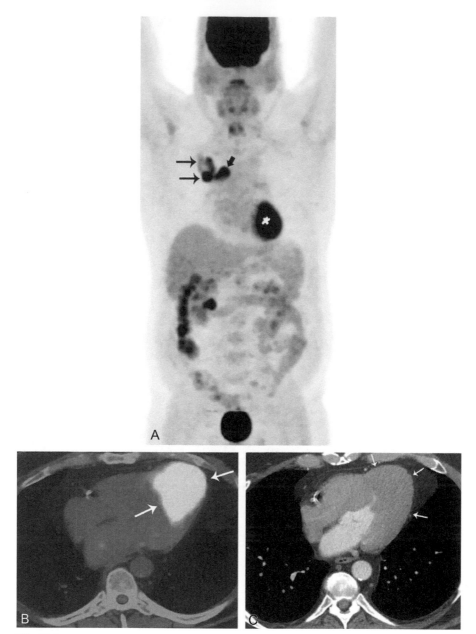

**FIG. 15.8**

Hypertrophic cardiomyopathy. Marked $^{18}$F-FDG accumulation in the left ventricle (*asterisk*) in a patient with apical hypertrophic cardiomyopathy (*white arrows*), who was referred for staging of nonsmall cell lung cancer. Primary cancer is shown by long arrows and ipsilateral hilar lymph node involvement is shown by short arrow. Maximum intensity projection (MIP) image (A), fused axial PET/CT image (B), and the corresponding slice of contrast-enhanced CT component of the study (C).

*Adapted from Cuellar SLB, Palacio D, Benveniste MF, Carter BW, Gladish G. Pitfalls and misinterpretations of cardiac findings on PET/CT imaging: a careful look at the heart in oncology patients. Curr Prob Diagn Radiol. 2019;48(2):172–183; with permission.*

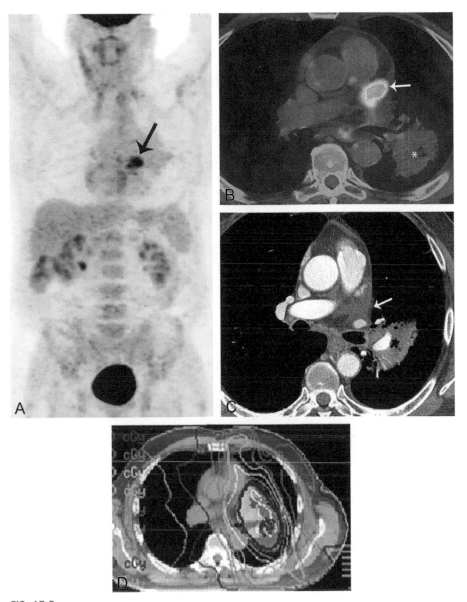

**FIG. 15.9**

Postradiation pericarditis. The PET/CT images reveal increased $^{18}$F-FDG accumulation corresponding to the transverse pericardial recess (*arrows*) in a man with nonsmall cell lung carcinoma and history of radiation therapy 6 months earlier. No $^{18}$F-FDG avidity is noticed in the primary malignant site (*asterisk*). The contrast-enhanced CT component of the PET/CT study reveals fluid in the aforementioned region with Hounsfield unit (HU) of 6. Maximum intensity projection (MIP) image (A); fused axial PET/CT image (B); contrast-enhanced CT component of the PET/CT study (C); and radiation treatment plan (D).

*Adapted from Cuellar SLB, Palacio D, Benveniste MF, Carter BW, Gladish G. Pitfalls and misinterpretations of cardiac findings on PET/CT imaging: a careful look at the heart in oncology patients. Curr Prob Diagn Radiol. 2019;48(2):172–183; with permission.*

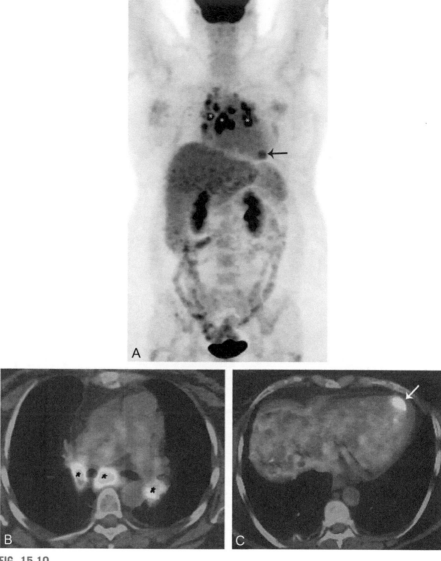

**FIG. 15.10**

Cardiac sarcoidosis. $^{18}$F-FDG accumulation in the left ventricular apex (*arrow*) as a result of cardiac sarcoidosis in a patient with suspected lymphoma. Multiple $^{18}$F-FDG-avid hilar and mediastinal adenopathy are present (*asterisks*). Maximum intensity projection (MIP) image (A), fused axial PET/CT image (B), and the corresponding slice of CT component of the study (C).

*Adapted from Cuellar SLB, Palacio D, Benveniste MF, Carter BW, Gladish G. Pitfalls and misinterpretations of cardiac findings on PET/CT imaging: a careful look at the heart in oncology patients. Curr Prob Diagn Radiol. 2019;48(2):172–183; with permission.*

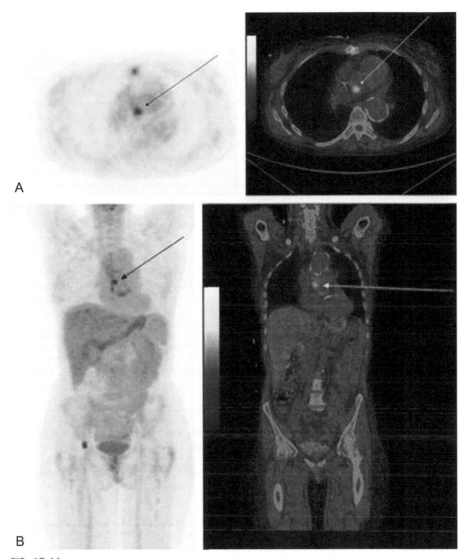

**FIG. 15.11**

Infective endocarditis. $^{18}$F-FDG accumulation at the region of the aortic valve in a patient with infective endocarditis. PET images in axial (*upper row*) and coronal (*lower row*) planes (*left side*) and corresponding fused axial PET/CT images (*right side*).

*Adapted from Bertagna F, Bisleri G, Motta F, Merli G, Cossalter E, Lucchini S, et al. Possible role of F18-FDG-PET/CT in the diagnosis of endocarditis: preliminary evidence from a review of the literature. Int J Cardiovasc Imaging. 2012;28(6):1417–1425; with permission.*

## Box 15.12 Cardiac and pericardial masses.

*Cardiac and pericardial masses encompass a heterogeneous broad spectrum of different entities, spanning from nonneoplastic to neoplastic processes of benign or malignant nature. In spite of rarity, they could pose significant diagnostic challenges [14]. Moreover, the hemodynamic alteration caused by cardiac masses including blood flow blockage, valvulopathy, embolic events, arrhythmias, and functional dysfunction secondary to myocardial infiltration, results in a wide variety of clinical presentations [15]. The patients' symptoms are, therefore, nonspecific and are mostly related to the tumor location versus tumor type. The majority of primary cardiac tumors are benign in nature, whereas the main source of cardiac malignant neoplastic involvement is metastatic lesions from extra-cardiac malignant tumors. On the other hand, primary cardiac neoplasms are more often of benign nature and include myxoma [16], fibroelastoma, lipoma, fibroma, rhabdomyoma, and hemangioma in descending prevalence [15,17]. $^{18}$F-FDG PET imaging has been found to be advantageous to differentiate malignant from benign cardiac tumors [2].*

| Tumor type | Description |
|---|---|
| *Myxoma* | Cardiac myxoma is known as the most common primary cardiac tumor with benign nature. This tumor typically arises from the left atrium. Incidental detection of cardiac myxoma is not infrequent as a result of routine use of echocardiography and widespread utilization of CT [18]. Cardiac myxoma can be detected with mild $^{18}$F-FDG uptake in PET imaging (Fig. 15.13) [2,16] |
| *Fibroma* | Cardiac fibroma is a fibroblast-derived benign connective tissue tumor which occurs predominantly in infants and young children. Cardiac fibroma is usually found in the septal and anterior walls of the left ventricle and might be visualized as cardiac masses of low to rather intense hyperactivity in PET images (Fig. 15.14) [19,20] |
| *Lipoma* | Cardiac lipomas are well-circumscribed encapsulated tumors which are mainly composed of mature fat cells. This tumor can arise from subendocardium, subpericardium, or endocardium and is more frequently in the left ventricle compared to the right one. Unlike lipomatous hypertrophy of interatrial septum which can appear as a focal hyperactive area in PET/CT imaging, cardiac lipoma is not a FDG-avid lesion and is visualized as fat attenuation mass with no FDG uptake [21,22] |
| *Hemangioma* | Cardiac hemangioma is a rare cardiac tumor that can occur in patients of all ages and at in any part of the heart. Hemangiomas are histologically classified as capillary, arteriovenous, and cavernous types. This tumor is usually visualized as mild FDG-avid mass in PET imaging (Fig. 15.15) [23,24] |

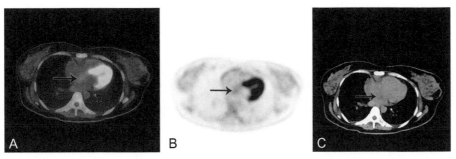

**FIG. 15.13**

Cardiac myxoma. Left atrial myxoma with mild [18]F-FDG accumulation, corresponding to the hypodense mass in CT image (*arrows*) in a patient with past history of gallbladder malignancy. Fused PET and CT (A), unfused PET (B), and CT (C) images in axial plane.

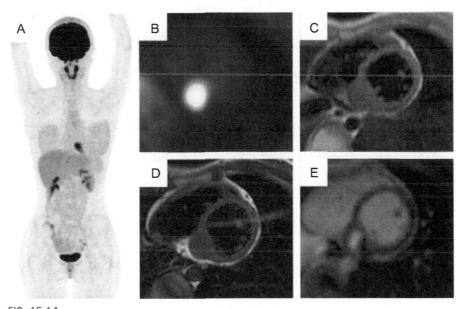

**FIG. 15.14**

Cardiac fibroma. Left ventricular fibroma with rather intense [18]F-FDG accumulation. The corresponding magnetic resonance (MR) images show isointense on T1WI, hypointense on T2WI, and hyperintense on LGE in the mass. PET maximum intensity projection (MIP) image (A); fused axial PET/CT image (B); T1-weighted MRI image (T1WI) (C); T2-weighted MRI image (T2WI) (D); and late gadolinium enhancement (LGE) image (E).

*Adapted from Masuda A, Osamu Manabe M, Oyama-Manabe N, Masanao Naya M, Obara M, Mamoru Sakakibara M, et al. Cardiac fibroma with high 18F-FDG uptake mimicking malignant tumor. J Nuclear Cardiol. 2017;24(1):323; with permission.*

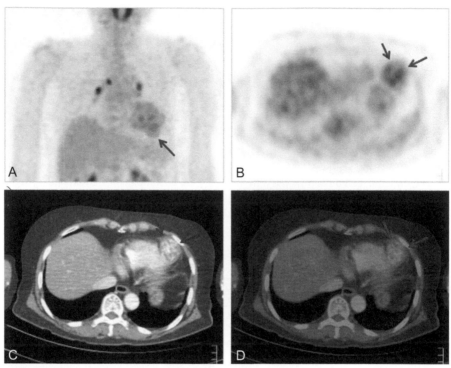

**FIG. 15.15**

Hemangioma. Pericardial hemangioma with mild $^{18}$F-FDG uptake (*arrows*). PET maximum intensity projection (MIP) image (A); axial nonfused PET image (B); axial CT image (C); and fused axial PET/CT image (D) of the same level.

*Adapted from Jeong YJ, Yoon HJ, Kang D-Y. Growing cardiac hemangioma on serial F-18 FDG PET/CT.*
*Nuclear Med Mol Imaging. 2012;46(3):223–226; with permission.*

# References

[1] Carter KR, Kotlyarov E. Common causes of false positive F18 FDG PET/CT scans in oncology. Braz Arch Biol Technol 2007;50(SPE):29–35.

[2] Rahbar K, Seifarth H, Schäfers M, Stegger L, Hoffmeier A, Spieker T, et al. Differentiation of malignant and benign cardiac tumors using 18F-FDG PET/CT. J Nucl Med 2012;53(6):856–63.

[3] Shao D, Tian R. Glucose transporters in cardiac metabolism and hypertrophy. Compr Physiol 2011;6(1):331–51.

[4] De Groot M, Meeuwis AP, Kok PJ, Corstens FH, Oyen WJ. Influence of blood glucose level, age and fasting period on non-pathological FDG uptake in heart and gut. Eur J Nucl Med Mol Imaging 2005;32(1):98–101.

[5] Cuellar SLB, Palacio D, Benveniste MF, Carter BW, Gladish G. Pitfalls and misinterpretations of cardiac findings on PET/CT imaging: a careful look at the heart in oncology patients. Curr Probl Diagn Radiol 2019;48(2):172–83.

[6] Kim S, Ding Y-G, Krynyckyi BR, MacHac J, Kim CK. Increased F-18 FDG uptake in the right auricle of a displaced heart: potential cause of a false-positive pathologic mediastinal node. Clin Nucl Med 2005;30(2):97–9.

[7] Fujii H, Ide M, Yasuda S, Takahashi W, Shohtsu A, Kubo A. Increased FDG uptake in the wall of the right atrium in people who participated in a cancer screening program with whole-body PET. Ann Nucl Med 1999;13(1):55–9.

[8] Fan C-M, Fischman AJ, Kwek BH, Abbara S, Aquino SL. Lipomatous hypertrophy of the interatrial septum: increased uptake on FDG PET. Am J Roentgenol 2005;184(1): 339–42.

[9] Pineda V, Cáceres J, Andreu J, Vilar J, Domingo ML. Epipericardial fat necrosis: radiologic diagnosis and follow-up. Am J Roentgenol 2005;185(5):1234–6.

[10] Minamimoto R. Series of myocardial FDG uptake requiring considerations of myocardial abnormalities in FDG-PET/CT. Jpn J Radiol 2021;39(6):540–57.

[11] Skali H, Schulman AR, Dorbala S. 18 F-FDG PET/CT for the assessment of myocardial sarcoidosis. Curr Cardiol Rep 2013;15(4):370.

[12] Teirstein AS, Machac J, Almeida O, Lu P, Padilla ML, Iannuzzi MC. Results of 188 whole-body fluorodeoxyglucose positron emission tomography scans in 137 patients with sarcoidosis. Chest 2007;132(6):1949–53.

[13] Bertagna F, Bisleri G, Motta F, Merli G, Cossalter E, Lucchini S, et al. Possible role of F18-FDG-PET/CT in the diagnosis of endocarditis: preliminary evidence from a review of the literature. Int J Cardiovasc Imaging 2012;28(6):1417–25.

[14] Bussani R, Castrichini M, Restivo L, Fabris E, Porcari A, Ferro F, et al. Cardiac tumors: diagnosis, prognosis, and treatment. Curr Cardiol Rep 2020;22(12):1–13.

[15] Bernhard D, Gräni C. 18F-FDG PET/CT imaging in the workup of cardiac and pericardial masses. Springer; 2021.

[16] Agostini D, Babatasi G, Galateau F, Grollier G, Potier JC, Bouvard G. Detection of cardiac myxoma by F-18 FDG PET. Clin Nucl Med 1999;24(3):159–60.

[17] Hoffmeier A, Sindermann JR, Scheld HH, Martens S. Cardiac tumors-diagnosis and surgical treatment. Dtsch Arztebl Int 2014;111(12):205.

[18] Colin GC, Gerber BL, Amzulescu M, Bogaert J. Cardiac myxoma: a contemporary multimodality imaging review. Int J Cardiovasc Imaging 2018;34(11):1789–808.

[19] Masuda A, Osamu Manabe M, Oyama-Manabe N, Masanao Naya M, Obara M, Mamoru Sakakibara M, et al. Cardiac fibroma with high 18F-FDG uptake mimicking malignant tumor. J Nucl Cardiol 2017;24(1):323.

[20] Liu E, Zhang X, Sun T, Chen Z, Dong H, Liu C, et al. Primary cardiac fibroma with persistent left superior vena cava in a young adult: contrast-enhanced CT and 18 F-FDG PET/CT finding. J Nucl Cardiol 2020;27(5):1837–40.

[21] Ismail I, Al-Khafaji K, Mutyala M, Aggarwal S, Cotter W, Hakim H, et al. Cardiac lipoma. J Community Hosp Intern Med Perspect 2015;5(5):28449.

[22] Maurer AH, Burshteyn M, Adler LP, Steiner RM. How to differentiate benign versus malignant cardiac and paracardiac 18F FDG uptake at oncologic PET/CT. Radiographics 2011;31(5):1287–305.

[23] Li Z, Li X, Wu Q. PET-CT diagnosis of cardiac cavernous hemangioma with large pericardial effusion. Eur Rev Med Pharmacol Sci 2014;18(21):3256–9.

[24] Jeong YJ, Yoon HJ, Kang D-Y. Growing cardiac hemangioma on serial F-18 FDG PET/CT. Nucl Med Mol Imaging 2012;46(3):223–6.

# PET in malignant cardiac tumors: Diagnosis, approach, and follow up

# 16

**Nahid Yaghoobi and Hadi Malek**

*Rajaie Cardiovascular Medical and Research Center, Iran University of Medical Sciences, Tehran, Iran*

## Key points

- In spite of the fact that cardiac tumors are a very rare entity, their diagnosis and clinical management are of paramount importance in the field of cardio-oncology. In addition, confronting with cardiac and paracardiac masses, including neoplastic and nonneoplastic lesions, is not an uncommon diagnostic dilemma in practical cardiology [1,2].
- As a general rule in oncology, early accurate diagnosis of tumors could have a great impact on patients' outcome by selecting a well-timed, appropriate, and efficient treatment. As a result, defining an accurate noninvasive diagnostic imaging modality with high specificity to introduce pertinent criteria for malignancy and differentiate it from the benign and especially from nonneoplastic lesions is of extreme clinical importance in terms of selecting the best therapeutic strategy to achieve the best prognosis and outcome [3–5].
- Clinical presentations of cardiac tumors constitute a broad range from an incidental finding during diagnostic imaging evaluation of an irrelevant clinical concern to critical manifestations including systemic embolization or those induced by mass effect such as arrhythmia, syncope, and cardiac tamponade, which are in part dependent on their locations and dimensions and could result in hampering the contractile function regardless of their histopathology [4,6,7].
- Although the histopathological results derived from biopsy are the point of reference for final diagnosis, considering the technical hazards, a presumptive identification of the lesion to precisely localize and to assess its relation to the cardiac structures is of great value. Furthermore, differentiation of malignancy from benignancy, if possible, could have a vital role in planning the forthcoming therapy and management [4,6,7].
- Considering the low incidence, there is not an established diagnostic imaging strategy for suspected cardiac masses. Echocardiography is widely available as the initial modality to detect cardiac masses with a high sensitivity. Nevertheless, several limitations either technically (such as poor acoustic window or difficulty

Multimodal Imaging Atlas of Cardiac Masses. https://doi.org/10.1016/B978-0-323-84906-7.00027-3

in obese patients) or inherently, in particular for tumor assessment (such as lack of capability to tissue characterization), have been introduced for this modality. As the next step, when the echocardiography findings are inadequate or suspicious, however, cardiac magnetic resonance imaging (MRI), using different sophisticated techniques, is considered as the preferred and reference noninvasive diagnostic method to provide meticulous information on the size and location, structural details, histopathological characterization, and accurate estimation of extent of the mass; nevertheless, even this pivotal modality is susceptible to some limitations such as claustrophobia or contraindication of gadolinium administration in some patients [2,5,7,8]. As an alternative method to MRI and an excessive part of morphological evaluation in some certain individuals, for example in whom with possibility of direct involvement of coronary arteries to define preferable surgical approach, cardiac computerized tomography (CT) enjoying excellent spatial resolution and fast acquisition time with capability to exhibit calcification and fat could be of help in tissue characterization along with providing useful morphologic information about cardiac masses [2,8].

- Positron emission tomography (PET) using tumor-targeted radiopharmaceuticals is widely accepted as an invaluable modality of molecular imaging to noninvasively assess variety of oncology issues, introducing acknowledged clinical indications such as tumor diagnosis, prognostic evaluation, clinical management, initial staging, restaging, differentiating benign from malignant lesions (Fig. 16.1), tailoring therapy, detection of recurrence, therapy response assessment, and patient's outcome study, every one of which depends on the histopathology and clinical status of certain types of cancers [9–12]. Additionally, by merging molecular information of PET with morphologic data

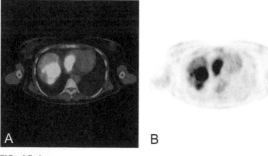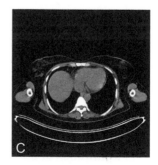

**FIG. 16.1**

Differentiation between neoplastic from nonneoplastic thrombus in patients with positive history of malignancy. Based on the metabolic rate of glucose and as an in vivo biological marker, FDG-PET can reflect the molecular functional state of tissues, which supplies additional information to anatomical imaging [9]. (A) Fused PET/CT; (B) PET; and (C) CT images in a known case of melanoma and liver metastases accompanied with tumor thrombosis through the inferior vena cava up to the right atrium. *CT,* computed tomography; *FDG,* fluorodeoxyglucose; *PET,* positron emission tomography.

by CT or MRI, the hybrid imaging modalities, PET/CT and PET/MRI, can provide an accurate and efficient tool for many clinical applications of different scenarios in the field of oncology [13,14].

- Despite the fact that a number of specific tracers have been introduced for some specified clinical and research issues, the radiolabeled glucose analogue, F18-fluorodeoxyglucose ($^{18}$F-FDG), is the most recognized PET radiopharmaceutical in clinical oncology to evaluate the disease and even to change the management decisions and therapeutic courses in many common cancers [10,13]. Based on the metabolic rate of glucose and as an in vivo biological marker, FDG-PET can reflect the molecular functional state of tissues, which supplies additional information to anatomical imaging and has been reported to be more sensitive than morphological changes while monitoring the treatment [9] (see Boxes 16.2, 16.4, and 16.5).

---

### Box 16.2 FDG-PET/CT in cardiac masses.

- Notwithstanding the fundamental role of FDG-PET/CT in general oncology, given the limited amount of evidence, the clinical contribution of this key imaging modality has not yet been firmly established in the imaging workup of cardiac tumors. Nevertheless, the cumulative body of literature, albeit few in number of cases, has been indicative of incremental value of functional molecular imaging in diagnosis, treatment, and clinical management of this group of rare and complex entity [5,14–16].

- Apart from qualitative and visual assessment of metabolic activity, which per se is of ultimate clinical importance in evaluation of tumors, capability of quantification of metabolic activity is the distinctive characteristic of molecular imaging using FDG-PET. Measuring the glucose metabolic activity of lesions could provide valuable data to clarify different aspects of diagnosis, management, and therapy. Standardized uptake value (SUV) is an objective method of metabolic activity quantification in PET imaging, which has most commonly been used in practice so far. This method of quantitative study and its derivatives such as SUVmax, which are practically available in common software, have been widely investigated with excellent results in terms of interoperator reproducibility; these methods of quantification have also provided good results concerning sensitivity and specificity in differentiating malignant from benign lesions [3,9].

- The practicality and effectiveness of quantitative metabolic assessment in cardiac masses have been initiated to define the histopathological status of the lesion for planning the treatment strategy as well as for demarcating the target volume in radiation therapy, monitoring early therapeutic response for better estimation of the final results as complete or partial response, stable disease or progression, and ultimately for more accurate estimation of patients' outcome [3,9].

- A universal cutoff value to distinguish benign from malignant lesions has not yet been established, even though different cutoff values for SUVmax have been proposed [2,3,16].

- According to literature, FDG-PET can differentiate benign from malignant cardiac tumors, which could prevent unnecessary biopsies and therapies. Furthermore, it has been used for estimation of the tumor burden as well as for staging the disease, detection of accompanied primary or metastatic extracardiac tumors, assessment of recurrence of tumor (Fig. 16.3), identification of posttreatment residue, evaluation of response to therapy, and finally prediction of patients' outcome [3,4,8,17–19].

---

### Box 16.4 Cardiac uptake of [18]F-FDG.

- For more accurate evaluation of cardiac tumors employing FDG-PET, understanding the mechanism of physiologic uptake and normal distribution pattern of FDG by the heart is crucial. It should be considered that the level of blood glucose as well as that of plasma insulin is the key to proportion of glycolysis and free fatty acid metabolism by the myocardium. To be specific, in a fasting state there is a decrease in myocardial glycolytic metabolism, resulting in diminished [18]F-FDG uptake by the myocytes. Needless to say, the reverse occurs when the blood level of glucose is high, demonstrating high myocardial [18]F-FDG uptake. As a result, to clearly display FDG uptake at the site of neoplastic lesions, a 6-hour fasting is mandatory in order to prevent normal background myocardial uptake as an interfering phenomenon [17].
- Cardiac [18]F-FDG uptake could normally illustrate a broad spectrum of variants from lack of activity (at fasting state) to focal, regional, or diffuse (in nonfasted and even fasted patients) pattern of myocardial activity. The atria and papillary muscles as well as the basal and anteroapical regions of the left ventricle are responsible for normal focal increased radiotracer uptake of the heart in FDG-PET imaging, while regional cardiac uptake could be attributed to physiologic normal increased activity in posterolateral wall and base of the left ventricle. Moreover, nonneoplastic etiologies could be associated with focal or regional increased [18]F-FDG uptake in the heart, of which atrial fibrillation, prominent crista terminalis, lipomatous hypertrophy of the interatrial septum, epicardial and pericardial fat, cardiac sarcoidosis, endocarditis, myocarditis, and pericarditis have been well known [1,17].

---

### Box 16.5 Cardiac tumors.

Neoplastic masses are generally categorized into two major groups of primary and secondary tumors with a far greater prevalence for the latter (about 20–40 times more common than the primaries) [7].

| Metastatic tumors | • Secondary tumors of the heart are estimated to comprise 15%–20% of all cardiac masses. Even though these malignant lesions are not common, by advancing in diagnostic modalities and therapeutic strategies, which is resulting in longer life expectancy of the patients suffering from cancer, the prevalence of secondary tumors is predicted to be increased [6]. While cardiac and pericardial metastatic lesions could originate from almost any malignant tumor (Fig. 16.6), they are mainly arising from melanoma (Fig. 16.7) and carcinoma of the lung (Fig. 16.8), breast, and esophagus as well as from hematologic cancers, leukemia and lymphoma [6,7]. |
|---|---|
| | • Owing to the fact that metastatic cardiac tumors are commonly in association with widespread metastases and that diagnosis of accompanied extracardiac lesions is crucial in clinical management of patients with cancer, FDG-PET could be of help to |

---

**Box 16.5 Cardiac tumors—Cont'd**

| | |
|---|---|
| | evaluate either the cardiac masses in question or the other expected disseminated lesions, simultaneously. Congruently, FDG-PET which is acknowledged for initial staging and evaluation of response to therapy in lymphoma could concurrently disclose the accompanied cardiac involvement, which is not uncommon in non-Hodgkin lymphoma [3,17]. |
| | • Although malignant melanoma has a significant proclivity for the heart, it is rarely seen in living patients and tumors are often detected in autopsy. The cardiac melanomas usually occur at chambers, more commonly involving the right atrium. They are generally discovered in transthoracic echocardiography (TTE); nevertheless, in some cases TTE fails to recognize the tumor, in which MRI or FDG-PET is supposed to help [20]. |
| Primary tumors | • Primary cardiac tumors are very rare, more than three-quarters of which are benign in nature originating from the myocardium or pericardium with myxoma as the most common primary cardiac neoplasm. Evidently, malignant primary tumors are exceedingly rare, incorporating a smaller proportion of this rare entity. Sarcomas of different types compose the leading histopathology followed by lymphoma (Fig. 16.9) and mesothelioma (Fig. 16.10) in descending order of occurrence [4,7,16,21]. Sarcomas generally demonstrate high $^{18}$F-FDG uptake (Fig. 16.11–16.19); these aggressive tumors comprise approximately two-thirds of all malignant primaries [7,17]. |
| | • Paragangliomas are rare neuroendocrine tumors of paraganglionic cells arising from an extraadrenal location. Histopathologically, malignant lesions are not distinguishable from the benign; only local invasion or distant metastases define the malignancy (Fig. 16.20). |

Primary cardiac lymphoma, comprising up to 2% of all primary tumors, is defined as non-Hodgkin predominantly diffuse large B-cell lymphomas, with predilection specifically for patients with impaired immune system. Although nonspecific systemic complaints are generally part of clinical manifestation, by definition, heart-related symptoms such as arrhythmia, chest pain, heart failure, or even restrictive cardiomyopathy are the main manifestations. Presence of multifocal lesions is not uncommon. Right side of the heart, the right atrium, in particular, is more susceptible to be involved, although lymphoma could occur in other chambers as well. The intensity of FDG uptake is proportionate to the metabolic activity, which means it could roughly estimate the magnitude of cell proliferation, i.e. malignancy, in the tumor. $^{18}$F-FDG has also been used as guidance for biopsy site, staging, restaging, and monitoring treatment response in patients with lymphoma [7,22,23].

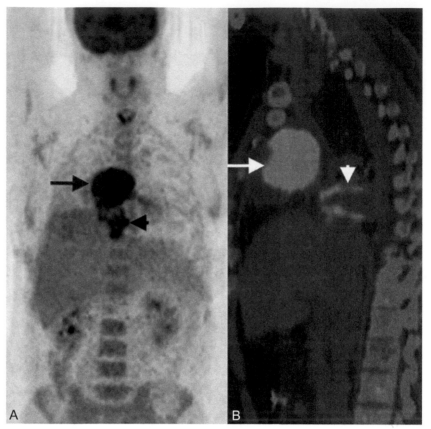

**FIG. 16.3**

Recurrence of tumor. Integrated FDG-PET/CT image: MIP (A) and sagittal section (B), hyperintense $^{18}$FDG uptake illustrating cardiac hypermetabolic lesions (*arrows*) in the left atrium and the anterior mediastinum representing recurrent tumor in a known case of myxofibrosarcoma. *CT*, computed tomography; *FDG*, fluorodeoxyglucose; *MIP*, maximum intensity projection; *PET*, positron emission tomography.

Adapted from Erdoğan EB, et al. Appearance of recurrent cardiac myxofibrosarcoma on FDG PET/CT. Clin Nucl Med. 2014;39(6):559–560 with permission.

Primary pericardial mesothelioma, the leading primary pericardial malignancy, is extremely rare with poor prognosis. The clinical manifestations are nonspecific with pericardial effusion with or without tamponade in most cases, exhibiting constrictive pericarditis. Although pericardial effusion is generally detected by echocardiography and despite the fact that cardiac MRI and CT clearly disclose pericardial masses encasing the pericardial space, FDG-PET/CT could have a vital role in diagnostic workup, staging, and decision-making for therapy in patients suffering from pericardial mesothelioma with measuring the metabolic glucose activity in the

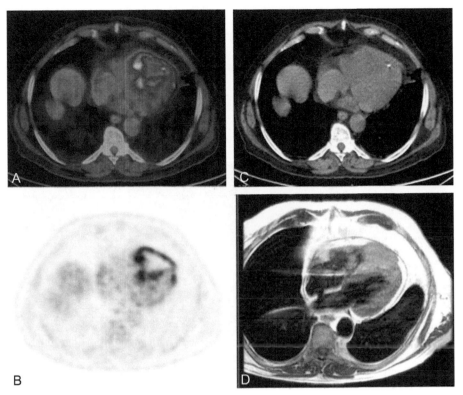

**FIG. 16.6**

Metastatic cardiac tumor originated from urothelial carcinoma. Transaxial images of (A) integrated FDG-PET/CT, (B) FDG-PET, (C) CT, and (D) MRI of a case of metastatic cardiac tumor originated from urothelial carcinoma. The right ventricle is involved, demonstrating intense [18]FDG uptake with SUVmax of 12 surrounding the lesion. The central necrosis of the tumor is evident in the CT image as a hypodense area inside the mass. MRI is clearly illustrating the tumor. *CT*, computed tomography; *FDG*, fluorodeoxyglucose; *MRI*, magnetic resonance imaging; *PET*, positron emission tomography; *SUV*, standardized uptake value.

*Adapted from Saponara M, et al. 18F-FDG-PET/CT imaging in cardiac tumors: illustrative clinical cases and review of the literature. Ther Adv Med Oncol. 2018;10:1758835918793569 with permission.*

neoplastic tissue and by providing whole body survey to illustrate potential distant metastases [7,24].

Sarcomas of different histopathologies are the leading primary malignancy of the heart and generally demonstrate high [18]F-FDG uptake; these aggressive tumors comprise approximately two-thirds of all malignant primaries [7,17].

Approximately 40% of all cardiac sarcomas are angiosarcomas (Figs. 16.12–16.14). This aggressive tumor has a predilection for the right atrium, consisting of almost 75% of cases, with symptoms secondary to right heart failure as the cardinal

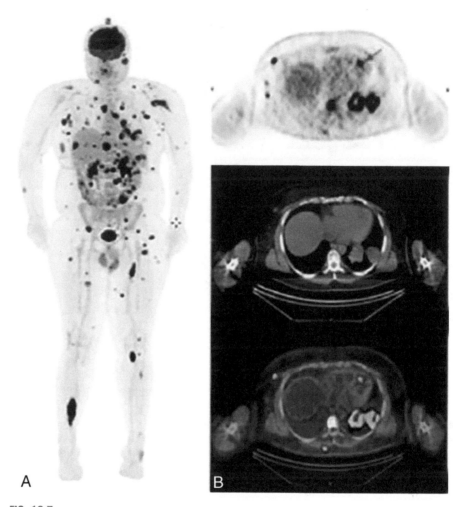

A

B

**FIG. 16.7**

Metastatic cardiac tumor originated from melanoma. A 37-year-old man, known case of melanoma for a few years. (A) Total body FDG-PET scan, demonstrating innumerous metastases as multiple foci of subcutaneous intense FDG uptake all over the body and (B) transaxial section of PET, CT, and hybrid PET/CT (top to bottom) images of thoracic region illustrating a focal metastasis as intense uptake (SUVmax: 8.7) corresponding to the apicoseptal segment of the left ventricle. *CT*, computed tomography; *FDG*, fluorodeoxyglucose; *PET*, positron emission tomography; *SUV*, standardized uptake value.

*Adapted from Brandão SCS, Dompieri LT. PET-CT 18F-FDG applications in cardiac tumors. CEP. 50750:400 with permission.*

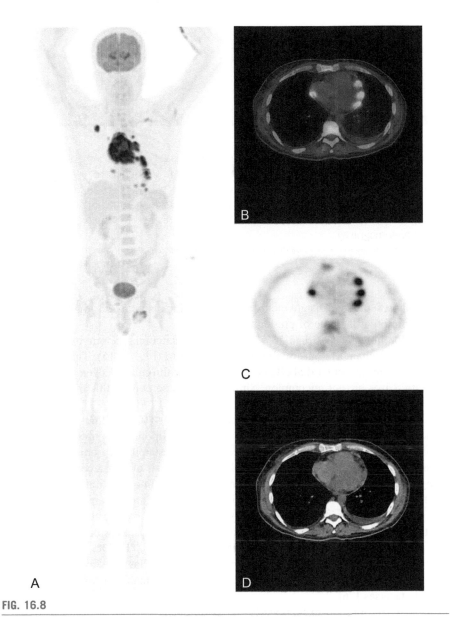

**FIG. 16.8**

Metastatic pericardial nodules originated from lung cancer. FDG-PET/CT images in a case of metastatic lung cancer to the pericardium. (A) MIP image; (B) fused PET and CT transaxial images; (C) PET only; and (D) CT image of the corresponding level. *CT*, computed tomography; *FDG*, fluorodeoxyglucose; *MIP*, maximum intensity projection; *PET*, positron emission tomography.

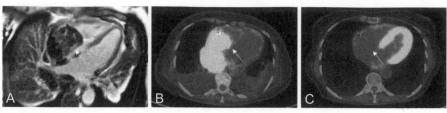

**FIG. 16.9**

Primary cardiac lymphoma. Primary cardiac lymphoma involving the right atrium and right ventricle with complete metabolic response to treatment. (A) A cardiac mass with heterogeneous enhancement on MRI; (B) very intense [18]FDG uptake on FDG-PET/CT transaxial image before treatment; and (C) low FDG uptake after therapy. *CT*, computed tomography; *FDG*, fluorodeoxyglucose; *MRI*, magnetic resonance imaging; *PET*, positron emission tomography.

*Adapted from Tyeball S, et al. Cardiac tumors: JACC CardioOncology state-of-the-art review. Cardio Oncol. 2020;2(2):293–311 with permission.*

clinical presentation. Distant metastases and local invasion to the adjacent structures are common at the time of presentation [7,22].

Accounting for less than 10% of all cardiac sarcomas, leiomyosarcoma could occur in all chambers but usually in the left atrium (Fig. 16.15). They can present with arrhythmia, pericardial effusion, and vascular thrombosis, even though asymptomatic cases are not uncommon. Similar to other sarcomas, this malignant tumor has a dismal prognosis [7,25].

Liposarcoma is exceptionally rare, accounting for 1% of primary malignant cardiac tumors (Figs. 16.16 and 16.17). In contrast to lipoma, this mesenchymal neoplastic lesion contains lipoblasts instead of macroscopic fat components, which makes its definite diagnosis difficult. Clinical diagnosis of liposarcoma is also challenging as its clinical presentation is nonspecific including constitutional symptoms, arrhythmia, and shortness of breath. Similar to other cardiac tumors, the first-line diagnostic modality is echocardiography; nevertheless, for more accurate evaluation of the disease and better assessment of the extent of invasion, other modalities play an essential role. Because of high metabolic activity, [18]F-FDG shows increased uptake in the tumor and could help with differential diagnosis as well as precise assessment of tumor extension; it could also provide valuable information on potential metastases [26].

Osteosarcoma is an exceptionally rare cardiac sarcoma manifesting as arrhythmia and heart failure (Fig. 16.18). Elements of osteoid, bone, and chondroid could exist in the tumor. Whereas the metastatic osteosarcoma shows tendency to the right atrium, the primary type of the tumor has a predilection to the left side. With regard to propensity for calcification and ossification, hybrid bone scintigraphy using technetium 99 m-methylene diphosphonate could be of help to reveal the histopathology of the tumor [7,27].

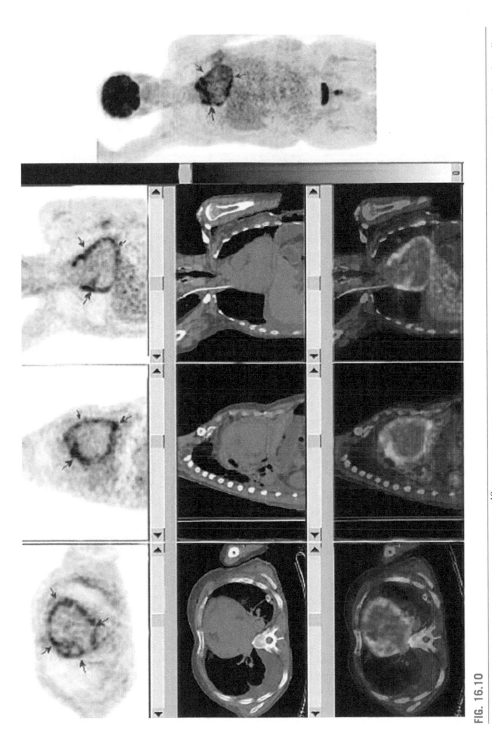

**FIG. 16.10**

Malignant pericardial mesothelioma. Intense $^{18}$FDG uptake (SUVmax: 7.5) surrounding the heart corresponding to the thickened pericardium representing malignant mesothelioma. (*Left*) FDG-PET (*upper row*), CT (*middle row*), integrated FDG-PET/CT (*lower row*); (*Right*) maximum intensity projection of PET image. *CT*, computed tomography; *FDG*, fluorodeoxyglucose; *PET*, positron emission tomography; *SUV*, standardized uptake value.

*Adapted from Sivrikoz IA, et al. F-18 FDG PET/CT images of a rare primer cardiac tumor: primary pericardial mesothelioma. Anat J Cardiol. 2016;16(8):635 with permission.*

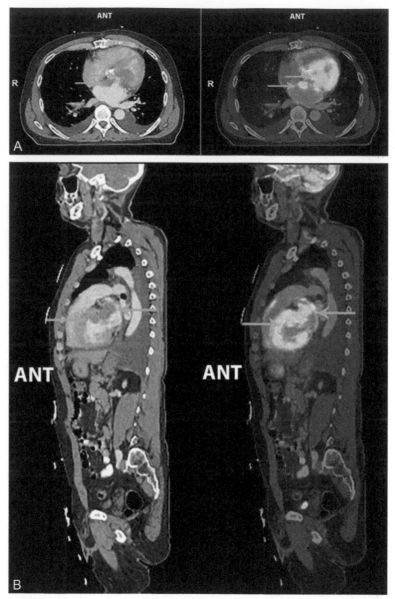

**FIG. 16.11**

Primary cardiac intimal sarcoma. CT (*left*) and integrated PET/CT with [18]FDG (*right*),
(A) transaxial and (B) sagittal views. The intracardiac masses in the left atrium and left
ventricle are demonstrating intense FDG uptake with SUVmax of 21.2, reflecting high glucose
metabolic activity, which is interpreted as a malignant tumor. The immunohistochemical
profile and pathology revealed cardiac intimal sarcoma. No distant metastasis was detected.
*CT*, computed tomography; *FDG*, fluorodeoxyglucose; *PET*, positron emission
tomography; *SUV*, standardized uptake value.

*Adapted from Andersen KF, et al. Primary cardiac intimal sarcoma visualized on 2-[18F] FDG PET/CT.*
*Diagnostics 2020;10(9):718 with permission.*

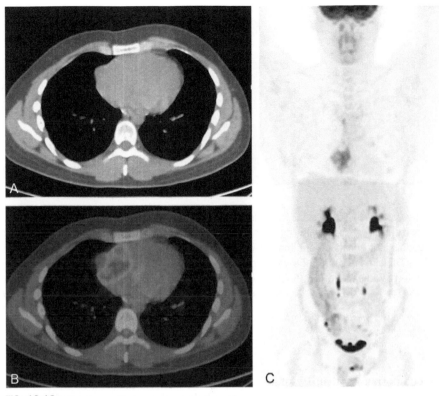

**FIG. 16.12**

Primary cardiac angiosarcoma. A 23-year-old patient with angiosarcoma involving the right atrium. On the left, (A) transaxial CT and (B) integrated FDG-PET/CT, on the right: MIP image. The heterogeneous intense [18]FDG with SUVmax of 12.3 is in favor of malignancy. Angiosarcoma was confirmed in transbronchial biopsy. *CT*, computed tomography; *FDG*, fluorodeoxyglucose; *MIP*, maximum intensity projection; *PET*, positron emission tomography; *SUV*, standardized uptake value.

*Adapted from Saponara M, et al. 18F-FDG-PET/CT imaging in cardiac tumors: illustrative clinical cases and review of the literature. Ther Adv Med Oncol. 2018;10:1758835918793569 with permission.*

By definition, undifferentiated is a term belonging to a group of sarcomas with uncertain immunohistological characters and with very poor prognosis (Fig. 16.19). These invasive tumors have a tendency to the left atrium and account for about one-quarter of sarcomas. Like other sarcomas, [18]F-FDG shows high uptake in undifferentiated type [7,28].

Paragangliomas are rare neuroendocrine tumors of paraganglionic cells arising from an extraadrenal location. When located in the heart, which is extremely rare

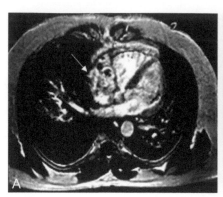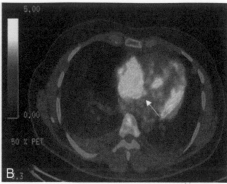

**FIG. 16.13**

Primary cardiac angiosarcoma. Representative of transaxial images; a heterogeneous hypervascular large mass in the right atrium with evidence of hemorrhage and necrosis on the late gadolinium enhancement image (A) and with hyperintense [18]FDG uptake in the FDG-PET/CT image (B) in a 58-year-old man with primary cardiac angiosarcoma. *CT, computed tomography; FDG, fluorodeoxyglucose; PET, positron emission tomography.*

*Adapted from Tyebally S, et al. Cardiac tumors: JACC CardioOncology state-of-the-art review. Cardio Oncol. 2020;2(2):293–311 with permission.*

and composing less than 1% of all cardiac tumors, they originate from ganglia associated with either the arteries (intrapericardial) or the atrium (intracardiac), most commonly at the left atrium. Histopathologically, malignant lesions are not distinguishable from the benign; only local invasion or distant metastases define the malignancy. Depending on the catecholamine secretory state, cardiac paraganglioma can be either symptomatic with clinical manifestation of excessive sympathetic excretion (palpitation, flushing, hypertension, etc.) or often clinically silent until the mass effect induces angina or dyspnea [7,29–31]. Nuclear imaging utilizing different methods and various radiotracers has played a significant role in detection and localization of neuroendocrine tumors and the distant metastases. Hybrid single photon emission computerized tomography by applying two different categories of radiotracers, one as an analogue of norepinephrine, [123]I-metaiodobenzylguanidine (MIBG), and the other, [111]In-octreotide by binding to somatostatin receptors expressed by paragangliomas, can sensitively localize neuroendocrine tumors by two disparate mechanisms [32]. Furthermore, PET can display the molecular metabolic state of the tumors by employing glucose analogue, [18]F-FDG, or exhibit the somatostatin receptors by 68Ga-DOTATATE [2,33].

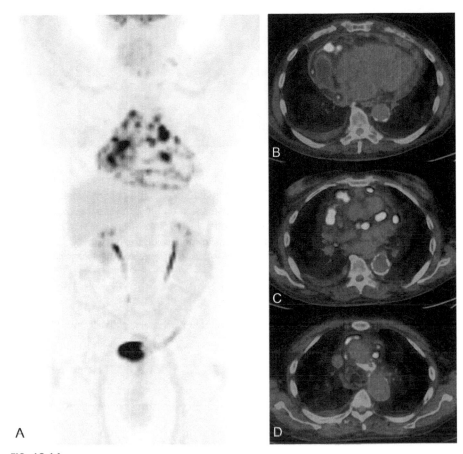

**FIG. 16.14**

Primary cardiac angiosarcoma. (A) MIP, (B–D) integrated FDG-PET/CT transaxial images of a case of poorly differentiated angiosarcoma with significant necrosis proved by surgical biopsy. Heterogeneous intense ¹⁸FDG uptake is evident in the heart involving right atrium (A) with pericardial infiltration (B) and prevascular lymph nodes (C), SUVmax: 34.7. *CT*, computed tomography; *FDG*, fluorodeoxyglucose; *MIP*, maximum intensity projection; *PET*, positron emission tomography; *SUV*, standardized uptake value.

*Adapted from Saponara M, et al. 18F-FDG-PET/CT imaging in cardiac tumors: illustrative clinical cases and review of the literature. Ther Adv Med Oncol. 2018;10:1758835918793569 with permission.*

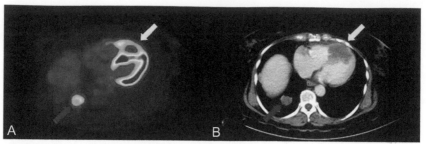

**FIG. 16.15**

Leiomyosarcoma. Transaxial images of FDG-PET (A) and CT (B) in a case of metastatic leiomyosarcoma is demonstrating FDG uptake in a donut-shaped pattern representing central necrosis corresponding to the hypodense lesion on the CT (*yellow arrows*). Lung metastasis is also obvious in both images, depicting FDG uptake (*red arrows*). *CT*, computed tomography; *FDG*, fluorodeoxyglucose; *PET*, positron emission tomography.

*Adapted from Dencker M, Valind S, Stagmo M. Right ventricular metastasis of leiomyosarcoma. Cardiovasc Ultrasound. 2009;7(1):1–3 with permission.*

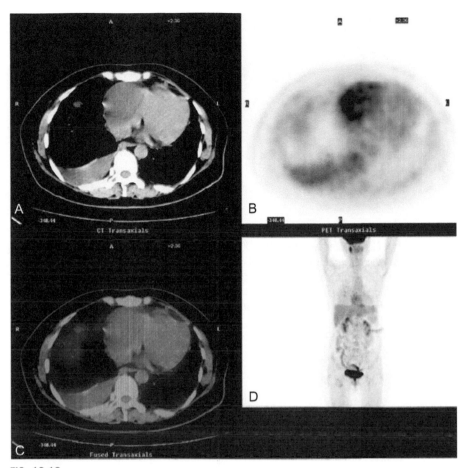

**FIG. 16.16**

Cardiac liposarcoma. Liposarcoma in a 61-year-old woman; transaxial images of CT (A), FDG-PET (B), integrated PET/CT (C), as well as MIP image (D). Increased metabolic activity (SUVmax: 3.2) is noticeable in the large mass corresponding to the right pericardium spreading to the right ventricle and right atrium. *CT*, computed tomography; *FDG*, fluorodeoxyglucose; *MIP*, maximum intensity projection; *PET*, positron emission tomography; *SUV*, standardized uptake value.

*Adapted from Miao Zhang M, Biao Li M, Jiang X. PET/CT imaging in a case of cardiac liposarcoma. J Nucl Cardiol. 2008;15(3):473 with permission.*

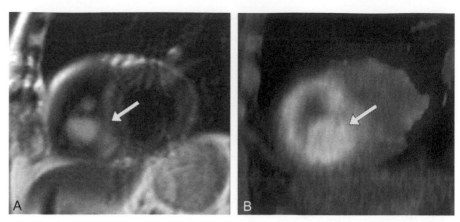

**FIG. 16.17**

Liposarcoma. T2-weighted MRI (A) and FDG-PET/CT (B). Intense [18]FDG uptake representing a hypermetabolic malignant tumor in a 71-year-old man with liposarcoma involving the right ventricle adhered to the septum (*arrow*). *CT*, computed tomography; *FDG*, fluorodeoxyglucose; *PET*, positron emission tomography.

*Adapted from Rahbar K, et al. Differentiation of malignant and benign cardiac tumors using 18F-FDG PET/CT. J Nucl Med. 2012;53(6):856–863 with permission.*

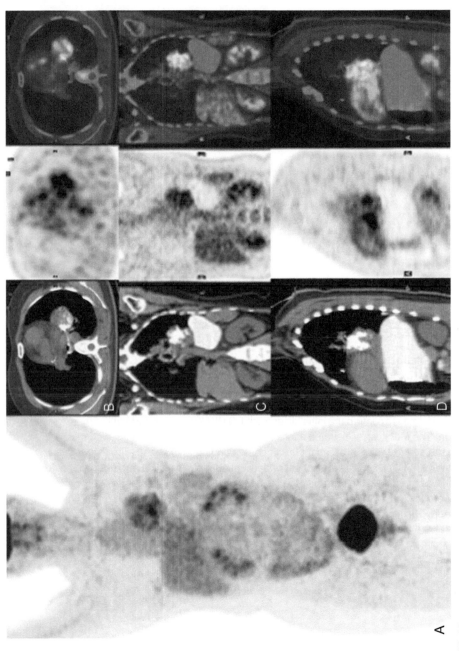

**FIG. 16.18**

Primary pericardial osteosarcoma. Primary pericardial osteosarcoma in an asymptomatic 38-year-old woman with abnormal chest X-ray in her routine exam. (A) MIP image of FDG-PET scan, (B) transaxial, (C) coronal, and (D) sagittal images of CT (*left column*), FDG-PET (*middle column*), and integrated FDG-PET/CT (*right column*). There is heterogeneous [18]FDG uptake reflecting malignancy corresponding to the paracardiac tumor visualized on the CT scan as a large calcified lesion adhered to the heart. Otherwise, no abnormal FDG uptake is noticeable in the whole body PET scan. *CT*, computed tomography; *FDG*, fluorodeoxyglucose; *MIP*, maximum intensity projection; *PET*, positron emission tomography.

*Adapted from Wang Q, et al. Primary pericardial osteosarcoma on FDG PET/CT. Clin Nucl Med. 2013;38(8):e326-8 with permission.*

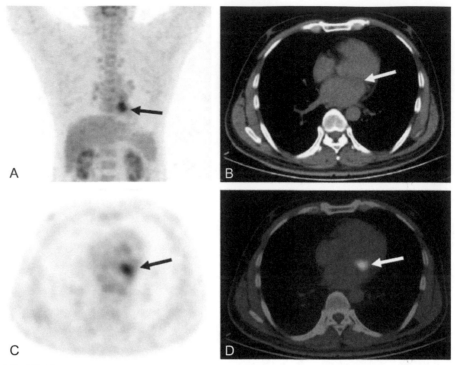

**FIG. 16.19**

Undifferentiated cardiac sarcoma. MIP image (A) and transaxial slices of CT (B), PET (C), and hybrid image (D) of FDG-PET/CT scan in a 52-year-old man admitted for recent shortness of breath and chest discomfort. The patient first underwent chest CT and then cardiac MRI, both with and without contrast (not shown). The anatomical imaging depicted findings in favor of cardiac myxoma. To confirm the initial diagnosis FDG PET/CT was performed before surgical operation. The MIP image illustrated a focal intense [18]FDG uptake indicating high metabolic activity and suggestive of a malignant lesion corresponding to the atrial mitral valve in the hybrid image (SUVmax: 5.8). The patient underwent surgical resection and undifferentiated sarcoma was reported in the postoperative histopathologic exam. *CT*, computed tomography; *FDG*, fluorodeoxyglucose; *MRI*, magnetic resonance imaging; *PET*, positron emission tomography; *SUV*, standardized uptake value.

*Adapted from Wang, R., G. Shen, and R. Tian, Primary atrial undifferentiated sarcoma found on FDG PET/CT mimicking cardiac myxoma. Clin Nucl Med. 2020;45(10):833–835 with permission.*

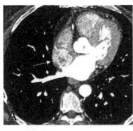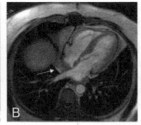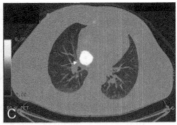

**FIG. 16.20**

Paraganglioma. Transaxial images of cardiac CT (A), SSFP image of cardiac MRI (B), and FDG-PET/CT (C) of a case of paraganglioma. The patient presented with flushing and palpitations. An enhanced heterogeneous mass on cardiac CT at the superior-septal aspect of the right atrium with compression effect on the right upper pulmonary vein presented as heterogeneity on SSFP image and revealed intense FDG uptake on FDG-PET/CT at right atrium corresponding to the tumoral lesion. *CT*, computed tomography; *FDG*, fluorodeoxyglucose; *MRI*, magnetic resonance imaging; *PET*, positron emission tomography; *SSFP*, steady-state free precession.

*Adapted from Tyebally S, et al. Cardiac tumors: JACC CardioOncology state-of-the-art review. Cardio Oncol. 2020;2(2):293–311 with permission.*

## References

[1] Maurer AH, et al. How to differentiate benign versus malignant cardiac and paracardiac 18F FDG uptake at oncologic PET/CT. Radiographics 2011;31(5):1287–305.

[2] Lopez-Mattei JC, Lu Y. Multimodality imaging in cardiac masses: to standardize recommendations, the time is now! Washington, DC: American College of Cardiology Foundation; 2020. p. 2412–4.

[3] Meng J, et al. Assessment of cardiac tumors by 18 F-FDG PET/CT imaging: histological correlation and clinical outcomes. J Nucl Cardiol 2020;1–11.

[4] Qin C, et al. 18 F-FDG PET/CT in diagnostic and prognostic evaluation of patients with cardiac masses: a retrospective study. Eur J Nucl Med Mol Imaging 2019;1–11.

[5] Saponara M, et al. 18F-FDG-PET/CT imaging in cardiac tumors: illustrative clinical cases and review of the literature. Ther Adv Med Oncol 2018;10:1–9.

[6] Burazor I, et al. Metastatic cardiac tumors: from clinical presentation through diagnosis to treatment. BMC Cancer 2018;18(1):1–9.

[7] Tyebally S, et al. Cardiac tumors: JACC CardioOncology state-of-the-art review. Cardio Oncol 2020;2(2):293–311.

[8] Andersen KF, et al. Primary cardiac intimal sarcoma visualized on 2-[18F] FDG PET/CT. Diagnostics 2020;10(9):718.

[9] Hirata K, Tamaki N. Quantitative FDG PET assessment for oncology therapy. Cancer 2021;13(4):869.

[10] Mahajan A, Cook G. Clinical applications of PET/CT in oncology. In: Basic science of PET imaging. Springer; 2017. p. 429–50.

[11] Reske SN, Kotzerke J. FDG-PET for clinical use. Eur J Nucl Med 2001;28(11):1707–23.

[12] Fathala A, Abouzied M, AlSugair A-A. Cardiac and pericardial tumors: a potential application of positron emission tomography-magnetic resonance imaging. World J Cardiol 2017;9(7):600.

[13] Becker J, Schwarzenböck SM, Krause BJ. FDG PET hybrid imaging. In: Molecular imaging in oncology. Springer; 2020. p. 625–67.

[14] Nensa F, et al. Integrated 18F-FDG PET/MR imaging in the assessment of cardiac masses: a pilot study. J Nucl Med 2015;56(2):255–60.

[15] Bernhard B, Gräni C. 18F-FDG PET/CT imaging in the workup of cardiac and pericardial masses. Springer; 2021. p. 1–3.

[16] Liu E-T, et al. Combined PET/CT with thoracic contrast-enhanced CT in assessment of primary cardiac tumors in adult patients. EJNMMI Res 2020;10(1):1–13.

[17] Brandão SCS, Dompieri LT. PET-CT 18F-FDG applications in cardiac tumors. CEP 2019;50750:309–17.

[18] Erdoğan EB, et al. Appearance of recurrent cardiac myxofibrosarcoma on FDG PET/CT. Clin Nucl Med 2014;39(6):559–60.

[19] Rahbar K, et al. Differentiation of malignant and benign cardiac tumors using 18F-FDG PET/CT. J Nucl Med 2012;53(6):856–63.

[20] Tse CS, et al. Cardiac melanoma: retrospective review of a rare disease at the Mayo clinic (1988–2015). Int J Cardiol 2017;249:383–6.

[21] Guazzaroni M, et al. Evaluation of a cardiac sarcoma with CT multislice contrast-enhanced and 18FDG-PET/TC. Radiol Case Rep 2019;14(3):368–71.

[22] Burke A, Tavora F. The 2015 WHO classification of tumors of the heart and pericardium. J Thorac Oncol 2016;11(4):441–52.

[23] Lee JC, et al. Positron emission tomography combined with computed tomography as an integral component in evaluation of primary cardiac lymphoma. Clin Cardiol 2010; 33(6):E106–8.

[24] Sivrikoz İA, et al. F-18 FDG PET/CT images of a rare primer cardiac tumour: primary pericardial mesothelioma. Anatol J Cardiol 2016;16(8):635.

[25] Dencker M, Valind S, Stagmo M. Right ventricular metastasis of leiomyosarcoma. Cardiovasc Ultrasound 2009;7(1):1–3.

[26] Miao Zhang M, Biao Li M, Jiang X. PET/CT imaging in a case of cardiac liposarcoma. J Nucl Cardiol 2008;15(3):473.

[27] Wang Q, et al. Primary pericardial osteosarcoma on FDG PET/CT. Clin Nucl Med 2013;38(8):e326–8.

[28] Wang R, Shen G, Tian R. Primary atrial undifferentiated sarcoma found on FDG PET/CT mimicking cardiac myxoma. Clin Nucl Med 2020;45(10):833–5.

[29] Patrianakos AP, et al. Cardiac paraganglioma: multimodality imaging of a rare tumor. Case Rep 2021;3(2):273–5.

[30] Khan MF, et al. Cardiac paraganglioma: clinical presentation, diagnostic approach and factors affecting short and long-term outcomes. Int J Cardiol 2013;166(2):315–20.

[31] Elder EE, et al. The management of benign and malignant pheochromocytoma and abdominal paraganglioma. Eur J Surg Oncol 2003;29(3):278–83.

[32] Semionov A, Sayegh K. Multimodality imaging of a cardiac paraganglioma. Radiol Case Rep 2016;11(4):277–81.

[33] Skoura E, et al. The impact of Ga-68 DOTATATE PET/CT imaging on management of patients with paragangliomas. Nucl Med Commun 2020;41(2):169–74.

# Benign masses: Macroscopic and microscopic evaluation

# 17

**Kambiz Mozaffari and Mahshid Hesami**

*Surgical and Clinical Pathology, Rajaie Cardiovascular Medical and Research Center, Iran University of Medical Sciences, Tehran, Iran*

## Key points

- Cardiac tumors in adults are rare and most of them are benign.
- The benign cardiac tumors include cardiac myxoma, fibroma, rhabdomyoma, papillary fibroelastoma, hemangioma, lipoma, hamartoma, teratoma, and paraganglioma/pheochromocytoma. By far, the most frequent benign neoplasm in the adult population consists of cardiac myxoma.

  Cardiac neoplasms are rare in infants and children and most of them are benign and primary. Rhabdomyoma is the most common primary cardiac neoplasm in children. The second most common tumor of the heart in this age group is cardiac fibroma [1,2].

## Benign cardiac tumors

Cardiac tumors are rare and about 90% of primary cardiac tumors are benign. Cardiac myxomas are the most common benign primary cardiac tumors in adults [17]. The other benign tumors include rhabdomyoma, fibroma, papillary fibroelastoma, hemangioma, pericardial cyst, benign fatty tumors (lipoma and lipomatous hypertrophy of the interatrial septum), hamartoma, teratoma, and benign neural neoplasm (paraganglioma/pheochromocytoma, neurofibroma, and schwannoma) [18]. Pediatric cardiac tumors are extremely rare; they are categorized into primary and secondary (or metastatic). Primary cardiac tumors are more common, and most of them are benign. Rhabdomyoma is the most common primary cardiac neoplasm in children. The second most common tumor of the heart in children after rhabdomyoma is cardiac fibroma (see Tables 17.1 and 17.2) [1,2].

Multimodal Imaging Atlas of Cardiac Masses. https://doi.org/10.1016/B978-0-323-84906-7.00022-4

**Table 17.1** Tumor-like lesion (reactive cardiac masses, pseudotumors, and ectopias).

| Tumor-like lesion | Description |
|---|---|
| Intramural thrombus | **Gross:**<br>Atrial appendage and ventricular endocardium are common sites for mural thrombi. Most of them occur with underlying heart disease. Atrial thrombi most occur in mitral valvular disease and atrial fibrillation. Ventricular thrombi particularly occur in ischemic heart disease or cardiomyopathy (see Fig. 17.3A) [1].<br>**Histopathology:**<br>Histopathology reveals layers of fibrin containing some leukocytes and erythrocytes. Fibrosis, proliferation of endothelial cells, and recanalization at the different phases of thrombus formation were seen. It is useful to evaluate the underlying myocardium to make a specific diagnosis (see Fig. 17.3B) [1]. |
| Cardiac calcified amorphous tumor (CAT) | **Gross:**<br>Cardiac calcified amorphous tumor (CAT) is a recently described nontumoral lesion with a clinical demonstration, undistinguishable from other heart tumors such as myxomas. Of great importance is the fact that cardiac masses potentially cause obstruction or embolization and prove fatal. Such masses were formerly called "pseudotumors," and a majority of them were termed thrombi (see Fig. 17.4A) [3–6].<br>**Histopathology:**<br>The lesion revealed multiple calcium deposits within a dense fibrocollagenous background; nevertheless, no malignant cells are seen. Other causes of calcification include myxomas, which present as mobile masses in the heart and could become calcified in about 20% of cases in the left atrium. Fibromas may also have a calcified appearance; nonetheless, they are usually located in the left ventricle with an intramyocardial location. Last but not least, vegetations, echinococcal cysts, tuberculomas, and calcified thrombi are to be borne in mind (see Fig. 17.4B) [3–6]. |
| Ectopic thyroid tissue | **Gross**:<br>It is defined that thyroid tissue is not located in its normal anatomical position. Intracardiac is a rare finding and common location is right ventricle. Paracardiac location with attachment to the ascending aorta has also been reported [7,8].<br>**Histopathology:**<br>Histologically, composed of colloid filled follicles with flat cuboidal cells and uniformly small nuclei resembling normal thyroid tissue (see Fig. 17.5) [7]. |

**Table 17.1** Tumor-like lesion (reactive cardiac masses, pseudotumors, and ectopias)–cont'd

| Tumor-like lesion | Description |
|---|---|
| Cardiac Tuberculoma | **Gross:**<br>Pericardial involvement is relatively common; however, myocardial tuberculosis has been reported in not more than 0.3% of all tuberculosis patients postmortem. Tuberculoma shows a well-circumscribed, solid, and creamy egg-shaped appearance with a lobulated surface. It is found in all cardiac chambers, most commonly in the right atrium. Most cases are solitary [4,9,10].<br>**Histopathology:**<br>The histopathological study shows multiple well-formed granulomas with multinucleated giant cells and extensive caseous necrosis compatible with a tuberculoma; however, the Ziehl-Neelsen stain helps reveal the acid-fast bacilli (see Fig. 17.6) [4,9,10]. |
| Hydatid cyst | **Gross:**<br>Hydatid cyst of the heart is uncommon. Any part of the heart may be affected but the most common location is the free wall of left ventricle. Single to multiple cysts with varying size were seen. In general the cysts were soft and filled with clear to slightly turbid fluid (see Fig. 17.7A) [11].<br>**Histopathology.**<br>The cyst consists of three layers: (1) outer fibrous layer, (2) middle hyaline and acellular laminated layer, and (3) inner germinative layer which consists of daughter cysts and brood capsules with scolices (see Fig. 17.7B) [12]. |
| Foregut Cyst | **Gross**<br>The cyst is predominantly unilocular with a thin fibrotic wall and contains homogeneous gelatinous material. Grossly, it consists of soft and creamy-gray fragments. The average size is about 3–4 cm [13–16].<br>**Histopathology**<br>It is usual to see ciliated columnar epithelium and foci of squamous metaplasia. Other endodermal and mesodermal elements may exist. The wall may contain hyaline cartilage, smooth muscle, bronchial glands, and nerve trunks (see Fig. 17.8) [13–16]. |

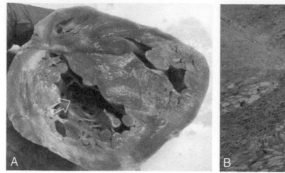
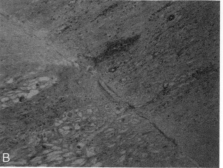

**FIG. 17.3**

Mural thrombus. Mural thrombus in apex of right ventricle in an 18-year-old man with hypertrophic cardiomyopathy. (A) Right ventricular endocardium shows attached brown colored fragile lesion M: 2 × 1 cm *(arrowhead)*. (B) Microscopic examination shows organizing mural thrombus. Underlying myocardium with hypertrophic and vacuolar changes is seen.

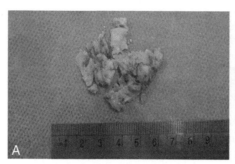
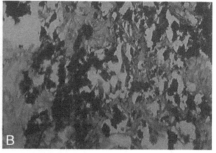

**FIG. 17.4**

Calcified amorphous tumor (CAT). Left atrial mass: (A) creamy-yellow firm to hard fragmented pieces. (B) Multiple calcium deposits in a dense fibrocollagenous background (H&E ×400).

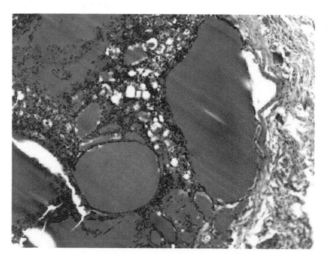

**FIG. 17.5**

Ectopic thyroid tissue. A 58-year-old woman who underwent cardiac surgery for bypass grafting was incidentally found to have an "irregularly shaped mass on aorta M: 1.5 × 1 × 0.5 cm." Sections show well-differentiated follicles with cuboidal epithelium and colloid material.

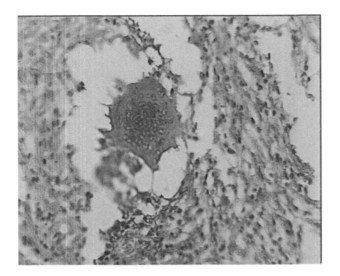

**FIG. 17.6**

Tuberculoma. Microscopic examination shows scattered Langhans giant cells, lymphocytes, plasma cells, and the characteristic caseous necrosis in tuberculoma (H&E, ×400).

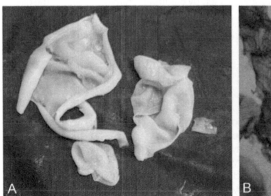
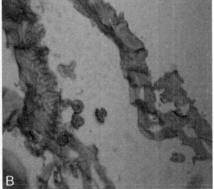

**FIG. 17.7**

Hydatid cyst. Pulmonary and interventricular septum hydatid cyst in a 50-year-old man.
(A) Gross examination shows white sheet-like structures (perforated cystic wall).
(B) Histopathology of the cyst showed outer lamellated acellular layers and inner germinal layer with protoscolices.

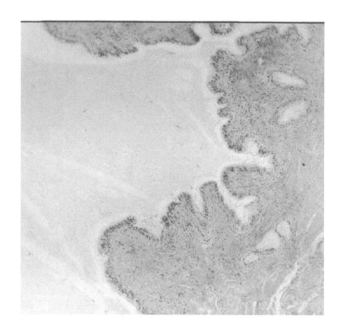

**FIG. 17.8**

Foregut cyst. Fibrous tissue forms a cyst wall, lined by columnar epithelium with some ciliated cells (H&E, ×100).

**Table 17.2** Benign cardiac tumors.

| Tumor type | Description |
| --- | --- |
| Cardiac myxoma | **Gross:**<br>Most frequently seen in the left atrium near fossa ovalis but it may occur in any cardiac chamber. Myxoma is usually pedunculated with a short stalk or may be sessile. Consistency varies from a soft, gelatinous, papillary mass to a firm, smooth tumor. The cut surface shows a variegated appearance, frequently with areas of hemorrhage and cyst formation. Calcification may be focal or extensive (see Fig. 17.9) [2,4,14,19,20].<br><br>**Histopathology:**<br>The tumor is composed of polygonal, bipolar, or stellate myxoma or lepidic cells that have round to oval nuclei with inconspicuous nucleoli, eosinophilic cytoplasm, and indistinct borders. Cells may be scattered singly, aggregate in small nests or cords, or form rings surrounding vascular channels. Minimal pleomorphism and mitoses are seen. Background typically consists of myxoid and loose fibrous tissue with scattered lymphocytic and histiocytic infiltrate, especially hemosiderin-laden macrophages. Surface thrombus may be identified. Rarely, ossification and mucinous glands may be seen (see Fig. 17.10) [2,4,14,19,20]. |

**Table 17.2** Benign cardiac tumors–cont'd

| Tumor type | Description |
|---|---|
| Cardiac Fibroma | **Gross**:<br>Cardiac fibroma is a firm, white mass which appears circumscribed [1]. They have a whorled cut surface (see Fig. 17.11) [21]. It may occur anywhere in the heart but usually involves the ventricles with a predilection for the ventricular septum [1]. Calcification is common (see Fig. 17.12C). Cardiac fibromas are classically single, but multifocal tumors have been reported [22].<br><br>**Histopathology:**<br>These tumors show bland spindle cells with fibroblastic cytologic features in a collagenous background, with variable numbers of elastic fibers (see Fig. 17.12A and B). The margins of the tumor are histologically infiltrative and more cellular in infants and children (see Fig. 17.12D) [23,24]. |
| Rhabdomyoma | **Gross:**<br>This tumor constitutes 50 to 90% of primary heart tumors in children and is usually noted in infancy. Valve obstruction or protrusion into heart chambers may occur. They are well-circumscribed, small but firm, gray-white masses. The size is 3–4 cm or may reach up to 10 cm (see Fig. 17.13A) [4,24–27].<br><br>**Histopathology:**<br>The large rounded polygonal cells which are clear (due to dissolution of glycogen during the H and E staining) are known as spider cells. The cytoplasmic vacuoles are separated by strands of cytoplasm extending between cell membrane and nucleus but no mitotic activity is seen. In adults, rhabdomyomas are more cellular with fewer spider cells and more cellular proliferation (see Fig. 17.13B) [4,24–27]. |
| Hemangioma | **Gross:**<br>Most hemangiomas are small, endocardial nodules ranging from 0.2 to 3.5 cm in diameter, either polypoid or sessile, and without evidence of infiltration (see Fig. 17.14A). The most frequent locations are the anterior wall of the right ventricle, the lateral wall of the left ventricle, and the interventricular septum, and sometimes the right ventricular outflow tract is involved [28].<br><br>**Histopathology:**<br>Composed of variably sized blood vessels containing bland endothelial cells. They are histologically classified as capillary (small capillary-like vessels), cavernous (large cystically dilated vessels with thin walls), and intramuscular cardiac hemangioma (heterogeneous vessel types) [29]. The capillary type tends to be circumscribed whereas the cavernous and intramuscular types tend to be infiltrative (see Fig. 17.14B and C) [1,30]. |

*Continued*

**Table 17.2** Benign cardiac tumors–cont'd

| Tumor type | Description |
|---|---|
| Papillary fibroelastoma | **Gross:** <br> Arborizing, thin strands of tan-white tissue, usually arising from a common stalk. The papillary fibroelastoma has been compared to a "sea anemone," an appearance heightened by placing the specimen in a bowl of water [1,29] (see Fig. 17.15A). Generally they are around 1.0 cm in diameter, but range in size from 0.2 to 7 cm [28]. Their most common location is the aortic valve, followed by the mitral and tricuspid valves, pulmonary valve, and endocardial surfaces [1]. <br><br> **Histopathology** <br> Avascular papillary fronds lined by endothelial cells. The papillary cores contain a proteoglycan-rich stroma, and layers of elastic fibers and collagen are prominent near the base of the lesion. It may show hydropic change (see Fig. 17.15B and C) [1,18]. |
| Lipomatous hypertrophy | **Gross:** <br> Lipomatous hypertrophy consists of an unencapsulated accumulation of mature adipose tissue within the interatrial septum. Fossa ovalis is generally spared, giving it a characteristic "dumbbell" shape. The atrial septum may measure between 2 cm and 8 cm in thickness (see Fig. 17.16A) [1,18,31,32]. <br><br> **Histopathology:** <br> It has a distinctive histological appearance marked by the presence of abundant multivacuolated lipocytes and hypertrophied myocytes (see Fig. 17.16B) [18,31]. |

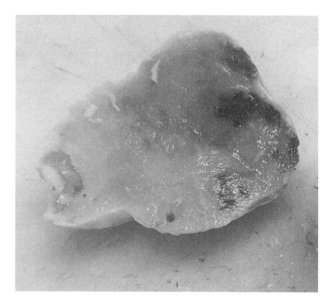

**FIG. 17.9**

Cardiac myoma (Gross). Large left atrial myxoma with a smooth cut surface and areas of hemorrhage and calcification.

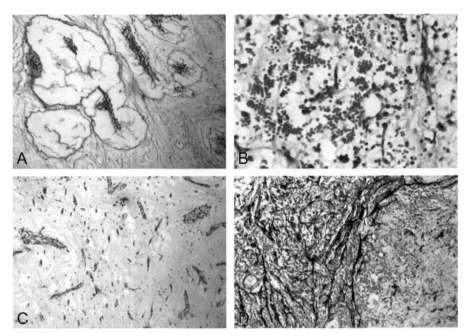

**FIG. 17.10**

Cardiac myxoma (Histopathology). (A) Concentrically arranged layers of elongated neoplastic cells around blood vessels and cords of tumor cells in abundant eosinophilic stroma are seen. (B) Scattered inflammatory cells, fresh hemorrhage, and vascular channels in a myxoid background. (C) Smooth muscle and stellate cells with some inflammatory cells. (D) Lacy calcification with fresh hemorrhage and vascular channels (H & E ×400).

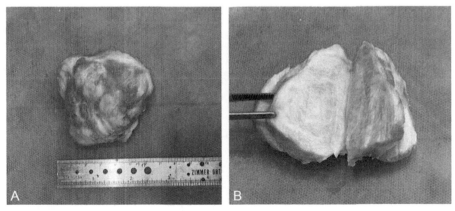

**FIG. 17.11**

Cardiac fibroma (Gross). Cardiac fibroma of right ventricular free wall in a 12-year-old boy. (A) A creamy-whitish mass with lobulated surface and firm consistency M: 6.5 × 6 × 4 cm. (B) Cut sections were solid and white with a whorled appearance. Hemorrhage or necrosis was not seen.

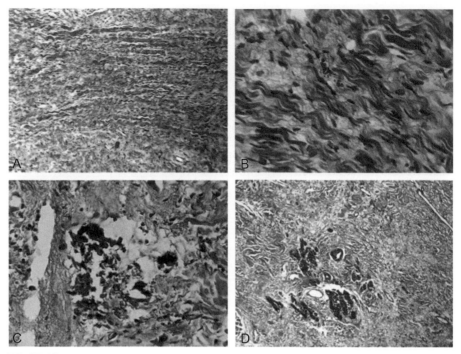

**FIG. 17.12**

Cardiac fibroma (Histopathology). Cardiac fibroma of the right ventricular free wall in a 12-year-old boy. (A) Microscopic examination (H&E, ×100) shows bland spindle cells in a collagenous background. (B) Higher magnification (H&E, ×400) shows relatively uniform spindle cells, without mitotic activity. (C) Foci of calcification are seen. (D) Trichrome stain shows infiltration of the collagenous tumor into the cardiac muscle.

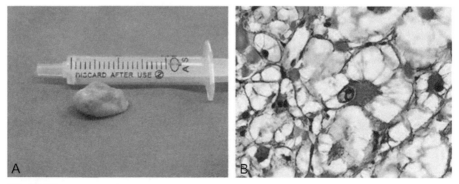

**FIG. 17.13**

Rhabdomyoma. Left atrial mass in a 2-year-old boy. (A) Well-defined creamy-whitish solid mass measuring 2 × 1 cm. (B) Spider cells are seen as large and clear cells with cytoplasmic vacuoles and central nuclei.

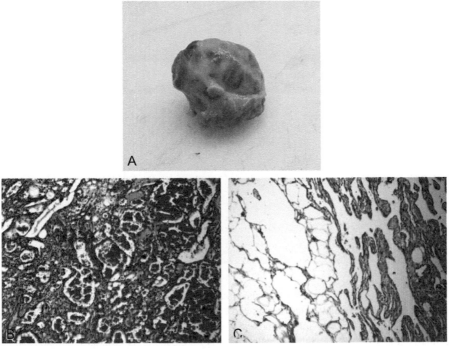

**FIG. 17.14**

Cardiac hemangioma. Right atrial hemangioma in a 50-year-old man. (A) Gross examination shows a well circumscribed oval grayish mass with soft consistency M· 2.5 × 2.5 × 1.5 cm. (B) Microscopic examination shows dilated thin walled vascular channels and capillary structures lined by flat endothelial cells without cellular atypia, necrosis, or mitoses. (C) Mature adipose and fibrous tissues also are seen.

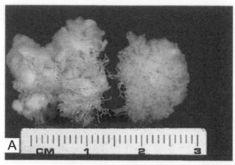

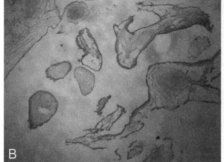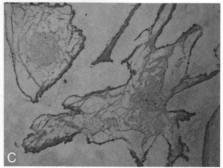

**FIG. 17.15**

Papillary fibroelastoma. Papillary fibroelastoma. (A) Typical gross appearance when placed in water. Mass with multiple small fronds and sea anemone appearance in a bowl of water. (B) and (C) Right atrium papillary fibroelastoma attached to anterior tricuspid valve annulus. Microscopic examination shows multiple papillary projections consisting of paucicellular avascular fibroelastic tissue lined by a single layer of endocardium with foci of hydropic changes.

*Adapted with permission from Buja LM, Butany J. Cardiovascular pathology. 2015. Academic Press.*

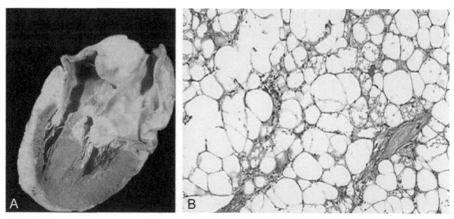

**FIG. 17.16**

Lipomatous hypertrophy. Lipomatous hypertrophy, atrial septum. (A) Gross picture of the heart with lipomatous hypertrophy of the interatrial septum, bulging into the right atrium. (B) Histological examination shows abundant multivacuolated lipocytes and hypertrophied myocytes.

*Adapted with permission from Buja LM, Butany J. Cardiovascular pathology. 2015. Academic Press.*

# References

[1] Ladich E, Virmani R. Tumors of the cardiovascular system: heart and blood vessels. In: Cardiovascular pathology. Elsevier; 2016. p. 735–72.

[2] Moradian M, Hejazi Zadeh B, Rashidi Ghader F, Khorgami MR, Mozaffari K, Mohammad Sadeghi F, et al. Primary cardiac tumors in children: an 8-year-experience in a single center. Iran J Pediatr 2020;30(6).

[3] Kambiz M, Hassan Mirmohammad S, Mozhgan P. What do we know about the cardiac CAT? [a case report]; 2011.

[4] Silver MD, Gotlieb AI, Schoen FJ. Cardiovascular pathology; 2001.

[5] Reynolds C, Tazelaar HD, Edwards WD. Calcified amorphous tumor of the heart (cardiac CAT). Hum Pathol 1997;28(5):601–6.

[6] Pietro DA, Parisi AF, Intracardiac masses. Tumors, vegetations, thrombi, and foreign bodies. Med Clin North Am 1980;64(2):239–51.

[7] Comajuan SM, Ayerbe JL, Ferrer BR, Quer C, Camazón NV, Sistach EF, et al. An intracardiac ectopic thyroid mass. Eur J Echocardiogr 2009;10(5):704–6.

[8] Noussios G, Anagnostis P, Goulis DG, Lappas D, Natsis K. Ectopic thyroid tissue: anatomical, clinical, and surgical implications of a rare entity. Eur J Endocrinol 2011; 165(3):375.

[9] Mozaffari K, Behzadnia N. Different histopathological appearances of cardiac tuberculosis: presentation of a rare case with review of literature; 2011.

[10] Chang B-C, Ha J-W, Kim J-T, Chung N, Cho S-H. Intracardiac tuberculoma. Ann Thorac Surg 1999;67(1):226–8.

[11] Firouzi A, Borj MNP, Ghavidel AA. Cardiac hydatid cyst: a rare presentation of echinococcal infection. J Cardiovascu Thorac Res 2019;11(1):75.

[12] Sultana N, Hashim TK, Jan SY, Malik T, Shah W. Primary cervical hydatid cyst: a rare occurrence. Diagn Pathol 2012;7(1):1–5

[13] Mozaffari K, Khajali Z, Givtaj N, Bakhshandeh H. Intracardiac foregut cyst, in a 42-year-old woman with partial atrioventricular septal defect, a rare incidental finding. Res Cardiovasc Med 2018;7(3):152.

[14] Rosai J. Rosai and Ackerman's surgical pathology e-book. Elsevier Health Sciences; 2011.

[15] Huang JH, Rudzinski ER, Minette MS, Langley SM. First case of intracardiac foregut cyst occurring in the left-ventricular outflow tract. Pediatr Cardiol 2013;34(8):2060–2.

[16] Chen C-C. Bronchogenic cyst in the interatrial septum with a single persistent left superior vena cava. J Chin Med Assoc 2006;69(2):89–91.

[17] Singhal P, Luk A, Rao V, Butany J. Molecular basis of cardiac myxomas. Int J Mol Sci 2014;15(1):1315–37.

[18] Hejna P, Mary N. Sheppard: practical cardiovascular pathology. Springer; 2012.

[19] Rafi Khourgami M, Ershad A, Mozaffari K. Left atrial myxoma misdiagnosis as infective endocarditis: a case report. Archives of pediatric infectious diseases; 2021 [in press].

[20] Reynen K. Cardiac myxomas. N Engl J Med 1995;333(24):1610–7.

[21] Basso C, Valente M, Thiene G. Cardiac tumor pathology. Springer Science & Business Media; 2012.

[22] Grunau GL, Leipsic JA, Sellers SL, Seidman MA. Cardiac fibroma in an adult AIRP best cases in radiologic-pathologic correlation. Radiographics 2018;38(4):1022–2026.

[23] Burke AP, Rosado-de-Christenson M, Templeton PA, Virmani R. Cardiac fibroma: clinicopathologic correlates and surgical treatment. J Thorac Cardiovasc Surg 1994; 108(5):862–70.

[24] Goldblum JR, Lamps LW, McKenney JK, Myers JL. Rosai and Ackerman's surgical pathology e-book. Elsevier Health Sciences; 2017.

[25] Mozaffari K, Baghaei TR, Moradian M, Totonchi MZ. A one-year old infant with multiple cardiac masses and congenital heart disease (a case report); 2011.

[26] Chopra P, Ray R, Saxena A. Illustrated textbook of cardiovascular pathology. CRC Press; 2013.

[27] Moradian M, Fard MZ, Mozaffari K. Atrial rhabdomyoma: a case report. Iran Heart J 2014;15(2):39–42.

[28] Suvarna S. Cardiac pathology: a guide to current practice. Springer Science & Business Media; 2012.

[29] Grebenc ML, Rosado de Christenson ML, Burke AP, Green CE, Galvin JR. Primary cardiac and pericardial neoplasms: radiologic-pathologic correlation. Radiographics 2000;20(4):1073–103.

[30] Li W, Teng P, Xu H, Ma L, Ni Y. Cardiac hemangioma: a comprehensive analysis of 200 cases. Ann Thorac Surg 2015;99(6):2246–52.

[31] O'Connor S, Recavarren R, Nichols LC, Parwani AV. Lipomatous hypertrophy of the interatrial septum: an overview. Arch Pathol Lab Med 2006;130(3):397–9.

[32] Moinuddeen K, Marica S, Clausi RL, Zama N. Lipomatous interatrial septal hypertrophy: an unusual cause of intracardiac mass. Eur J Cardiothorac Surg 2002;22(3):468–9.

# Malignant masses: Macroscopic and microscopic evaluation

18

**Kambiz Mozaffari and Mahshid Hesami**

*Surgical and Clinical Pathology, Rajaie Cardiovascular Medical and Research Center, Iran University of Medical Sciences, Tehran, Iran*

## Key points

- Cardiac neoplasms are rare and most of the malignancies in this organ are metastatic in origin.
- The most important primary cardiac malignancies include angiosarcomas, rhabdomyosarcomas, malignant fibrous histiocytoma, leiomyosarcoma, and primary cardiac lymphoma.
- Metastatic sarcomas to the heart involve the myocardium more often than the pericardium. All types of sarcomas and carcinomas metastasize to this organ and this occurs via the hematogenous route.

**Table 18.1** Malignant cardiac tumors.

| Tumor | Description |
| --- | --- |
| Angiosarcoma | *Gross*<br>They are large, hemorrhagic (red to dark brown), and infiltrative masses, mostly occurring in the right atrium. They involve the myocardium and pericardium. Invasion into the tricuspid valve and vena cava is also seen. The size ranges from 2.0 to 17 cm in greatest dimension (see Fig. 18.2) [1–3]<br><br>*Histopathology*<br>Histopathological findings range from a pattern so well differentiated vascular channels resembling benign hemangioma to poorly differentiated solid areas [4]. The anastomosing vascular channels lined by atypical endothelial cell with spindle to plump and epithelioid shapes [5]. Extravascular erythrocytes and the identification of vacuoles with red blood cells may help in the diagnosis. Hemorrhage and necrosis are common (see Fig. 18.3) [1] |

*Continued*

Multimodal Imaging Atlas of Cardiac Masses. https://doi.org/10.1016/B978-0-323-84906-7.00031-5

**Table 18.1** Malignant cardiac tumors—Cont'd

| Tumor | Description |
|---|---|
| Malignant fibrous histiocytoma | *Gross*<br>Most of them arise in the left atrium, most commonly the posterior wall and atrial septum. They are endocardial based and may be soft or firm polypoid lesions, sometimes distending the left atrium (see Fig. 18.4A) [1,6,7]<br>*Histopathology*<br>They are malignant undifferentiated mesenchymal tumors of fibroblastic or myofibroblastic differentiation [1]. They are characterized by proliferation of spindle shape and epithelioid cells with variable degrees of atypia, mitotic activity, including atypical forms, necrosis, and nuclear polymorphism with storiform and whorled patterns (see Fig. 18.4B) [1,2] |
| Leiomyosarcoma | *Gross*<br>Most cardiac leiomyosarcomas occur in left atrium followed by the right atrium. They are homogeneous firm white to tan masses with variable necrosis (see Fig. 18.5) [7]<br>*Histopathology*<br>Tumor composed fascicles of spindle-shaped cells, with oval blunt nuclei. The cytoplasm is often vacuolated. Area of necrosis, myxoid changes, more pleomorphic tumor cells, and high mitotic activity also are present (see Fig. 18.5) [2,6,8] |
| Rhabdomyosarcoma | *Gross*<br>Approximately 5% of cardiac sarcomas. Either atrium or ventricle may be the primary site. These are bulky, invasive tumors that may exceed 10 cm in the greatest diameter (see Fig. 18.6A) [5,9]<br>*Histopathology*<br>The majority is of the embryonal type and may be well differentiated with numerous tadpole-shaped rhabdomyoblasts. Extensive sheets of myxoid areas and small round cells are seen. The tumor is arranged as moderately cellular to hypocellular foci. This hypercellularity is more prominent at the periphery of the lesion, reminiscent of the cambium layer. Considerable tumoral necrosis may also be noted (see Fig. 18.6B) [5,9] |
| Primary cardiac lymphoma | *Gross*<br>It accounts for only 1.6% of cardiac neoplasms, predominantly arising from the right chamber and is primarily of B-cell origin. No association has thus far been established with viruses. There is usually no trace of lymphadenopathy or organomegaly. Multiple firm whitish-yellow nodules are seen grossly with a solid appearance and firm to fragile consistency [10]<br>*Histopathology*<br>Infiltration of myocardium is seen by discohesive sheets of malignant round cells that have a high N/C ratio, scanty cytoplasm, and a coarse chromatin pattern. Because these tumors are mainly diffuse large B-cell lymphomas according to the lymphoma classification, one expects IHC markers such as CD 45 and CD 20 to be positive (see Fig. 18.7) [10] |

**Table 18.1** Malignant cardiac tumors—Cont'd

| Tumor | Description |
|---|---|
| Metastatic carcinoma (metastatic papillary thyroid carcinoma) | *Gross*<br>Most metastatic carcinomas involve the pericardium followed by the myocardium [1]. Carcinoma of the lung, breast, thyroid, and kidney cancers has the highest rates of spread to the heart [1,11]. Metastatic deposits can be large, solitary, bulky masses; can consist of multiple smaller masses; or rarely can be present only microscopically [7]<br><br>*Histopathology*<br>Pathological evaluation remains the most definite method for differentiating neoplastic from nonneoplastic cardiac masses [12]. Papillary thyroid carcinomas show papillary structures with branching lined by epithelium with characteristic nuclear features (nuclear enlargement and overlapping, chromatin clearing, ground glass nuclei, irregular nuclear contour, nuclear grooves, and nuclear pseudoinclusions). There are different morphological variants such as follicular variant, diffuse sclerosing variant, oncocytic variant, and papillary microcarcinoma (see Fig. 18.8) [5] |
| Metastatic malignant melanoma | *Gross*<br>Malignant melanoma is well known to have a propensity to metastasize to the heart. Patients may present with multiple or single nodular masses in the heart chambers as well as bloody effusions that may lead to cardiac tamponade. Multiple mobile, large masses in left atrium (LA), left ventricle (LV), and right atrium (RA) may be seen [13,14]<br><br>*Histopathology*<br>As well as the masses mentioned before, it may give rise to effusions. The cytological examination reveals a bloody background with clusters and nests of malignant cells. The tumoral cells have a high nucleocytoplasmic (N/C) ratio and moderate pleomorphism. Their cytoplasmic spaces are laden with coarse and fine dark brown melanin pigment (see Fig. 18.9) [13,14] |
| Metastatic osteosarcoma | *Gross*<br>Metastatic sarcomas to the heart involve the myocardium more often than the pericardium. All types of sarcomas metastasize to this organ and this occurs via the hematogenous route. Bilateral or diffuse involvement is seen in 30% to 35% of cases. Another extremely uncommon feature noted is its occurrence as an isolated lesion. It is usually large in size and often intracavitary in location [9,15,16]<br><br>*Histopathology*<br>Morphological findings reveal a pleomorphic round cell sarcoma with foci of hemorrhage and necrosis. Plump and large clear cells are seen with pleomorphic round nuclei (see Fig. 18.10) [9,15,16] |

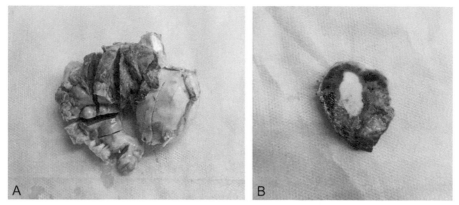

**FIG. 18.2**

Angiosarcoma (gross). Right atrial angiosarcoma in a 49/Y woman: (A) Gross examination shows an irregular creamy-brownish mass with firm consistency M: 8.5 × 5 × 4.5 cm. (B) Cut section shows a heterogeneous dark-brown surface with areas of necrosis.

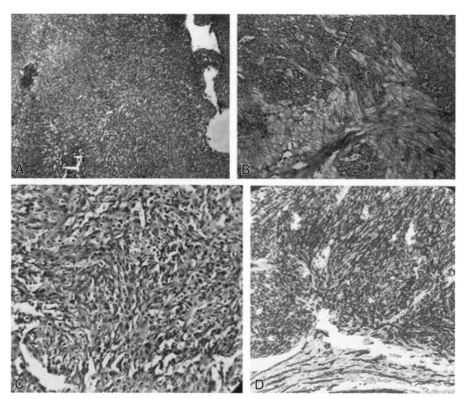

**FIG. 18.3**

Angiosarcoma (histopathology). Histopathology of right atrial angiosarcoma: (A) Microscopic examination shows anastomosing vascular channels lined by atypical spindled endothelial cells and areas of solid growth pattern. (B) Tumor infiltration into the cardiac myocytes is seen. (C) High power magnification shows vascular proliferation lined by endothelial cells with large hyperchromatic nuclei and prominent nucleoli. (D) The neoplastic cells show diffuse and strong immunoreaction with CD31.

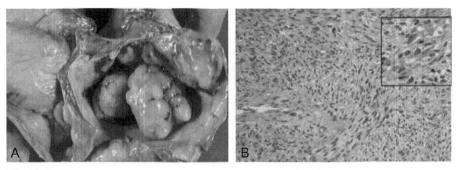

**FIG. 18.4**

Malignant fibrous histiocytoma. (A) Polypoid mass at left atrium. (B) Histological examination shows neoplastic tissue composed of spindle cells with fibrohistiocytic appearance, marked pleomorphism and storiform pattern.

*Reproduced with permission from Buja LM. Tumors of cardiovascular system heart and blood vessels. In: Cardiovascular pathology. Elsevier; 2016. p. 735–72.c.*

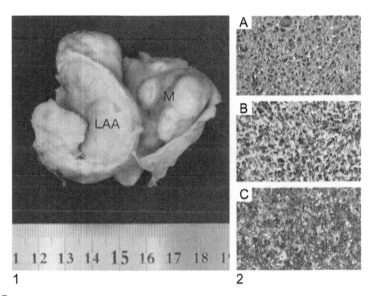

**FIG. 18.5**

Leiomyosarcoma. Left atrial leiomyosarcoma in a 39/Y old woman. (1) Gross examination shows a white mass with a smooth surface (M: mass, LAA: left atrial auricle)
(2) (A) Microscopic examination (H&E × 400) shows sheets of spindle cells with hyperchromatic nuclei and moderate pleomorphism. Immunochemical studies show tumoral cells reactivity with (B) vimentin and (C) α-smooth muscle actin. MIB-1 labeling index is 44.1%.

*Reproduced with permission from Nakashima K, Inatsu H, Kitamura K. Primary cardiac leiomyosarcoma: a 27-month survival with surgery and chemotherapy. Intern Med 2017;56(16):2145–9.*

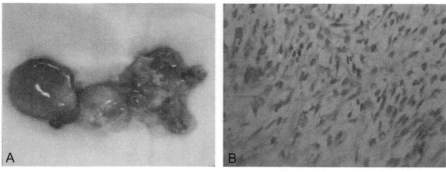

**FIG. 18.6**

Rhabdomyosarcoma. (A) Gross examination shows multiple creamy and lobulated, soft to firm masses with foci of necrosis and hemorrhage. (B) Relatively cellular tumor with pleomorphic round to spindle cells in a myxoid background (H & E ×400).

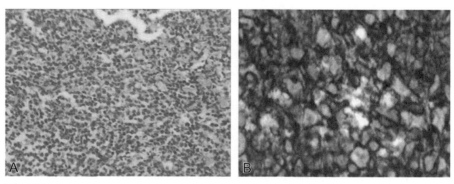

**FIG. 18.7**

Primary cardiac lymphoma. (A) Diffusely infiltrated tissue showing large atypical lymphocytes with round or irregular nuclei (hematoxylin and eosin staining; magnification, ×400). (B) Immunohistochemical study staining is positive for CD20 (magnification, ×400).

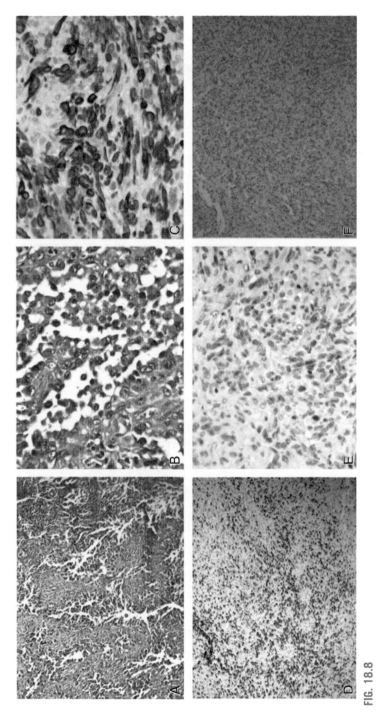

**FIG. 18.8**

Metastatic papillary thyroid carcinoma. A 50 Y/O man with history of papillary thyroid carcinoma presenting with very large nonhomogeneous mass in right ventricle with extension to right ventricular outflow tract and RV apex. (A and B) Microscopic examination (H&E) reveals neoplastic tissue arranged in sheets and focal papillary structures composed of pleomorphic neoplastic cells with vesicular nuclei, eosinophilic cytoplasm, and prominent nucleoli. Increased mitotic figures with areas of massive necrosis are noted. Immunochemical (IHC) study shows tumoral cells reactivity with CK7 (C) and TTF1 (D). The tumoral cells show negative reaction to CK 20 (E) and NAPSIN A (F).

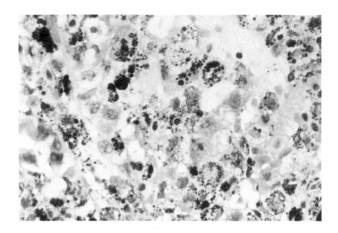

**FIG. 18.9**

Metastatic malignant melanoma cells in the pericardial fluid filled with melanin pigment and revealing pleomorphism (Giemsa method ×400).

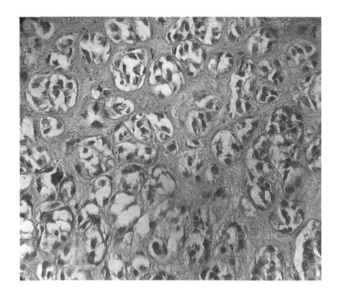

**FIG. 18.10**

Metastatic osteosarcoma. Plump and large clear cells are seen with pleomorphic round nuclei (H & E ×400).

# References

[1] Ladich E, Virmani R. Tumors of the cardiovascular system: heart and blood vessels. In: Cardiovascular pathology. Elsevier; 2016. p. 735–72.

[2] Hejna P, Mary N. Sheppard: practical cardiovascular pathology. Springer; 2012.

[3] Suvarna S. Cardiac pathology: a guide to current practice. Springer Science & Business Media; 2012.

[4] Patel SD, Peterson A, Bartczak A, Lee S, Chojnowski S, Gajewski P, et al. Primary cardiac angiosarcoma—a review. Med Sci Monit 2014;20:103.

[5] Goldblum JR, Lamps LW, McKenney JK, Myers JL. Rosai and Ackerman's surgical pathology e-book. Elsevier Health Sciences; 2017.

[6] Basso C, Valente M, Thiene G. Cardiac tumor pathology. Springer Science & Business Media; 2012.

[7] WHO. WHO classification of tumours of the lung, pleura, thymus and heart. WHO/IARC Classification of Tumours; 2015. p. 7.

[8] Nakashima K, Inatsu H, Kitamura K. Primary cardiac leiomyosarcoma: a 27-month survival with surgery and chemotherapy. Intern Med 2017;56. 6965-15.

[9] Chopra P, Ray R, Saxena A. Illustrated textbook of cardiovascular pathology. CRC Press; 2013.

[10] Mozaffari K, Kargar F, Azami H. Primary cardiac lymphoma in a 62-year-old man. Iran Heart J 2008;9:47–9.

[11] Sheppard M. Practical cardiovascular pathology. CRC Press; 2011.

[12] Burazor I, Aviel-Ronen S, Imazio M, Goitein O, Perelman M, Shelestovich N, et al. Metastatic cardiac tumors: from clinical presentation through diagnosis to treatment. BMC Cancer 2018;18(1):1–9.

[13] Samiei N, Farahani MM, Sadeghipour A, Mozaffari K, Maleki M. Intracardiac metastasis of malignant melanoma. Eur J Echocardiogr 2008;9(3):393–4.

[14] Mozaffari K, Samiei N, Abdolrahimi S. Malignant melanoma in the heart, with focus on the histopathological diagnosis: review of our two cases in a five-year period. Iran Heart J 2011;12:50–5.

[15] Maleki M, Mozaffari K, Givtaj N, Tatina A, Bahadorian B. Metastatic osteosarcoma and heart: a rare involvement in an unusual cardiac location. Heart Asia 2013;5(1):120–1.

[16] Silver MD, Gotlieb AI, Schoen FJ. Cardiovascular pathology. Churchill Livingstone Publishers; 2001.

# Surgical features of benign cardiac masses

# 19

**Sven Z.C.P. Tan[a], Joaquin Alfonso Palanca[a], Sidhant Singh[a], L. Maximillian Buja[b,c],
Idhrees Mohammed[d], Saeid Hosseini[e], and Mohamad Bashir[f]**

*[a]Barts and The London School of Medicine and Dentistry, Queen Mary University of London,
London, United Kingdom [b]Department of Pathology and Laboratory Medicine, McGovern Medical
School, The University of Texas Health Science Center at Houston (UTHealth), Houston, TX,
United States [c]Cardiovascular Pathology, Texas Heart Institute, Houston, TX, United States
[d]Institute of Cardiac and Aortic Disorders, SRM Institutes for Medical Science, Vadapalani,
Chennai, India [e]Rajaie Cardiovascular Medical and Research Center, Tehran, Iran [f]Vascular and
Endovascular Surgery, Health Education and Improvement Wales, Nantgarw, Wales, United
Kingdom*

## Key points

- Benign cardiac masses are exceedingly rare, and the underlying pathophysiological mechanisms behind their emergence are poorly understood
- Most patients are asymptomatic unless the mass exerts an effect over cardiac mechanics, hemodynamics, or depolarization, or if cardioembolism results from the mass
- An understanding of the surgical features of cardiac masses is essential for the diagnosis and successful excision thereof (Boxes 19.1 and 19.2)

---

### Box 19.1  Introduction

Cardiac tumors are rare and, when they occur, they are most frequently benign. The autopsy incidence of primary cardiac tumors ranges from 0.001% to 0.3%. Metastatic tumors, on the other hand, are the most common tumors of the heart with the reported ratio of cardiac metastases to primary cardiac tumors ranging from 100:1 to 1000:1. More than three-fourths of primary cardiac tumors are benign, with the cardiac myxoma representing the majority of these neoplasms. The most common cardiac tumor in children is the rhabdomyoma. This chapter details the surgical features, investigations, and manifestations associated with key examples of benign cardiac tumors.

---

Multimodal Imaging Atlas of Cardiac Masses. https://doi.org/10.1016/B978-0-323-84906-7.00014-5

**Box 19.2 There are a range of known benign cardiac masses, the majority of which are benign tumors that are exceedingly rare in modern practice. Hence, an appreciation of their surgical features (namely, presentation, approach to imaging, visual appearance, and tissue characterization) is beneficial.**

| Entity | Description |
|---|---|
| Myxoma<br>Figs. 19.3–19.6 | **Overview**<br>Cardiac myxomas are the most common form of cardiac tumors, though to account for up to 50% of all adult cardiac tumors. It affects primarily 40- to 60-year-olds and is associated with a female-male ratio of 3 [1]. The majority of cases are thought to be sporadic. Though the underlying pathogenesis remains unclear, autosomal dominant transmission has been identified in familial atrial myxoma (less than 10% of cases) [1]. Cardiac myxomas mostly arise from remnants of subendocardial or multipotent mesenchymal cells, around the fossa ovalis—75% of cases are attached to the left fossa ovalis [1].<br><br>**Presentation**<br>Though many patients with cardiac myxoma may be asymptomatic, some present with symptomatology and signs on examination consistent with mitral valve obstruction (e.g., syncope, dyspnea/orthopnea, and pulmonary congestion) and may exhibit embolic manifestations in later stages. Sudden death, weight loss, fatigue, pyrexia of unknown origin, and anemia have also been associated with cardiac myxoma [2].<br><br>Clinical examination of a patient with an indwelling cardiac myxoma should reveal [2]:<br>- Tumor plop: a low-pitched diastolic sound produced by the tumor prolapsing into the left ventricle<br>- Systolic murmur (in 50% of cases), loud S1 (32% of cases), opening snap (26% of cases), or diastolic murmur (15% of cases) [3]<br>- Peripheral stigmata of embolic phenomena, varying depending on the affected vasculature (neurological deficit, acute coronary syndrome, bowel or peripheral ischemia)<br><br>**Investigations**<br>Apart from the usual investigations undertaken when there is suspicion of cardiac pathologies (e.g., 12-lead ECG, routine bloods, troponin, etc.), the mainstay of diagnosis and detection of cardiac myxoma remains imaging and biopsy if needed. Transthoracic or transesophageal echocardiography (TTE and TEE, respectively) allows for the detection and localization of intracavitary masses, while further imaging techniques such as |

**Box 19.2 There are a range of known benign cardiac masses, the majority of which are benign tumors that are exceedingly rare in modern practice. Hence, an appreciation of their surgical features (namely, presentation, approach to imaging, visual appearance, and tissue characterization) is beneficial—Cont'd**

| Entity | Description |
|---|---|
| | computed tomography (CT) or cardiac magnetic resonance (CMR) should be employed to discern and delineate the extent of the intracardiac mass, provide information on involvement of extracardiac structures, and provide information for preoperative planning [3,4]. If imaging-based investigations are ambiguous, biopsy (guided by TEE) may be indicated to differentiate between tumors suitable for resection and metastatic tumors, as well as enabling histopathological analysis [4]. |
| | Differentials such as mitral stenosis, infective endocarditis, connective tissue disorders, and other cardiac tumors must be ruled out for a diagnosis of cardiac myxoma to be made. |
| | **Surgical Features**<br>On visualization, cardiac myxomas typically are yellowish-brown and are frequently covered with thrombi. Size may vary from 1 cm to 15 cm, and 15–180 g [1,5]. The surface of a cardiac myxoma is usually smooth, but cases in which myxoma have developed villous or papillary surfaces are also documented in literature. Unsurprisingly, spontaneous fragmentation of such papilla or villi poses increased embolic risk, and as such care should be taken during surgical resection [3]. |
| | Surgical resection of cardiac myxoma usually proceeds via the biatrial approach (under cardiopulmonary bypass and through median sternotomy) to afford the surgeon with optimal visualization and access to the lesion [4]. The transseptal and unilateral left atrial approaches may also be taken. Once the myxoma stalk and underlying endocardium are resected, repair and closure of the excision site is required (as in up to 83% of cases) with autopericardium or prosthetic materials [4]. |
| | Lifelong follow-up is indicated as 5%–14% of cases are thought to feature recurrence; however, overall prognosis following successful tumor resection is good: 87% survival at 13 years. Tumors with irregular/friable surfaces are associated with increased risk of embolic complications [2]. |
| | **Tissue Characterization**<br>Myxomas are composed generally of myxoma cells—which arise from subendothelial vasoformative reserve cells and endothelial progenitors—as well as endothelial cells and smooth muscle |

*Continued*

**Box 19.2 There are a range of known benign cardiac masses, the majority of which are benign tumors that are exceedingly rare in modern practice. Hence, an appreciation of their surgical features (namely, presentation, approach to imaging, visual appearance, and tissue characterization) is beneficial—Cont'd**

| Entity | Description |
|---|---|
| | fibers. Notably, the neoplastic cells are immunoreactive to S100, calretinin, vimentin, and nonspecific enolase [6]. |
| Papillary fibroelastoma Fig. 19.7 | **Overview** Cardiac papillary fibroelastoma (CPF) is the second most common type of benign cardiac tumor following cardiac myxoma [7]. Similarly, the majority of patients with CPF are asymptomatic on presentation, however may present with manifestations secondary to cardioembolism (such as stroke, transient ischemic attack (TIA), myocardial infarct (MI), and angina) [8]. CPF are usually found in the perivalvular area, arising from the papillary muscles. Unlike cardiac myxoma, CPF is slightly more common in men, who account for around 55% of CPF patients. The mainstay of treatment is successful surgical excision, and this is associated with excellent prognostic outlook [7]. |
| | **Presentations** Clinical manifestations in patients symptomatic with CPF depend on the size, location, and extent of the tumor. Up to 30% of CPF are identified incidentally or on autopsy of patients without previous symptoms or findings suggestive of CPF [7]. Overt clinical signs and symptoms in CPF are typically due to embolization of CPF fragments or associated thrombi, and therefore it is unsurprising that the most commonly associated clinical syndromes include stroke, TIA, syncope, angina, MI, and sudden cardiac death. Though the risk factors and underlying pathogenesis associated with CPF remain elusive, it is thought that CPF results from acquired rather than congenital processes, such as viral or traumatic causes [7,9]. |
| | Physical examination of a patient with CPF is unlikely to reveal any telltale signs; however, if cardioembolism secondary to CPF has occurred, stigmata of neurological, peripheral vascular, coronary, or mesenteric ischemia may result. It is likely that on investigation of the underlying cause of such manifestations CPF may then be identified and subsequently managed [10]. |
| | **Investigations** Bearing in mind the rarity of CPF, and the fact that CPF patients may present with more "urgent" syndromes, it is more likely that CPF is uncovered incidentally during investigations during follow-up for, for example, a stroke or MI. |

> **Box 19.2 There are a range of known benign cardiac masses, the majority of which are benign tumors that are exceedingly rare in modern practice. Hence, an appreciation of their surgical features (namely, presentation, approach to imaging, visual appearance, and tissue characterization) is beneficial—Cont'd**

| Entity | Description |
|---|---|
| | It is perhaps because of this paradox that echocardiography is the most commonly used imaging modality for the detection of CPF—not only is it widely indicated in patients presenting with such syndromes, but it also allows robust assessment of CPF location, attachment point, mobility, and morphology [11]. |
| | CPF tumors are, on average, 12.1 × 9.0 mm, but this ranges from 1 × 1 mm to 21 × 17 mm [12]. Due to their relatively small size, initial identification on TTE should be followed up with TEE and specialist imaging modalities such as CMR [13]. TTE for CPF, though perhaps useful as a first-line screening tool, is associated with suboptimal sensitivity as it fails to detect up to 38% of cases, while TEE on the other hand detects 15% more cases and misses only 23.4% thereof [7]. On echocardiography, CPF appears with speckled echolucencies and simmers when intracardiac blood brushes against the tumor [7]. |
| | CT and CMR can subsequently characterize the tumor. On CMR, CPF is usually seen as a small, well-defined mobile nodule (notably the small size and mobility of CPF attenuates the efficacy of plain MRI in its diagnosis) and should appear similar in color to nearby myocardium on T1/T2-weighted imaging [14]. |
| | **Surgical features** <br> Successful surgical resection of CPF is usually curative as recurrence is rare. Tumors >10 mm, overt symptoms, previous embolic events, and excessive tumor mobility are indications for open surgical excision. The role of anticoagulation in the management of CPF remains unclear [7]. |
| | The surgical appearance of CPF grossly features a centralized core with extensive radiating fronds, composed of a myxomatous core with elastic tissue [7]. |
| Lipoma | **Overview** <br> Cardiac lipoma is a rare entity that mostly effects patients between the ages of 40 and 60 years old. It features proliferation of mature adipocytes, which then infiltrate into the myocardium and lead to downstream problems, for example refractory arrhythmias and sudden death [15]. Approximately half of all cardiac lipoma cases are thought to originate from the subendocardium, while the remaining 50% are thought to arise |

*Continued*

**Box 19.2 There are a range of known benign cardiac masses, the majority of which are benign tumors that are exceedingly rare in modern practice. Hence, an appreciation of their surgical features (namely, presentation, approach to imaging, visual appearance, and tissue characterization) is beneficial—Cont'd**

| Entity | Description |
|--------|-------------|
| | from either the subepicardium or the myocardium itself. Cardiac lipomas are most often found in either the right atrium or left ventricle [16]. |

**Presentation**

The majority of patients with cardiac lipoma lack overt symptoms, therefore identification is usually incidental. Depending on the size and location of the neoplasm, cardiovascular symptoms such as chest tightness, dyspnea, or orthopnea may manifest, and ECG changes such as premature complexes, ventricular arrhythmias, or junctional rhythms may also be observed [15]. On auscultation a tumor plop may be heard, similar to that which might be heard in cases of atrial myxoma.

**Investigations**

TTE remains the imaging modality of choice for invasive lipoma and can detect the size, shape, location, boundaries, and mobility of the tumor. In addition, the investigating physician should bear in mind the propensity for cardiac lipoma to cause associated aneurysmal dilation as well as its relationship with surrounding tissues. Hemodynamic changes resulting from cardiac lipoma may also be observed on TTE; however, TTE cannot conclusively differentiate between cardiac lipomas and other primary tumors such as LHIS [15,17].

TEE provides the clinician with enhanced view and should be done prior to intervention to confirm findings on TTE, and thereby further aid in surgical decision making.
CMR can be used to provide tissue characterization: increased T1-weighted signaling with septations within the mass should be observed [15].

Further, TEE may guide biopsy which will enable differentiation between cardiac lipoma, LHIS, and more importantly, to rule out well-differentiated liposarcoma. Finally, preoperative CT angio is useful to determine the relationship between the cardiac lipoma and coronary vasculature [15,17].

**Histology**

Histologically, cardiac lipomas are usually composed of mature adipocytes within a lipomatous capsule, with the absence of soft

> **Box 19.2 There are a range of known benign cardiac masses, the majority of which are benign tumors that are exceedingly rare in modern practice. Hence, an appreciation of their surgical features (namely, presentation, approach to imaging, visual appearance, and tissue characterization) is beneficial—Cont'd**

| Entity | Description |
|---|---|
| | tissue components (which would suggest liposarcoma instead) and limited myocyte infiltration. Liposarcoma should also be ruled out by negative MDM2 gene amplification [18]. |
| Lipomatous hypertrophy Fig. 19.8 | **Overview**<br>Lipomatous hypertrophy of the interventricular septum (LHIS) is an extremely rare entity, distinct from cardiac lipoma. There have hitherto been only a few case reports available in the literature. The disease process involves aberrant hypertrophy of adipocytes within the interventricular septum, without the presence of a lipomatous capsule, and with marked muscle fiber involvement. Notably, the majority of such cases are diagnosed at the postmortem stage [19,20].<br><br>**Presentation**<br>Similar to almost all other benign cardiac masses, patients with LHIS are often asymptomatic and detection is incidental at postmortem. Unlike intracavitary masses such as CPF, the intramural nature of LHIS means that the likelihood of cardioembolic events is low, and symptomatology associated with LHIS more likely involves insult to cardiac mechanics and conduction. Unsurprisingly therefore, the most common manifestations of LHIS include atrial fibrillation, premature complexes, supraventricular arrhythmias, junctional arrhythmias, or mild orthopnea. In the absence of such signs, the detection of LHIS is usually incidental [20].<br><br>**Investigations**<br>Initial investigations may reveal signs consistent with diminished cardiac output, in cases where LHIS has led to in/outflow obstruction or restricts myocardial contractility. The 12-lead ECG often reveals Wolff-Parkinson-White patterns, as well as the previously mentioned arrhythmias [19]. This results from the neoplasm's injurious effect on the cardiac conduction system. TTE may reveal a hyperechogenic mass within the interventricular septum, with or without outflow tract obstruction. Delineation of said mass is usually achieved via CMR, providing good imaging data on the degree of mixing between adipose and muscular tissue. LHIS appears as a hyperintense mass on T1-weighted CMR [19,21]. |

*Continued*

**Box 19.2 There are a range of known benign cardiac masses, the majority of which are benign tumors that are exceedingly rare in modern practice. Hence, an appreciation of their surgical features (namely, presentation, approach to imaging, visual appearance, and tissue characterization) is beneficial—Cont'd**

| Entity | Description |
|--------|-------------|
| | Prior to surgical intervention, CT angiography should be undertaken to establish the relationship between the mass and coronary blood supply, and biopsy should be considered if CMR is not able to distinguish between LHIS and cardiac lipoma. Finally, preoperative TEE should also be done to confirm the location and extent of the neoplasm, and the effect thereof on cardiac mechanics [15]. |
| | **Surgical features**<br>Following median sternotomy and establishment of CPB, open excision may proceed via right atriotomy followed by ventriculotomy. It is not uncommon for LHIS tumors to be removed piece by piece, depending on the degree to which the adipose tissue and muscle tissue intermix. Reconstruction of the septum and valve repair are also likely to be required. Notably, resection can be avoided in patients without symptoms, or with low risk of malignancy [19–21]. |
| | **Tissue characterization**<br>The cardinal features of LHIS that differentiate it from cardiac lipoma are the absence of a capsule, and tendency for there to be a mixture of brown and white adipose tissue within the neoplasm, intermixed with hypertrophied myocytes and fibrous tissues [19]. |
| Rhabdomyoma Figs. 19.9 and 19.10 | **Overview**<br>Rhabdomyoma is considered the most common fetal cardiac tumor, accounting for up to 90% of tumors in the pediatric population [22]. Rhabdomyoma, although extremely rare in the general population, is commonly found in those with the autosomal genetic condition tuberous sclerosis complex (TSC). Some studies have found that nearly 90% of children with TSC will have several rhabdomyomas [23,24]. Rhabdomyomas are seen readily after 20 weeks of gestation and enlarge significantly during the second half of pregnancy [24]. The majority of cardiac rhabdomyomas are asymptomatic and have a natural history of spontaneous regression. They are typically found in the ventricles, where they can compromise ventricular function and outflow [24,25]. Due to asymptomatic nature and natural history |

---

**Box 19.2 There are a range of known benign cardiac masses, the majority of which are benign tumors that are exceedingly rare in modern practice. Hence, an appreciation of their surgical features (namely, presentation, approach to imaging, visual appearance, and tissue characterization) is beneficial—Cont'd**

| Entity | Description |
|--------|-------------|
|  | of the condition, surgery is commonly reserved for symptomatic patients with significant hemodynamic obstruction [26].<br><br>**Presentation**<br>Rhabdomyomas are generally asymptomatic and therefore do not cause symptoms or hemodynamic compromise in the vast majority of patients [24]. Clinical symptoms are largely related to the tumor size and location within the heart [26]. Tumors of the ventricles can compromise ventricular function by obstructing inflow and outflow in addition to interfering with valvular function [25]. Arrhythmias, common in patients suffering from TSC, may result from rhabdomyoma tumor tissue connecting atria to ventricle [24,27]. Clinically, the presentation of arrhythmia in these patients can be extremely varied but may include fatigue, syncope (commonly confused with "drop seizures"), bradycardia, and palpitations [24].<br><br>**Investigations**<br>Prenatal ultrasound can be used as an important imaging modality. It can detect the presence of rhabdomyomas commonly after 20 weeks of gestation. Rhabdomyomas are thought to develop earlier than this; however, we are currently limited by the technical limits of ultrasonography [24,28]. Echocardiography, however, is the imaging modality of choice for assessing cardiac involvement in TSC [24]. It has high sensitivity with studies showing 75%–80% of rhabdomyomas satisfy criteria for TSC postnatally [28,29]. Typically, rhabdomyomas are seen as multiple, echogenic, nodular masses which appear homogenous and hyperechoic compared with normal myocardium. Doppler echocardiography can also be used to assess the hemodynamic gradient across outflow tracts. This is an important tool for indicating surgery. MRI can also be used as an adjunct to echocardiography when and where the diagnosis of rhabdomyoma using echocardiography is unclear. Ultrasound is not commonly used; however if used, rhabdomyomas may be seen as solid hyperechoic masses [24].<br><br>**Surgical features**<br>Due to the natural history of spontaneous regression and asymptomatic nature of the tumor, surgical resection is not required in the vast majority of infants. Surgery is often reserved only for symptomatic patients with significant hemodynamic obstruction, with only a proportion of the 2%–5% of patients who |

*Continued*

| Box 19.2 There are a range of known benign cardiac masses, the majority of which are benign tumors that are exceedingly rare in modern practice. Hence, an appreciation of their surgical features (namely, presentation, approach to imaging, visual appearance, and tissue characterization) is beneficial—Cont'd | |
|---|---|
| **Entity** | **Description** |
| | present with heart failure requiring surgery [26,30]. The goal of surgical excision is to provide immediate relief to acute outflow obstruction [26]. Tumors are equally distributed between left, right, and septal myocardium [24,26]. Surgical treatment for right ventricular outflow obstruction can be achieved via access through the tricuspid valve or via a right ventriculostomy if adequate resection through tricuspid valve is unattainable. Treatment of left ventricular outflow is more surgically challenging as the approach through aortic valve is limited by size of aortic annulus [26,31–33]. Having said this, excellent short- and long-term results have been reported in multiple papers, suggesting the strength of surgical intervention [26,34,35]. |
| | **Tissue characteristics**<br>Macroscopically, rhabdomyomas are yellow-tan in color, solid, well circumscribed, and nonencapsulated lesions. These cells are derived from embryonal myoblast [36]. Immunochemistry shows skeletal muscle differentiation with desmin and myoglobin and occasionally these cells may also express alpha smooth muscle actin or s100 receptor [37]. Microscopically rhabdomyomas have a pathognomonic spider cell-like appearance with cytoplasmic strands of glycogen extending into the plasma membrane [24,36]. Fetal rhabdomyomas show no obvious nuclear atypia and necrosis in contrast to adult rhabdomyomas [37]. |
| Rhabdomyoma Figs. 19.9 and 19.10 | **Overview**<br>Fibroma is the second most common primary cardiac tumor in children, after rhabdomyomas [38]. Fibroma is a fibroblast-rich tumor with intervening collagen and connective tissue, which is often extremely large in size. These tumors most commonly arise in the left ventricular free wall but they also can be found in the interventricular septum or right ventricular free wall [39]. These tumors are rarely asymptomatic and do not regress spontaneously unlike rhabdomyomas.<br><br>**Presentation**<br>Patients can present asymptomatically or symptomatically. Common symptoms include dyspnea, syncope, fatigue, chest pain, angina, and palpitations [39,40]. |

> **Box 19.2 There are a range of known benign cardiac masses, the majority of which are benign tumors that are exceedingly rare in modern practice. Hence, an appreciation of their surgical features (namely, presentation, approach to imaging, visual appearance, and tissue characterization) is beneficial—Cont'd**

| Entity | Description |
|---|---|
|  | On clinical examination, arrhythmias such as ventricular fibrillation and ventricular tachycardia are commonly observed in these patients [38,41]. This is seen when the tumor involves the interventricular septum, inducing conduction defects [42]. Cardiac fibromas are occasionally hemodynamically significant, obstructing ventricular inflow and outflow, resulting in valvular dysfunction, congestive heart failure, and sudden death. Heart murmurs are also commonly observed in this subgroup of patients [38,40,42,43]. In contrast to myxoma and fibroelastoma, cardiac fibromas rarely cause embolic phenomena and rarely regress spontaneously unlike rhabdomyoma [41,44].<br><br>**Investigations**<br>TTE, CT, or MRI can be used as initial diagnostic modality depending on initial presentation as TTE (echocardiography) is a noninvasive, fast, and less expensive tool which is often used in the initial diagnosis of fibromas. In addition to providing information on tumor size, location, and surrounding structures, it can also provide information on ventricular and valvular function [45]. MRI and CT help define tissue characteristic and extent of tissue involvement [40]. On T1-weighted images the tumor appears isointense and hypointense (fibrous nature) on T2-weighted imaging, a distinct feature of fibroma, uncommon in other cardiac tumors [46–48]. In CT imaging, cardiac fibromas appear as homogenous soft tissue masses, with calcification seen in approximately 25% of cases, another key finding which may further suggest fibroma [46]. As a result of the avascular nature of the tumor, fibromas show late hyperenhancement, 7–10 min after administration of contrast, during perfusion imaging [48].<br><br>**Surgical features**<br>Fibromas are classically single tumors and range from 2 to 10 cm in size [46]. Surgical resection is currently recommended in symptomatic fibromas; however, there is growing consensus that this should be extended to asymptomatic patients [45]. Surgical resection is a curative treatment that has been shown to alleviate the need for defibrillator and long-term antiarrhythmic medications [38]. Resection is associated with low operative morbidity and mortality and excellent mean survival [38,49]. Median sternotomy using CPB with aortic cross clamping creates a bloodless operative field. An incision is then created on |

*Continued*

> **Box 19.2 There are a range of known benign cardiac masses, the majority of which are benign tumors that are exceedingly rare in modern practice. Hence, an appreciation of their surgical features (namely, presentation, approach to imaging, visual appearance, and tissue characterization) is beneficial—Cont'd**

| Entity | Description |
| --- | --- |
| | the ventricular wall, allowing access to the tumor. The borders of fibroma can be easily identified, allowing a plane to be readily developed by sharp dissection. After resection of the tumor, the defect can either be closed by primary repair (small defects) or by patch repair (suitable for larger defects). Patch repair prevents distortion of tissue and excessive reduction of ventricular cavity, which may cause heart failure [40,45]. |
| | **Tissue characteristics** |
| | Fibromas are well defined, solitary, firm gray-white neoplasms that are often partially calcified and without a tumor. Microscopically, they feature collections of spindle-shaped fibroblasts interspersed with abundant collagen and elastic fibers. Fibromas have low cellularity and therefore have large extracellular spaces [45,46]. Fibromas, unlike other primary cardiac tumors, have no foci of cystic change or necrosis with occasional aggregates of lymphocytes and sparse inflammation at the junction between tumors and uninvolved myocardium [38,50]. These cells show myofibroblast differentiation and are positive for vimentin and smooth muscle actin. However, they are negative for CD34, S100, and HMB45 [43,51]. |

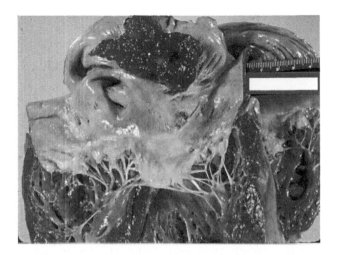

**FIG. 19.3**

Cardiac myxoma in left atrium attached to the mid-interatrial septum in the fossa ovalis region by a narrow stalk. The tumor can prolapse into the mitral orifice during diastolic phase of each cardiac contractile cycle. The mitral valve is normal.

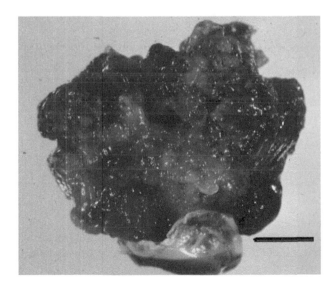

**FIG. 19.4**

Left atrial myxoma excised with segment of interatrial septum encompassing the attachment site of the narrow stalk of the pedunculated lesion. Magnification bar equals 1 cm.

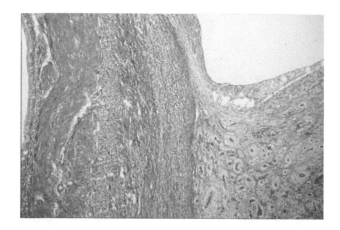

**FIG. 19.5**

Low magnification photomicrograph showing attachment of narrow base of myxoma to interatrial septum.

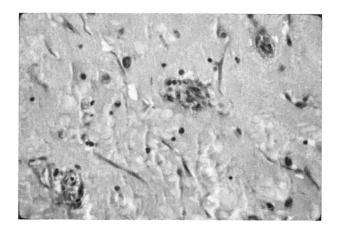

**FIG. 19.6**

High magnification photomicrograph showing typical cytological features of myxoma featuring myxoma cells (lepidic cells) as single cells and nests in abundant myxoid stroma. (Hematoxylin and eosin-stained sections).

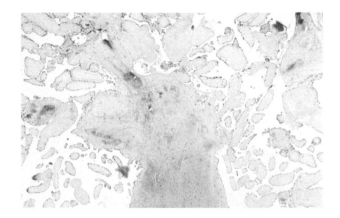

**FIG. 19.7**

Papillary fibroelastoma of the aortic valve: note the central stalk giving rise to multiple papillary fronds composed of collagen and elastin *(dark areas)*. Stained for elastic tissue.

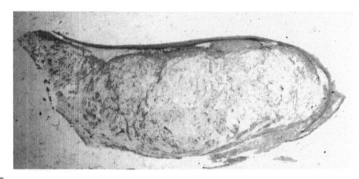

**FIG. 19.8**

Resected portion of a lipomatous hypertrophy of the interatrial septum. The interatrial septum here is thickened greatly by adipocytes.

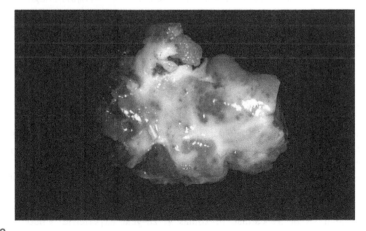

**FIG. 19.9**

Cardiac rhabdomyoma: a hamartoma that occurs exclusively in the heart as single or multiple nodules composed of altered cardiac myocytes with large vacuoles and abundant intracellular glycogen. Strongly associated with TSC.

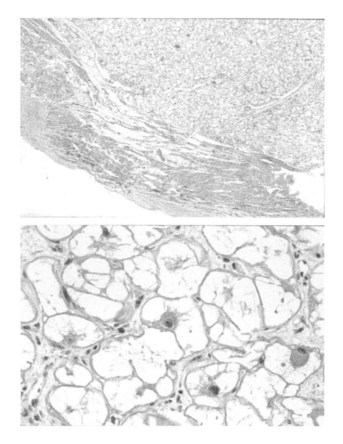

**FIG. 19.10**

Photomicrographs of cardiac rhabdomyoma. The mass is composed of large vacuolated "spider cells" which are aberrant cells of striated muscle origin. At higher magnification, these spider cells exhibit central nucleus and strands of sarcoplasm between large glycogen-rich vacuolated areas. Low and high magnification photomicrographs. Hematoxylin and eosin-stained sections.

## References

[1] Edwards A, Bermudez C, Piwonka G, Berr ML, Zamorano J, Larrain E, Franck R, Gonzalez M, Alvarez E, Maiers E. Carney's syndrome: complex myxomas. Report of four cases and review of the literature. Cardiovasc Surg 2002;10(3):264–75.

[2] Pinede L, Duhaut P, Loire R. Clinical presentation of left atrial cardiac myxoma: a series of 112 consecutive cases. Medicine 2001;80(3):159–72.

[3] Acebo E, Val-Bernal JF, Gomez-Roman JJ, Revuelta JM. Clinicopathologic study and DNA analysis of 37 cardiac myxomas: a 28-year experience. Chest 2003;123(5):1379–85.

[4] Lee KS, Kim GS, Jung Y, Jeong IS, Na KJ, Oh BS, Ahn BH, Oh SG. Surgical resection of cardiac myxoma—a 30-year single institutional experience. J Cardiothorac Surg 2017;12(1):1–6.

[5] McAllister HA, Fenoglio JJ. Tumors of the cardiovascular system. Washington: Armed Forces Institute of Pathology; 1978.

[6] Robins SL, Cotran RS, Kumar V. Pathologic basis of disease. Philadelphia, London and Toronto: WB Saunders Company; 1979. p. 1333.

[7] Lak HM, Kerndt CC, Unai S, Maroo A. Cardiac papillary fibroelastoma originating from the coumadin ridge and review of literature. BMJ Case Rep 2020;13(8), e235361.

[8] Sung JP, Asher CR, Yang XS, Cheng GG, Scalia GM, Massed AG. Clinical and echocardiographic characteristics of papillary fibroelastomas. Circulation 2001;103: 2687–93.

[9] Lodhi AM, Nguyen T, Bianco C, Movahed A. Coumadin ridge: an incidental finding of a left atrial pseudotumor on transthoracic echocardiography. World J Clin Cases 2015;3(9):831.

[10] Lestuzzi C. Primary tumors of the heart. Curr Opin Cardiol 2016;31(6):593–8.

[11] Gowda RM, Khan IA, Nair CK, Mehta NJ, Vasavada BC, Sacchi TJ. Cardiac papillary fibroelastoma: a comprehensive analysis of 725 cases. Am Heart J 2003;146(3):404–10.

[12] Klarich KW, Enriquez-Sarano M, Gura GM, Edwards WD, Tajik AJ, Seward JB. Papillary fibroelastoma: echocardiographic characteristics for diagnosis and pathologic correlation. J Am Coll Cardiol 1997;30(3):784–90.

[13] Akay MH, Sciffert M, Ott DA. Papillary fibroelastoma of the aortic valve as a cause of transient ischemic attack. Tex Heart Inst J 2009;36(2):158.

[14] Hoey ET, Shahid M, Ganeshan A, Baijal S, Simpson H, Watkin RW. MRI assessment of cardiac tumours: part 1, multiparametric imaging protocols and spectrum of appearances of histologically benign lesions. Quant Imaging Med Surg 2014;4(6):478.

[15] D'Souza J, Shah R, Abbass A, Burt JR, Goud A, Dahagam C. Invasive cardiac lipoma: a case report and review of literature. BMC Cardiovasc Disord 2017;17(1):1–4.

[16] Ismail I, Al-Khafaji K, Mutyala M, Aggarwal S, Cotter W, Hakim H, Khosla S, Arora R. Cardiac lipoma. J Community Hosp Intern Med Perspect 2015;5(5):28449.

[17] Barbuto L, Ponsiglione A, Del Vecchio W, Altiero M, Rossi G, De Rosa D, Pisani A, Imbriaco M. Humongous right atrial lipoma: a correlative CT and MR case report. Quant Imaging Med Surg 2015;5(5):774.

[18] Kashima T, Halai D, Ye H, Hing SN, Delaney D, Pollock R, O'donnell P, Tirabosco R, Flanagan AM. Sensitivity of MDM2 amplification and unexpected multiple faint alphoid 12 (alpha 12 satellite sequences) signals in atypical lipomatous tumor. Mod Pathol 2012;25(10):1384–96.

[19] Vaidya Y, Green G. Lipomatous hypertrophy of the interventricular septum. J Card Surg 2020;35(7):1740–2.

[20] Heyer CM, Kagel T, Lemburg SP, Bauer TT, Nicolas V. Lipomatous hypertrophy of the interatrial septum: a prospective study of incidence, imaging findings, and clinical symptoms. Chest 2003;124(6):2068–73.

[21] Rocha RV, Butany J, Cusimano RJ. Adipose tumors of the heart. J Card Surg 2018;33(8):432–7.

[22] Grebenc M, Rosado de Christenson M, Burke A, Green C, Galvin J. Primary cardiac and pericardial neoplasms: radiologic-pathologic correlation. Radiographics 2000;20(4): 1073–103.

[23] Harding C, Pagon R. Incidence of tuberous sclerosis in patients with cardiac rhabdomyoma. Am J Med Genet 1990;37(4):443–6.

[24] Hinton R, Prakash A, Romp R, Krueger D, Knilans T. Cardiovascular manifestations of tuberous sclerosis complex and summary of the revised diagnostic criteria and surveillance and management recommendations from the international tuberous sclerosis consensus group. J Am Heart Assoc 2014;3(6).

[25] Geva T, Santini F, Pear W, Driscoll S, Van Praagh R. Cardiac rhabdomyoma. Chest 1991;99(1):139–42.

[26] Black M, Kadletz M, Smallhorn J, Freedom R. Cardiac rhabdomyomas and obstructive left heart disease: histologically but not functionally benign. Ann Thorac Surg 1998;65 (5):1388–90.

[27] Venugopalan P, Babu J, Al-Bulushi A. Right atrial rhabdomyoma acting as the substrate for Wolff-Parkinson-white syndrome in a 3-month-old infant. Acta Cardiol 2005;60 (5):543–5.

[28] Tworetzky W, McElhinney D, Margossian R, Moon-Grady A, Sallee D, Goldmuntz E, et al. Association between cardiac tumors and tuberous sclerosis in the fetus and neonate. Am J Cardiol 2003;92(4):487–9.

[29] Bader R, Chitayat D, Kelly E, Ryan G, Smallhorn J, Toi A, et al. Fetal rhabdomyoma: prenatal diagnosis, clinical outcome, and incidence of associated tuberous sclerosis complex. J Pediatr 2003;143(5):620–4.

[30] Foster E, Spooner E, Farina M, Shaher R, Alley R. Cardiac rhabdomyoma in the neonate: surgical management. Ann Thorac Surg 1984;37(3):249–53.

[31] Luciani G, Faggian G, Consolaro G, Graziani S, Martignoni G, Mazzucco A. Pulmonary valve origin of pedunculated rhabdomyoma causing moderate right ventricular outflow obstruction: surgical-implications. Int J Cardiol 1993;41(3):233–6.

[32] Giamberti A, Giannico S, Squitieri C, Iorio F, Amodeo A, Carotti A, et al. Neonatal pulmonary autograft implantation for cardiac tumor involving aortic valve. Ann Thorac Surg 1995;59(5):1219–21.

[33] Jacobs J, Konstantakos A, Holland F, Herskowitz K, Ferrer P, Perryman R. Surgical treatment for cardiac rhabdomyomas in children. Ann Thorac Surg 1994;58(5):1552–5.

[34] Mda M, Gow R, Haney I, Mawson J, Williams W, Freedom R. Pediatric primary benign cardiac tumors: a 15-year review. Am Heart J 1997;134(6):1107–14.

[35] Takach TJ, Reul GJ, Ott DA, Cooley DA. Primary cardiac tumors in infants and children: immediate and long-term operative results. Ann Thorac Surg 1996;62(2):559–64. 8694623.

[36] El-Feky M, Weerakkody Y. Cardiac rhabdomyoma. Radiopaediaorg; 2009.

[37] Skeletal SR, Tumors M. Bone and soft tissue pathology; 2010. p. 131–45.

[38] Rajput FA, Bishop MA, Limaiem F. Cardiac fibroma. In: StatPearls. Treasure Island, FL: StatPearls Publishing; 2021. 30725766.

[39] Parmley L, Salley R, Williams J, Head G. The clinical spectrum of cardiac fibroma with diagnostic and surgical considerations: noninvasive imaging enhances management. Ann Thorac Surg 1988;45(4):455–65.

[40] Cho J, Danielson G, Puga F, Dearani J, McGregor C, Tazelaar H, et al. Surgical resection of ventricular cardiac fibromas: early and late results. Ann Thorac Surg 2003;76(6): 1929–34.

[41] Miyake C, Del Nido P, Alexander M, Cecchin F, Berul C, Triedman J, et al. Cardiac tumors and associated arrhythmias in pediatric patients, with observations on surgical therapy for ventricular tachycardia. J Am Coll Cardiol 2011;58(18):1903–9.

[42] Chen Y, Sun J, Chen W, Peng Y, An Q. Third-degree atrioventricular block in an adult with a giant cardiac fibroma. Circulation 2013;127(13).

[43] Zheng X, Song B. Left ventricle primary cardiac fibroma in an adult: a case report. Oncol Lett 2018;16:5463–5.

[44] Elderkin R, Radford D. Primary cardiac tumours in a paediatric population. J Paediatr Child Health 2002;38(2):173–7.

[45] Ikegami H, Lemaire A, Gowda S, Fyfe B, Ali M, Russo M, et al. Case report: surgical resection of right ventricular cardiac fibroma in an adult patient. J Cardiothorac Surg 2021;16(1).

[46] Grunau G, Leipsic J, Sellers S, Seidman M. Cardiac fibroma in an AdultAIRP best cases in radiologic-pathologic correlation. Radiographics 2018;38(4):1022–2026.

[47] Gravina M, Casavecchia G, Totaro A, Ieva R, Macarini L, Di Biase M, et al. Left ventricular fibroma: what cardiac magnetic resonance imaging may add? Int J Cardiol 2014;176(2):e63–5.

[48] Motwani M, Kidambi A, Herzog B, Uddin A, Greenwood J, Plein S. MR imaging of cardiac tumors and masses: a review of methods and clinical applications. Radiology 2013;268(1):26.

[49] ElBardissi A, Dearani J, Daly R, Mullany C, Orszulak T, Puga F, et al. Survival after resection of primary cardiac tumors. Circulation 2008;118(14_suppl_1).

[50] Humez S, Gibier J, Recher M, Leteurtre S, Leroy X, Devisme L. Le fibrome cardiaque: une cause rare de mort subite de l'enfant. Ann Pathol 2015;35(5):445–8.

[51] Cronin B, Lynch M, Parsons S. Cardiac fibroma presenting as sudden unexpected death in an adolescent. Forensic Sci Med Pathol 2014;10(4):647–50.

# Surgical features of malignant cardiac tumors

20

**Muath Bishawi and Edward P. Chen**
*Division of Cardiothoracic Surgery, Department of Surgery, Duke University Medical Center, Durham, NC, United States*

## Key points

- Differentiating primary benign vs malignant cardiac tumors can be done using multimodal imaging as well as tissue biopsy.
- Clinical features including rapid growth, involvement of multiple cardiac chambers or structures, and local invasion are all suggestive for a malignant cardiac tumor.
- Complete tumor resection may involve complex reconstruction or the potential need for cardiac explant, tumor resection, reconstruction, and then auto-transplantation.
- The prognosis is generally poor; however, there is a survival benefit for patients undergoing surgical resection compared to those patients who do not undergo resection.
- The goals of surgery may include both an R0 resection and tumor debulking for symptomatic improvement.

Less than 10% of primary cardiac tumors are malignant, and of those the majority (75%) are sarcomas [1]. There are several important factors to consider when evaluating a malignant cardiac tumor for surgical resection. In addition, patient comorbidities, tumor involvement of multiple cardiac structures, blood supply, rapid growth with presence of necrosis, metastatic disease, and goals of resection (R0 resection vs symptomatic improvement) are important considerations which influence clinical outcome.

Multimodal imaging (CT, Cardiac MR, and Echo) is a gold standard for diagnosis, staging, and surgical planning. It is important to not only characterize the tumor with preoperative imaging but also establish an accurate diagnosis, preferably with tissue biopsy. This is critical for (a) differentiating benign from malignant histology, and (b) identifying certain malignant tumors where optimal treatments may be nonsurgical such as cardiac lymphoma [2]. Adjuvant chemotherapy may be necessary in many of these patients. Survival is poor; however, there is a benefit of surgical resection for select patients.

Multimodal Imaging Atlas of Cardiac Masses. https://doi.org/10.1016/B978-0-323-84906-7.00007-8

Modern series on these tumors focus on the advantages of combined selected cardiac resection with systemic adjuvant therapy. In some cases, a complete resection might require cardiac auto-transplantation whereby the heart is explanted, to allow full access to the posterior structures of the heart and the posterior mediastinum. Ex vivo tumor resection is completed along with any required reconstruction, and the heart is then reimplanted into the mediastinum. One of the largest series reported on 34 patients who underwent this technique [3,4]. Of those, 26 were for primary cardiac sarcomas, Overall 1-year survival for primary malignant tumors was 46%, and two-year survival was a dismal 28%. Among patients with primary malignant tumors, 19 had isolated cardiac auto-transplantation and 7 had auto-transplantation plus pneumonectomy. Operative mortality was significantly higher for patients requiring pneumonectomy. Interestingly, for primary sarcomas, survival was not impacted by the presence of microscopically positive resection [3–5].

The most common location of primary malignant cardiac tumors is either the right or left atrium. If a malignant tumor is located in the right atrium, it is most commonly an angiosarcoma. Accurate imaging is necessary to better understand tumor involvement with the tricuspid valve as well as the right ventricle (Fig. 20.1) [6] and assess potential occlusion of blood flow from the IVC or SVC, which may ultimately require palliative resections and reconstruction. Reconstruction of the right atrium and, if necessary, the inferior or superior cava with an autologous pericardium patch may prevent narrowing of these structures at the time of resection.

Overall prognosis of primary cardiac angiosarcoma is poor and only marginally improved with surgical resection [7,8]. Most of the studies comparing surgery vs nonsurgical options involve small numbers of patients and are associated with a strong selection bias, since patients undergoing surgery usually were found to have more localized disease. A significant percentage of patients with angiosarcoma present with advanced disease, where complete surgical resection is not possible [9] and incomplete resection is associated with local recurrence [10,11]. In those instances, a combination of neoadjuvant chemo/radiation therapy has been demonstrated to reduce tumor size and allow for a more complete resection [7,12]. In select patients,

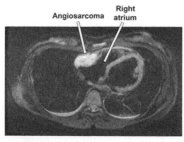 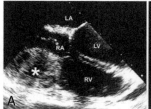 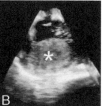

**FIG. 20.1**

MRI demonstrating an angiosarcoma in the right atrium. Further imaging with echo (A) and 3D echo (B) demonstrates possible involvement of the tricuspid valve.

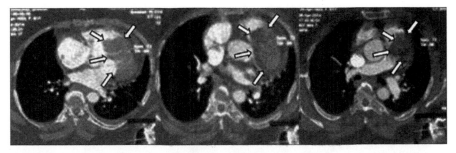

**FIG. 20.2**

CTA demonstrating a 4.3 × 3.6 cm large pleomorphic sarcoma in the right ventricle with adhesion extending into the RVOT and pulmonary artery.

an aggressive combination of resection, chemotherapy, radiation therapy, and even cardiac transplantation for nonresectable disease has been attempted [13].

In the left atrium, the most common malignant tumors are pleomorphic sarcomas [14] (malignant fibrous histiocytoma) and leiomyosarcoma [15] (Fig. 20.2). Leiomyosarcomas are extremely rare with only a limited number of cases reported in the literature. In one report, a 24-year-old patient was found to have a left atrial leiomyosarcoma involving both the interatrial septum and the right atrial free wall [15]. The patient underwent two surgical excisions followed by adjuvant radiation and chemotherapy resulting in a nearly 7-year survival (Fig. 20.3).

Rhabdomyosarcoma is another rare primary cardiac tumor and thought to be the most frequent cardiac malignancy in infants and children. It is aggressive and associated with rapid growth with involvement of multiple cardiac structures at the time

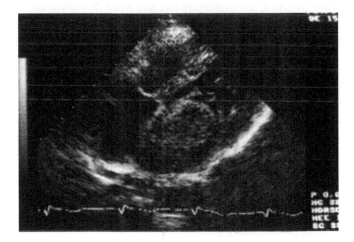

**FIG. 20.3**

Echocardiogram showing a 5 × 4.5 cm left atrial (LA) mass arising from the interatrial septum, occupying the atrial cavity and the mitral valve orifice.

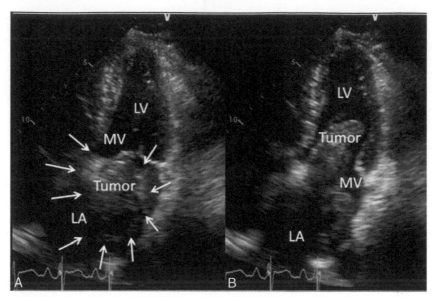

**FIG. 20.4**

(A) Echocardiography demonstrating a large mass in the left atrium. (B) Left atrial tumor involvement with the mitral valve orifice.

of presentation. In one recent case report, a 49-year-old patient underwent surgery for a biatrial cardiac rhabdomyosarcoma [16] and was found to have recurrence at eight months (Fig. 20.4). This patient then received salvage chemotherapy which was not tolerated and ultimately died 13 months after surgical resection.

Nonvascular sarcomas are even more rare and when diagnosed are generally very aggressive and invasive. Cardiac lymphomas are similarly rare, representing 5% of primary cardiac malignancies. Typical findings include a pericardial effusion upon diagnosis, and treatment is typically nonsurgical chemotherapy or radiation [17].

Finally, pericardial mesothelioma has been reported and generally presents as pericardial thickening, pericardial constriction, and pericardial effusion. In one case report, a 70-year-old woman presented with dyspnea and was found to have a large pericardial effusion on echo and a hyperenhancing mass in the pericardium [18]. Cardiac MRI and positron emission tomography/computed tomography showed invasion of the pericardial mass into the adjacent tissues and distant metastases (Fig. 20.5). In this patient, the diagnosis was confirmed by biopsy of a metastatic lesion. In another report, a 44-year-old patient presented with similar symptoms and was found to have constrictive pericarditis with a mass-like lesion [19] (Fig. 20.6). This patient underwent pericardiectomy and postoperative chemotherapy with a good early postoperative outcome.

Given the rarity of malignant cardiac tumors, it is difficult to fully establish guidelines or criteria to follow in determining which patients should undergo surgical resection vs nonsurgical management. Furthermore, retrospective series from large

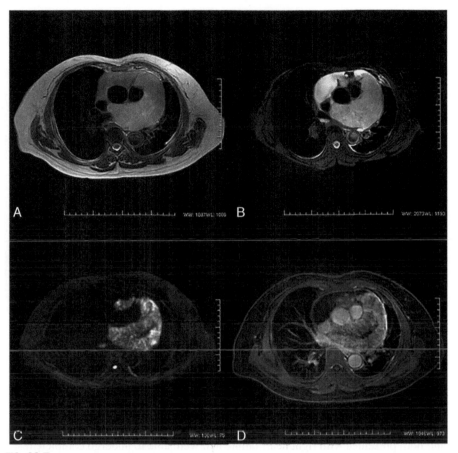

**FIG. 20.5**

Cardiac magnetic resonance imaging. (A) T2-weighted imaging showed an irregular mass in the pericardium. (B) The signal intensity of the mass was hyperintense on T2-weighted imaging with fat suppression. (C) The diffusion-weighted image was hyperintense. (D) The mass showed irregular enhancement with gadolinium injection on T1-weighted imaging.

medical centers typically combine malignant and nonmalignant primary cardiac tumors. As an example, Bossert and colleagues evaluated 77 patients who underwent surgical resection for primary cardiac tumors [20] and only 4 patients had malignant tumors (sarcoma). The overall outcomes of patients with malignant tumors were poor compared to those with a benign tumor. In this series, one patient with a malignant tumor was a 65-year-old female who presented with right heart failure due to a right ventricular sarcoma and died 4 days after incomplete resection. A second patient with a right atrial and right ventricular angiosarcoma had tumor invasion of the tricuspid valve requiring valve reconstruction at the time of resection. The patient also underwent chemotherapy and eventually passed from tumor progression

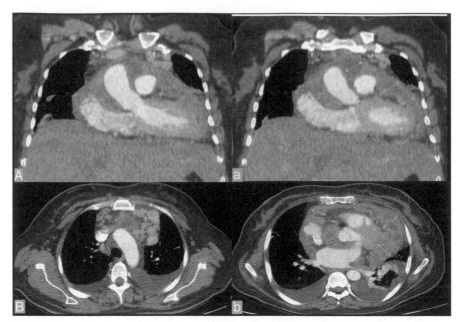

**FIG. 20.6**

Two reconstructed coronal computed tomography images (A, a) and thin section axial computed tomography images (B, b) revealed some large enhancing nodes in the left anterior mediastinum *(arrows)*, and nodular thickening of the pericardium *(double arrows)* with irregularity and enhancement associated with effusion compressing heart chambers.

after 15 months. The last two patients with malignant tumors had a leiomyosarcoma and both presented with right heart failure and were able to undergo complete resection. One patient died at 10 months from tumor progression and the other survived a 18-month follow-up period [20].

In another recent report by the Michigan group evaluating the outcomes of 39 patients with primary cardiac sarcoma [21], 14 had angiosarcoma, 10 with high-grade undifferentiated pleomorphic sarcoma, and 5 had leiomyosarcoma. The left ($n = 18$) and right ($n = 16$) atria were most commonly the primary location. At the time of presentation, 18 had metastases involving lung (10), bone (7), liver (5), and brain (4). Twenty-five patients underwent resection, and of those, an R0 resection was only achievable in 3 patients and almost all patients undergoing systemic therapy. Median overall survival was one year and there was improved survival in patients who underwent resection (14 months) compared to those who did not (8 months). Brain metastases occurred in a third of patients, and the majority of these (75%) were associated with left-sided tumors. Average survival with the presence of brain metastases was only 5.6 months [21].

In conclusion, primary malignant cardiac tumors are very rare, often presenting in a younger age population. The use of multiple imaging modalities combining echocardiography, CT, PET, and cardiac MRI is essential to characterize these tumors and evaluate the presence of metastatic disease which is often present frequent at the time of diagnosis. There appears to be a role of surgical resection combined with systemic therapy for select patients. Despite the overall poor survival of these patients, survival and symptoms appear to be improved with surgical intervention in select patients.

## References

[1] Tyebally S, Chen D, Bhattacharyya S, et al. Cardiac tumors: JACC CardioOncology state-of-the-art review. JACC CardioOncol 2020;2(2):293–311.

[2] Leja MJ, Shah DJ, Reardon MJ. Primary cardiac tumors. Texas Heart Inst J 2011;38 (3):261.

[3] Ramlawi B, Al-Jabbari O, Blau LN, et al. Autotransplantation for the resection of complex left heart tumors. Ann Thorac Surg 2014;98(3):863–8.

[4] Blackmon SH, Patel AR, Bruckner BA, et al. Cardiac autotransplantation for malignant or complex primary left-heart tumors. Texas Heart Inst J 2008;35(3):296.

[5] Reardon MJ, Malaisrie SC, Walkes JC, et al. Cardiac autotransplantation for primary cardiac tumors. Ann Thorac Surg 2006;82(2):645–50.

[6] Chen YC. Localization of angiosarcoma by peri-operative transesophageal echocardiography. Int J Card Imaging 2017;33(11):1749–51. Available from: https://link.springer.com/article/10.1007/s10554-017-1183-2.

[7] Patel SD, Peterson A, Bartczak A, et al. Primary cardiac angiosarcoma – a review. Med Sci Monit 2014;20:103.

[8] Elbardissi AW, Dearani JA, Daly RC, et al. Survival after resection of primary cardiac tumors: a 48-year experience. Circulation 2008;118(14 Suppl):S7–S15.

[9] Antonuzzo L, Rotella V, Mazzoni F, et al. Primary cardiac angiosarcoma: a fatal disease. Case Rep Med 2009;1–4. Available from: https://pubmed.ncbi.nlm.nih.gov/19724650/.

[10] Senthil Kumaran S, Asif AA, Hussain H, Chatterjee T. Pericardial angiosarcoma: a diagnostic challenge. Cureus 2021;13(5):e15350. Available from: http://www.ncbi.nlm.nih.gov/pubmed/34235027.

[11] Chaves VM, Pereira C, Andrade M, von Hafe P, Almeida JS. Cardiac angiosarcoma: from cardiac tamponade to ischaemic stroke – a diagnostic challenge. Eur J Case Rep Int Med 2019;6(4):001079. Available from http://www.ncbi.nlm.nih.gov/pubmed/31139583.

[12] Look Hong NJ, Pandalai PK, Hornick JL, et al. Cardiac angiosarcoma management and outcomes: 20-year single-institution experience. Ann Surg Oncol 2012;19(8):2707–15. Available from: https://pubmed.ncbi.nlm.nih.gov/22476752/.

[13] Centofanti P, Di Rosa E, Deorsola L, et al. Primary cardiac tumors: early and late results of surgical treatment in 91 patients. Ann Thorac Surg 1999;68(4):1236–41.

[14] Yadsar S, Abavisani M, Lakziyan R, Sarchahi Z. Right ventricular undifferentiated pleomorphic sarcoma: a case report. Ann Card Anaesth 2021;24(1):102.

[15] Pessotto R, Silvestre G, Luciani GB, et al. Primary cardiac leiomyosarcoma: seven-year survival with combined surgical and adjuvant therapy. Int J Cardiol 1997;60(1):91–4.

[16] Uchida T, Kuroda Y, Sadahiro M. Primary biatrial cardiac rhabdomyosarcoma. Braz J Cardiovasc Surg 2020;35(3):399–401. Available from: https://pubmed.ncbi.nlm.nih.gov/32549111/.

[17] Simpson L, Kumar SK, Okuno SH, et al. Malignant primary cardiac tumors. Cancer 2008;112(11):2440–6. Available from: https://onlinelibrary.wiley.com/doi/full/10.1002/cncr.23459.

[18] Liu J, Wang Z, Yang Y, et al. Multimodal diagnostic workup of primary pericardial mesothelioma: a case report. Front Cardiovasc Med 2021;8. Available from: https://pubmed.ncbi.nlm.nih.gov/34869673/.

[19] Savarrakhsh A, Vakilpour A, Davani SZN, et al. Malignant primary pericardial mesothelioma presenting as effusive constrictive pericarditis: a case report study. J Cardiothorac Surg 2021;16(1). Available from: https://pubmed.ncbi.nlm.nih.gov/34645482/.

[20] Bossert T, Gummert JF, Battellini R, et al. Surgical experience with 77 primary cardiac tumors. Interact Cardiovasc Thorac Surg 2005;4(4):311–5. Available from: https://academic.oup.com/icvts/article/4/4/311/894996.

[21] Siontis BL, Zhao L, Leja M, et al. Primary cardiac sarcoma: a rare, aggressive malignancy with a high propensity for brain metastases. Sarcoma 2019;2019. Available from: https://pubmed.ncbi.nlm.nih.gov/30962762/.

# Differential diagnosis of cardiac masses by operation view

## 21

**Sidhant Singh[a], Sven Z.C.P. Tan[a], Idhrees Mohammed[b], Saeid Hosseini[c], and Mohamad Bashir[d],***

[a]*Barts and The London School of Medicine and Dentistry, Queen Mary University of London, London, United Kingdom* [b]*Institute of Cardiac and Aortic Disorders, SRM Institutes for Medical Science, Vadapalani, Chennai, India* [c]*Rajaie Cardiovascular Medical and Research Center, Tehran, Iran* [d]*Vascular and Endovascular Surgery, Health Education and Improvement Wales, Nantgarw, Wales, United Kingdom*

## Key points

- Most patients with cardiac masses are asymptomatic; however, they may present with symptomatology and clinical signs suggestive of more common and rapidly debilitating syndromes such as angina, myocardial infarct, or cerebrovascular insufficiency. Therefore the presence of an intramural or intracavitary mass is usually detected on imaging undertaken to rule out other structural pathologies, such as valvular disease.
- A sequential approach to imaging that allows appropriate use of resources in a step-up fashion is usually undertaken, i.e., bedside modalities (such as transthoracic echocardiography) should be performed prior to more invasive and costly options such as transesophageal echocardiography or cardiac magnetic resonance imaging, as this may satisfactorily rule out the presence of such a mass.
- Each subsequent imaging modality provides useful information, which guides the decision on whether to excise the mass in question. Finally, biopsy or postexcision histopathological analysis may reveal the final diagnosis and tissue characterization.

## Box 21.1: Introduction

Cardiac masses represent a rare and complex entity that often result from metastatic cancers or more complicated disease processes. The diagnostic process often involves multidisciplinary approaches with careful multimodal imaging

---

*Senior author.

Multimodal Imaging Atlas of Cardiac Masses. https://doi.org/10.1016/B978-0-323-84906-7.00016-9

consultations. Cardiac masses can be broadly categorized into tumors, thrombi, vegetations, calcific lesions, and other rare conditions. Unlike other anatomical sites in the body, cardiac masses can have significant repercussions on blood flow obstructions, formation of emboli, and can result in electrical or mechanical dysfunction as a result of interference with the underlying anatomy. Presentations of such masses need to be viewed with a full diagnostic workup which involves clinical presentation imaging, invasive and noninvasive investigations, and long-term management considerations. These masses can be further divided into subcategories including benign and malignant primary and nonneoplastic tumors, or by the anatomical site that they occupy such as intracardial or pericardial tumors which fall under the category of cardiac masses [1].

The process of reaching a diagnosis surrounding a space occupying lesion or mass in the heart can be done as a result of symptomology or specific incidents. The majority of tumors found in the heart tend to be benign with over a 50% being a myxoma. Primary malignant tumors are very rare accounting for less than 25% of primary cardiac tumors, and in the majority of cases these would present as sarcomas. In studies performed on autopsy results, cardiac tumors are most commonly present as metastatic malignant tumors. The prevalence of first-degree cardiac tumors is 1 in 2000 whereas autopsies and autopsy studies show a ratio of 1 in 100 for metastatic tumors. This indicates a ratio of primary to secondary cardiac tumors in the range of 20 to 1. However, there is great variation among autopsy studies with ranges of the incidence of cardiac metastases from 2.3% to 18.3% in patients with extracardiac malignant tumors [1].

Multimodal cardiac imaging including transthoracic echocardiography, transesophageal echocardiography, cardiac magnetic resonance, cardiac computed tomography, and fluorodeoxypositron emission tomography have a complementary and reinforcing role in the evaluation of cardiac masses. Given the diverse range of cardiac masses that can be identified both on autopsy imaging and other forms of investigation, there are currently no strict guidelines or general consensus on the diagnostic algorithm or best diagnostic approach in identifying these masses [1].

This chapter aims to outline a classification-based approach to identifying and diagnosing each type of cardiac mass.

## Benign primary cardiac tumors

The most common type of benign cardiac tumors is myxomas which tend to present in early adulthood in the case of familial myxoma, and middle adulthood for all other types of myxoma. Myxomas are commonly located in the left atrium along the atrial septum. They are generally identified using echocardiography which shows a mildly lobar mass with heterogeneous echogenicity and are usually mobile. CT shows low attenuation with potential calcification, and CMR confirms heterogenicity. The main clinical manifestations for a myxoma include emboli, flow obstructions, and systemic symptoms [2].

Papillary fibroelastomas tend to present in middle or late adulthood and are commonly located on cardiac valves. Echocardiography tends to show a circular, pedunculated, nonprotruding mass which rarely interferes with valve function. CT also shows a smooth and pedunculated mass. CMR shows a highly mobile mass and could indicate the need for a TEE. Clinical manifestations include emboli; however, patients are usually asymptomatic [2].

Lipomas usually present during adulthood and at any site. Echocardiography shows a homogenous structure, with CT showing a smooth homogenous encapsulated structure with some fat attenuation. Clinical manifestations include arrhythmias and flow obstruction; however, most patients are usually asymptomatic [2].

Rhabdomyomas tend to present in infancy or early childhood on the ventricles or atrioventricular valves. Echocardiography will usually show a homogenous, slightly echogenic mass. CTs will show similar attenuation to intramural myocardium. Main clinical manifestations include flow obstruction, arrhythmias, and heart failure; however, patients are usually asymptomatic [2].

Fibromas tend to present in early childhood on the intraventricular septum or ventricle walls. Echocardiography shows a heterogeneous, echogenic, and noncontractible mass which can sometimes mimic hypertrophic cardiomyopathy. CT shows soft tissue attenuation with possible calcification. Patients tend to be asymptomatic; however, some may have arrhythmias [2].

Hemangiomas can present at any age and at any site. Echocardiography shows a highly echogenic mass which may resemble a cavity. CTs will show a heterogeneous mass with potential calcification and CMR confirms heterogenicity. Most patients are asymptomatic or experience low-grade dyspnea [2].

## Malignant primary cardiac tumors

Angiosarcomas tend to present during early adulthood in the right atrium or pericardium. Echocardiography shows a heterogeneous highly echogenic mass. CT confirms heterogenicity and shows low attenuation with CMR also confirming heterogenicity. Main clinical manifestations include constitutional symptoms, pericardial effusion, and heart failure [2].

Rhabdomyosarcomas usually present in childhood and in some cases very early adulthood. They can present at multiple sites but have a tendency to present in the ventricles. Echocardiography shows normal to high echodensity. CT shows irregular shape and low attenuation with CMR showing a homogenous mass. The main clinical manifestation is heart failure [2].

Myxofibrosarcomas tend to present in early to middle adulthood and can present anywhere. Echocardiography shows a heterogeneous mass with normal to high echodensity. CT and CMR confirm heterogenicity, with CT also highlighting low attenuation. The main clinical manifestations include flow obstruction, pericardial effusion, and metastases [2].

Lymphomas tend to present in adulthood on the right atrium and at other sites. Echocardiography can rarely differentiate size and shape. CT shows normal to low attenuation and a heterogeneous mass. The main clinical manifestations are pericardial effusion, flow obstruction, and heart failure [2].

Mesotheliomas tend to present in adulthood on the pericardium. Echocardiography and CMR show a heterogeneous mass and CT is able to outline the variable characteristics [2].

## Nonneoplastic cardiac masses

Clots usually occur in adulthood in the left atrial appendage and the left ventricle. Echocardiography shows low echodensity in acute clots and high echodensity in chronic clots, with CT showing possible calcification. The main clinical manifestation is an embolus [2].

Vegetations are usually found in adulthood on cardiac valves. Echocardiography shows a highly mobile, protruding mass and some valvular dysfunction. CT shows low attenuation, perivalvular extension, fistulas, and abscesses. CMR shows a highly mobile mass which may lead to consideration for TEE. Main clinical manifestations include valve dysfunction, emboli, and heart failure [2].

Nonneoplastic calcified masses usually present in adulthood and typically in the posterior mitral annulus. Echocardiography shows high echodensity, and CT shows heterogeneous calcification. Due to signal loss CMR is not useful and thus imaging is reliant on CT. Patients are usually asymptomatic [2].

Pericardial cysts are usually present in adulthood on the pericardium. Echocardiography shows low echodensity with CT showing the presence of wall and fluid attenuation. The main clinical manifestation is external compression; however, most patients are asymptomatic [2].

Lipomatous hypertrophy usually presents in late adulthood on the atrial septum. Echocardiography shows homogenous dumbbell appearance of the atrial septum, with CT showing fat attenuation. There are rarely any clinical manifestations, but some patients may experience arrhythmias [2].

## Box 21.2

The differential diagnosis by operative view of cardiac masses can be carried out using key investigations in a step-up approach. Essentially, upon initial presentation of a patient with manifestations possibly associated with an intracavitary or intramural mass, echocardiographic imaging may initially determine the presence or absence of said mass. Once the presence thereof is determined, subsequent imaging-based investigations are undertaken to explore further parameters concerning the mass, enabling the clinician to rule out other differentials in the process. Finally, once surgical intervention is undertaken, visual aspects of the mass and histopathological

Box 21.2   **321**

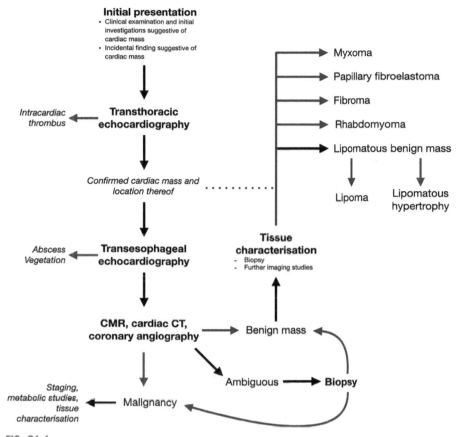

**FIG. 21.1**

Flow chart depicting the key steps in the differential diagnosis of cardiac masses via imaging modalities and biopsy. Differentiation between each benign mass is aided by history, examination, tumor location, size, and tissue characterization. Details on these individual features may be found in Chapters 19 and 20 (Native).

analysis then confirms the diagnosis. A detailed approach to each tumor's surgical and clinical features may be found in Chapters 19 and 20. Fig. 21.1 depicts a flow chart outlining the differential diagnostic approach in cardiac masses.

| Diagnostic step | Details |
|---|---|
| Initial presentation | It is crucial to bear in mind that though cardiac masses—both malignant and benign in nature—are exceedingly rare entities (for a number of reasons), they represent a considerable insult to the heart and potentiate a number of debilitating and potentially lethal adverse outcomes |

*Continued*

| Diagnostic step | Details |
|---|---|
|  | The presence or absence of clinical manifestations associated with benign and malignant cardiac masses depends primarily on the extent to which said mass effects cardiac mechanics' conduction or output. Such manifestations may include arrhythmias, pulmonary congestion, angina, dyspnea/orthopnea, or thromboembolic events [3]. Unsurprisingly, when faced with such manifestations, it is crucial to first treat the acute event prior to undertaking investigations to determine the underlying cause |
|  | As an example, patients with atrial myxoma (the most common benign cardiac mass) may exhibit clinical signs consistent with mitral valvular disease, such as pulmonary congestion, a systolic murmur (present in 50% of cases), loud S1 (in 32% of cases), diastolic murmur (15% of cases), or a "tumor plop"—a low-pitched, diastolic murmur heard as the tumor prolapses into the left ventricle [3–5]. Additionally, depending on the thrombogenicity of the tumor, patients with atrial myxoma may also exhibit stigmata of peripheral thromboembolism depending on the vasculature affected [4] |
|  | When faced with such findings, and once acute problems have either been managed or ruled out, various imaging modalities may be undertaken to confirm the presence or absence of a mass, and subsequently to determine its location, extent, effect on surrounding tissues, and to inform preoperative decision making |
| Transthoracic echocardiography (TTE) | TTE is one of the most common modalities used in the detection and diagnosis of cardiac masses, possibly because its use is widely indicated as part of the diagnosis or follow-up of cardiovascular and thromboembolic pathologies, from atrial fibrillation to valvular disease. The fact that it can be performed bedside and is relatively inexpensive, rapid, and nonirradiating (in comparison to more specialist modalities employed downstream) makes it even more useful [6] |
|  | For example, TTE allows robust assessment for patients with suspected cardiac papillary fibroelastoma (CPF), allowing the clinician to quickly establish the lesion's location, approximate size, attachment site, mobility, and morphology [7] |
|  | It should, however, be emphasized that TTE plays a facilitatory rather than determining role in the differential diagnosis of cardiac masses. It is insufficiently accurate to provide a definitive diagnosis or to fully inform surgical decision making: TTE is associated with suboptimal sensitivity—it fails to detect up to 38.1% of cases of CPF. However, TTE serves as a useful juncture to rule out acute cardiac masses (e.g., intracavitary thrombi that could |

*Continued*

Box 21.2    **323**

| Diagnostic step | Details |
|---|---|
| | readily embolize) or indeed to rule in certain comorbidities (in addition to a cardiac mass), such as heart failure or valvular disease, that may influence decisions around management and prognosis [6,7] |
| Transesophageal echocardiography (TEE) | Following the affirmative identification of an intracardiac mass, and having ruled out the presence of an intracavitary thrombus via TTE, following up with TEE may be useful to determine with more accuracy the parameters surrounding the mass in question |
| | For intracavitary masses such as CPF or atrial myxoma, TEE with contrast may elucidate the hemodynamic effects of mass, in addition to determining with greater confidence the size, mobility, and attachment point. For example, TEE is noted to detect 15% more cases of CPF, and reportedly only misses 23.4% of cases (compared to TTE, which misses up to 38.1% of cases) [7] |
| | TEE would also be useful in the identification of intramural masses, such as lipomatous hypertrophies of the interventricular septum (LHIS): septal hyperechogenicity on TEE would increase the likelihood of a patient's symptoms being caused by LHIS rather than mitral valve regurgitation or congenital outflow tract obstruction. Indeed, TEE helps to confirm the location of intramural masses and properly assess the extent to which the mass obstructs cardiac inflow/outflow [8,9] |
| | Notably, TEE-guided biopsy is particularly useful when faced with a lipomatous mass (seen on echocardiography as areas of hyperechogenicity). It is important to differentiate between LHIS and cardiac lipoma—the invasive (albeit benign) nature of LHIS puts patients at substantial risk of developing aberrant conduction or possibly obstructed outflow tracts [10] |
| Specialist imaging modalities | More specialist imaging modalities may be employed following TTE and TEE, primarily with a view of determining the extent of the cardiac mass, its delineations, relationship with surrounding tissues, and tissue characterization |
| | Cardiac magnetic resonance (CMR), for instance, provides optimal delineation of the intracardiac mass and the relationship between the mass and local myocardium—informing the decision on whether the mass can or should be excised, and what the optimal surgical approach would be. It would also inform the care team whether the mass is solid, fatty, or hemorrhagic [4]. In differentiating between cardiac lipoma and LHIS, CMR can provide useful information on the degree of mixing between adipose and muscle tissue, which would inform surgical decision making. Cardiac lipoma, for example, would show increased T1-weighted signaling on CMR and reveal the lipoma capsule and thin septations within the mass. In |

*Continued*

| Diagnostic step | Details |
|---|---|
| | contrast, LHIS would similarly appear hyperintense on CMR; however, LHIS would also feature invaginations of muscular tissue and the absence of a lipomatous capsule [9,11] Coronary angiography should similarly be undertaken preoperatively, for several reasons. Not only would it reveal the extent to which coronary circulation is compromised by the extent of the mass (allowing the care plan to be adjusted accordingly), but it would also reveal the route by which the mass is supplied by coronary circulation—allowing the surgical team to anticipate and prevent catastrophic hemorrhage during excision [8] |
| Operative view and histological analysis | Intraoperative visualization and successful excision of the cardiac mass facilitate pathological examination of the tumor, and in doing so provides definitive information tumor staging and tissue characterization For example, the characteristic appearance of a CPF with a centralized core of elastic tissue surrounded by an outer layer of radiating fronds, originating from the perivalvular papillary tissue, may well confirm the diagnosis of CPF [7,12]. However, further histochemical analysis may be required to rule out more malignant masses, for example liposarcoma should be ruled out in cases of suspected lipoma via gene amplification testing In malignant cases, functional metabolic imaging modalities may be undertaken as part of determining the malignancy's staging and aggressiveness, which would aid prognostication |

# References

[1] Basso C, Rizzo S, Valente M, Thiene G. Cardiac masses and tumours [internet]. BMJ 2021. [cited 1 November 2021]. Available from: https://heart.bmj.com/content/102/15/1230.short.

[2] Aggeli C, Dimitroglou Y, Raftopoulos L, Sarri G, Mavrogeni S, Wong J, et al. Cardiac masses: the role of cardiovascular imaging in the differential diagnosis. Diagnostics 2020;10(12):1088. Basso C, Rizzo S, Valente M, Thiene G. Cardiac masses and tumours [Internet]. BMJ. 2021 [cited 1 November 2021]. Available from: https://heart.bmj.com/content/102/15/1230.short.

[3] Pinede L, Duhaut P, Loire R. Clinical presentation of left atrial cardiac myxoma: a series of 112 consecutive cases. Medicine 2001;80(3):159–72.

[4] Edwards A, Bermudez C, Piwonka G, Berr ML, Zamorano J, Larrain E, Franck R, Gonzalez M, Alvarez E, Maiers E. Carney's syndrome: complex myxomas. Report of four cases and review of the literature. Cardiovasc Surg 2002 Jun;10(3):264–75.

[5] Acebo E, Val-Bernal JF, Gomez-Roman JJ, Revuelta JM. Clinicopathologic study and DNA analysis of 37 cardiac myxomas: a 28-year experience. Chest 2003;123 (5):1379–85.

[6] Akay MH, Seiffert M, Ott DA. Papillary fibroelastoma of the aortic valve as a cause of transient ischemic attack. Tex Heart Inst J 2009;36(2):158.

[7] Lak HM, Kerndt CC, Unai S, Maroo A. Cardiac papillary fibroelastoma originating from the coumadin ridge and review of literature. BMJ Case Reports CP 2020;13(8), e235361.

[8] Vaidya Y, Green G. Lipomatous hypertrophy of the interventricular septum. J Card Surg 2020 Jun;35(7):1740–2.

[9] Heyer CM, Kagel T, Lemburg SP, Bauer TT, Nicolas V. Lipomatous hypertrophy of the interatrial septum: a prospective study of incidence, imaging findings, and clinical symptoms. Chest 2003;124(6):2068–73.

[10] D'Souza J, Shah R, Abbass A, Burt JR, Goud A, Dahagam C. Invasive cardiac lipoma: a case report and review of literature. BMC Cardiovasc Disord 2017 Dec;17(1):1–4.

[11] Rocha RV, Butany J, Cusimano RJ. Adipose tumors of the heart. J Card Surg 2018 Aug;33(8):432–7.

[12] Sung JP, Asher CR, Yang XS, Cheng GG, Scalia GM, Massed AG. Clinical and echocardiographic characteristics of papillary fibroelastomas. Circulation 2001;103:2687–93.

# Oncologic essentials in benign cardiac masses (approach and follow-up)

# 22

## Seyyed Asadollah Mousavi and Mohammad Biglari

*Hematology-Oncology and Stem Cell Transplantation Research Center, Tehran University of Medical Sciences, Tehran, Iran*

## Key points

- Cardiac tumors consist of a diverse group of conditions with various characteristics, most of them being benign lesions
- Association of benign cardiac lesions with genetic syndromes mandates thorough evaluation of these patients
- Most common type of cardiac benign tumors is myxoma followed by fibroelastoma, rhabdomyoma, fibroma, lipoma, and other less common types
- Presentation and symptoms depend on the tumor location and histopathology, including constitutional symptoms, thromboembolism, obstructive symptoms, and arrhythmias
- Diagnosis is by echocardiography, and frequently cardiac MRI
- Treatment of benign tumors is mainly by excision or close observation

Multimodal Imaging Atlas of Cardiac Masses. https://doi.org/10.1016/B978-0-323-84906-7.00003-0

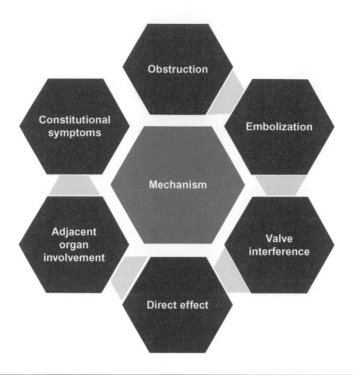

**FIG. 22.1**

Benign cardiac tumor symptom mechanisms.

Cardiac tumors cause symptoms by various means. Aortic valve and left atrial tumors are more likely to be complicated by embolization, which is mostly systemic [1]. Obstructing blood flow might result in heart failure symptoms. Valvular regurgitation is also possible if the tumor interferes with the heart valves. Though true invasion is less likely with benign tumors, direct pressure by the mass may lead to ventricular dysfunction, arrhythmias, or pericardial effusion. The pressure effect of tumor may also cause bronchogenic symptoms. Constitutional symptoms like fatigue, weakness, and light headedness are also noticeable.

**Table 22.2** Clinical manifestations of benign cardiac tumors by location [2–5].

| | Mechanism | Sign/symptom | Example |
|---|---|---|---|
| Left atrium | *Obstruction* | Dyspnea, pulmonary edema, fatigue, cough, orthopnea<br>Mitral regurgitation<br>Tumor plop<br>Stroke | Myxoma<br>Lipoma |
| | *Embolization* | | |
| Right atrium | *Obstruction* | Peripheral edema, hepatomegaly, ascites, fatigue<br>Tricuspid regurgitation<br>Pulmonary emboli | Myxoma<br>Lipoma |
| | *Embolization* | | |
| Left ventricle | *Obstruction*<br>*Embolization*<br>*Direct effect* | Heart failure<br><br>Arrhythmia | Fibroma<br>Rhabdomyoma |
| Right ventricle | *Obstruction* | Peripheral edema, hepatomegaly, ascites, syncope | Fibroma<br>Rhabdomyoma |
| Valves | *Valve interference* | Regurgitation | Fibroelastoma |

**Table 22.3** Causal association of benign cardiac tumors with genetic predispositions [6].

| Genetic syndrome | Gene involved | Inheritance | Tumor type | Association |
|---|---|---|---|---|
| Gorlin syndrome | *PTCH1* | AD | Fibroma | Nevoid basal cell carcinoma, skeletal abnormalities, medulloblastoma, meningioma |
| Carney complex | *PRKAR1A* | AD | Myxoma | Endocrine hyperfunction, skin pigmentation |
| Von Hippel–Lindau syndrome | *VHL* | AD | Paraganglioma | Renal cell carcinoma, pancreatic NET |
| Tuberous Sclerosis | *TSC1, TSC2* | AD | Rhabdomyoma | Hamartoma, brain tumors, angiomyolipoma, skin changes |

AD, *autosomal dominant;* NET, *neuroendocrine tumor.*

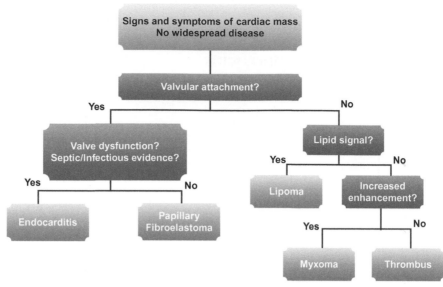

**FIG. 22.4**

Diagnostic approach to benign cardiac mass in adults [7].

*Adapted from Kilani S, Gaxotte V, Midulla M, Beregi JP. Cardiac mass: algorithms for an integrative diagnostic approach. ECR 2012; C-0729. 10.1594/ecr2012/C-0729; with permission.*

**Table 22.5** Diagnostic modalities in benign cardiac tumors [2,4,8–10].

| | Indication | Considerations |
|---|---|---|
| **Imaging** | | |
| Echocardiography | Initial study | • Direct visualization<br>• Transesophageal might be more informative<br> • Ionizing radiation |
| Cardiac CT | MRI unavailable<br>MRI prohibited | • Less expensive<br> • Slightly preferred to CT<br>• Provide clues to tumor type |
| Cardiac MRI | | • Differentiate thrombus<br>• Useful to rule out metastasis |
| PET scan | Functional assessment | |
| **Coronary angiography** | | |
| | Epicardial tumors | • Tumor blood supply delineation |
| **Biopsy** | | |
| | Unresectable or diffuse tumors | • Gold standard<br>• Risk of embolization (e.g. myxomas)<br>• Risk of perforation |

CT, *computed tomography;* MRI, *magnetic resonance imaging;* PET, *positron emission tomography.*

**Table 22.6** Benign cardiac tumor behavior in cardiac MRI [5].

| | T1 weighted | T2 weighted | LGE |
|---|---|---|---|
| Myxoma | Isointense[a] | Hyperintense | Heterogeneous |
| Lipoma | Hyperintense | Hyperintense | No uptake |
| Fibroma | Isointense | Hypointense | Hyper-enhanced |
| Rhabdomyoma | Isointense | Isointense | Minimal |

LGE, *late gadolinium enhancement;* MRI, *magnetic resonance imaging.*
[a]*Intensity compared to myocardium.*

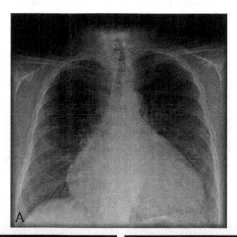

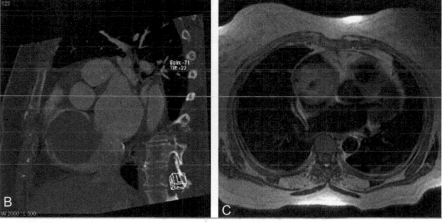

**FIG. 22.7**

Right atrial myxoma. Chest X-ray showing an enlarged cardiac silhouette accompanied by widening of the carina (A). Cardiac CT in arterial phase illustrating the enlarged heart with a low-density filling defect occupying almost the entire right atrium (B). A cardiac MRI sequence defining the intermediate intensity of the mass on T1-weighted image. This patient underwent a surgical resection and the diagnosis of atrial myxoma was established in histologic examination [11].

*Case courtesy of Assoc. Prof. Frank Gaillard, Radiopaedia.org, rID: 8544.*

Myxomas are by far the most common primary cardiac tumor and the most common benign mass of the heart. It appears as an intracavitary mass, frequently located in the left atrium and is mostly seen in middle-aged women. Diagnostic features of cardiac myxoma are thoroughly discussed in previous chapters (Chapters 8 and 14). Resection is required for a histological diagnosis but mainly to prevent major complications. Surgical intervention and simple resection is considered the only treatment and is well tolerated with an acceptable low mortality and favorable long-term prognosis. The only follow-up necessary is annual echocardiography for the first 5 years postoperatively, as nearly 10% of these tumors may reappear, typically at the primary site [5,12].

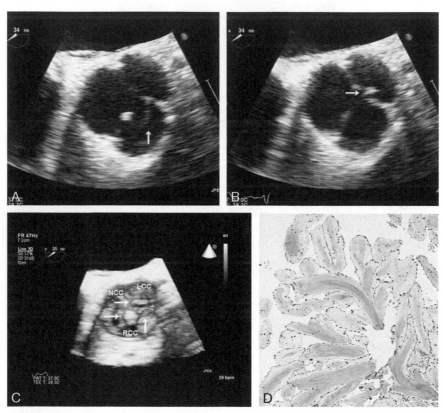

**FIG. 22.8**

Mitral valve papillary fibroelastoma. (A) Transesophageal short axis view demonstrating a hypoechoic mass adjacent to the right coronary cusp of the aortic valve (*arrow*).
(B) Transesophageal short axis view of another hyperechoic mass attached to the left coronary cusp of the aortic valve (*arrow*) in the same patient. (C) A 3D zoom transesophageal echocardiography of the aortic valve in the patient illustrating three masses attached to both noncoronary cusp and right coronary cusp of the aortic valve (*arrows*) [13]. (D) Medium power H&E stained pathology slide of fibroelastoma consisting of frondlike projections and an avascular core and a myxomatous outer region [6]. *LCC*, left coronary cusp; *RCC*, right coronary cusp; *NCC*, noncoronary cusp.

Papillary fibroelastoma is the most common tumor of heart valves and the second most common benign tumor of the heart mostly observed in the elderly. Their origin is not well understood, and their most important complication is embolization. Some experts recommend resection for all cases even the asymptomatic ones [12,14]; however, some suggest close follow-up as a reasonable approach for asymptomatic patients while the tumor is small and nonmobile with no embolic complications.

Another treatment approach is based on the location of fibroelastoma. Hence, left side tumors are generally considered for resection especially if larger than 1 cm and the patient is a good surgical candidate. On the other hand, right side tumors could be followed conservatively while they are asymptomatic and uncomplicated [5,15–17].

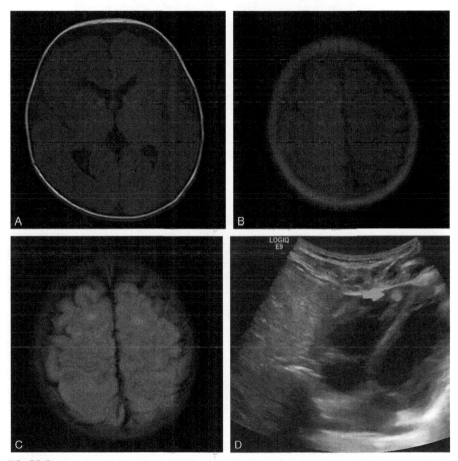

**FIG. 22.9**

Cardiac rhabdomyoma. A 3-year-old boy presented with stunted growth, seizure, and developmental delay later diagnosed with tuberous sclerosis. The axial T1W MRI sequence demonstrating multiple hyperintense subependymal nodules compatible with hamartomas (A). An axial T1W MRI sequence (B) and axial FLAIR sequence (C) showing cortical and subcortical high signal intensities defining tubers. Subxiphoid cardiac ultrasound window delineating a well-defined hyperechoic lesion attached to the right ventricular wall (D) [18].

*Case courtesy of Dr. Abdulmajid Bawazeer, Radiopaedia.org, rID: 70089.*

Rhabdomyomas are recognized as the most common primary cardiac tumor in children. It is unique in cardiac tumors because of a strong association between cardiac rhabdomyomas and tuberous sclerosis (80%). Most of these masses regress after infancy and do not require interventions. Nevertheless, rhabdomyomas with obstructive symptoms or arrhythmia have poorer prognosis and must be excised, even though complete resection might not be feasible according to their deep intramyocardial site. Serial echocardiography is essential to follow these tumors and may be the only required intervention needed [17].

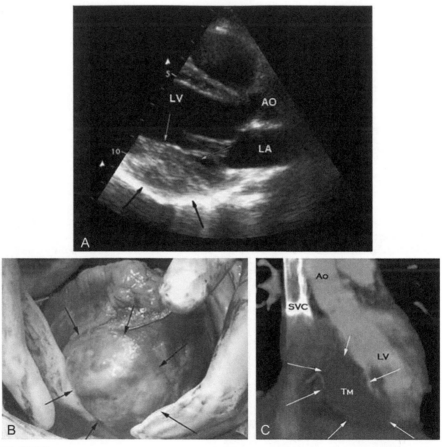

**FIG. 22.10**

Cardiac fibroma. Long axis parasternal echocardiographic view in a 21-year-old woman with no previous history and complaint of chest pain. The image shows the tumor compressing the left ventricle near to the mitral valve. *Arrows* indicate the tumor margins. (*Top*). Image of the left ventricular tumor (*bottom left*). Sagittal computed tomographic image of the tumor. The arrows demarcating the borders of the mass (*Bottom right*). *AO*, aorta; *LA*, left atrium; *LV*, left ventricle; *SVC*, superior vena cava; *TM*, tumor [19].

Fibroma is the second most prevalent primary tumor of the heart in children. They are consistently found in the ventricular myocardium. Fibromas are typically described as demarcated, hyperechoic, and solitary masses ranging from 1 to 10 cm in size [20]. They are usually symptomatic and due to the increased risk for fatal arrhythmias, surgical resection is the optimal treatment regardless of symptoms [17]. Echocardiography is recommended postoperatively, and the final outcome is generally good.

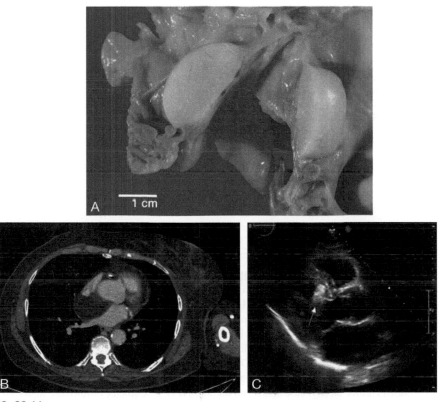

**FIG. 22.11**

Lipoma and lipomatous hypertrophy of interatrial septum. Cardiac lipoma. A gross photo of a well-demarcated yellow tumor in the right atrium with no obvious infiltration to the myocardium (A) [6]. An axial cardiac CT image with contrast showing a pericardial lipoma just next to the right heart chambers (B) [21]. An ovoid mass (*white arrow*) in the long axis view of transthoracic echocardiography in a 65-year-old man. Diagnosis of lipoma was later confirmed (C) [5]. *LA*, left atrium; *LV*, left ventricle; *RA*, right atrium; *RV*, right ventricle.

*Case courtesy of Dr. Bruno Di Muzio, Radiopaedia.org, rID: 15292.*

Lipomas are rare primary cardiac tumors of adults. They are more frequently seen in the pericardium, subendocardium, or interatrial septum. While they are mostly asymptomatic, large ones may produce cardiomegaly and dyspnea. Cardiac lipomas are well-defined, yellow and encapsulated masses of adipose tissue. Lipomatous hypertrophy, on the other hand, are nonencapsulated involving mostly the interatrial septum and seen in older patients.

The two conditions are characteristically incidental findings, and surgical intervention is required only in cases of valvular dysfunction, intractable arrhythmias, or unstable hemodynamics [12].

---

> **Box 22.12 Follow-up recommendations in benign cardiac tumors [22,23].**
>
> - Clinical examination and cardiology visit annually
> - Transthoracic echocardiography is endorsed every 2–5 years
> - Prophylactic antibiotics is recommended in case of
>   - Residual postoperative valvular dysfunction
>   - Implanted prosthetic valves or artificial materials
>   - Outflow tract obstruction

---

# References

[1] Elbardissi AW, Dearani JA, Daly RC, et al. Embolic potential of cardiac tumors and outcome after resection: a case-control study. Stroke 2009;40:156.

[2] Araoz PA, Mulvagh SL, Tazelaar HD, et al. CT and MR imaging of benign primary cardiac neoplasms with echocardiographic correlation. Radiographics 2000;20:1303.

[3] Wintersperger BJ, Becker CR, Gulbins H, et al. Tumors of the cardiac valves: imaging findings in magnetic resonance imaging, electron beam computed tomography, and echocardiography. Eur Radiol 2000;10:443.

[4] Pearman JL, Wall SL, Chen L, Rogers JH. Intracardiac echocardiographic-guided right-sided cardiac biopsy: case series and literature review. Catheter Cardiovasc Interv 2020.

[5] Tyebally S, Chen D, Bhattacharyya S, Mughrabi A, Hussain Z, Manisty C, Westwood M, Ghosh AK, Guha A. Cardiac tumors: JACC CardioOncology state-of-the-art review. JACC: CardioOncology 2020;2(2):293–311.

[6] Jain D, Maleszewski JJ, Halushka MK. Benign cardiac tumors and tumorlike conditions. Ann Diagn Pathol 2010;14(3):215–30. https://doi.org/10.1016/j.anndiagpath.2009.12.

[7] Kilani S, Gaxotte V, Midulla M, Beregi JP. Cardiac mass: algorithms for an integrative diagnostic approach. ECR 2012;C-0729. https://doi.org/10.1594/ecr2012/C-0729.

[8] Ren DY, Fuller ND, Gilbert SAB, Zhang Y. Cardiac tumors: clinical perspective and therapeutic considerations. Curr Drug Targets 2017;18(15):1805–9.

[9] Salcedo EE, Cohen GI, White RD, Davison MB. Cardiac tumors: diagnosis and management. Curr Probl Cardiol 1992 Feb;17(2):73–137.

[10] Pazos-Lopez P, Pozo E, Siqueira ME, et al. Value of CMR for the differential diagnosis of cardiac masses. JACC Cardiovasc Imaging 2014 Sep;7(9):896–905.

[11] Gaillard F. Atrial myxoma. Case study. Radiopaedia.org (accessed on 31 Oct 2021); 2021. https://doi.org/10.53347/rID-8544.

[12] Bruce CJ. Cardiac tumours: diagnosis and management. Heart 2010;97(2):151–60. https://doi.org/10.1136/hrt.2009.186320.

[13] Kurosawa K, Negishi K, Tateno R, Koitabashi N, Koike N, Mohara J, et al. Multiple papillary fibroelastomas of the aortic valve detected by real time three-dimensional transesophageal echocardiographic images. J Cardiol Cases 2013 Apr;8(1):e9–e12.

[14] Yandrapalli S, Mehta B, Mondal P, et al. Cardiac papillary fibroelastoma: the need for a timely diagnosis. World J Clin Cases 2017;5(1):9–13.

[15] Armstrong WF, Ryan T. Feigenbaum's echocardiography. 7th ed. Philadelphia, PA: Lippincott Williams and Wilkins; 2009.

[16] Bogaert J, Dymarkovski S, Taylor A, Muthurangu V. Clinical cardiac MRI. 2nd ed. Berlin: Springer; 2012.

[17] Pepi M, Evangelista A, Nihoyannopoulos P, et al. On behalf of the European Association of Echocardiography Recommendations for echocardiography use in the diagnosis and management of cardiac sources of embolism. Eur J Echocardiogr 2010;11:461–76.

[18] Bawazeer A. Cardiac rhabdomyoma—tuberous sclerosis. Case study. Radiopaedia.org (accessed on 31 Oct 2021); 2021. https://doi.org/10.53347/rID-70089.

[19] Gasparovic H, Coric V, Milicic D, Rajsman G, Burcar I, Stern-Padovan R, et al. Left ventricular fibroma mimicking an acute coronary syndrome. Ann Thorac Surg 2006;82(5):1891–2.

[20] Galiuto L, Badano L, Fox K, Sicari R, Zamorano JL. The EAE textbook of echocardiography. 1st ed. Oxford: Oxford University Press; 2011.

[21] Di Muzio B. Cardiac lipoma. Case study. Radiopaedia.org (accessed on 01 Nov 2021); 2021. https://doi.org/10.53347/rID-15292.

[22] Samanidis G, Khoury M, Balanika M, Perrea DN. Current challenges in the diagnosis and treatment of cardiac myxoma. Kardiol Pol 2020 Apr;78(4):269–77.

[23] [Guideline] Cheitlin MD, Alpert JS, Armstrong WF, et al. ACC/AHA guidelines for the clinical application of echocardiography. A report of the American College of Cardiology/American Heart Association task force on practice guidelines (Committee on Clinical Application of Echocardiography). Developed in collaboration with the American Society of Echocardiography. Circulation 1997 Mar;95(6):1686–744.

# Oncologic essentials in malignant cardiac masses (approach and follow-up)

# 23

**Sahar Parkhideh[a] and Seyyed Asadollah Mousavi[b]**

*[a]RIOHCT, TUMS, Tehran, Iran [b]Hematology-Oncology and Stem Cell Transplantation Research Center, Tehran University of Medical Sciences, Tehran, Iran*

## Key points

- Malignant tumors are extremely rare.
- 25% of primary cardiac tumors are malignant.
- Most malignant cardiac tumors are metastatic (from breast, lung, melanoma, soft tissue sarcoma, etc.).
- Sarcoma, lymphoma, and malignant pericardial mesothelioma are three main primary malignant cardiac tumors.
- Usual imaging studies consist of TTE, CMR, and contrast TTE that are helpful noninvasive tools to diagnose suspicious cardiac masses.
- Generally, despite multimodal treatment strategies, prognosis of malignant cardiac tumors is poor.

## Epidemiology and classification

Malignant cardiac tumors are extremely rare (0.001%–0.03% in most autopsy series) and account for 10%–25% of primary cardiac masses [1–7].

Multimodal Imaging Atlas of Cardiac Masses. https://doi.org/10.1016/B978-0-323-84906-7.00019-4

**Table 23.1** Major outlines of the 2015 WHO classification of tumors of the heart and pericardium [4].

| |
|---|
| Benign tumors and tumor-like conditions |
| Tumors of uncertain biologic behavior |
| Germ cell tumors |
| Malignant tumors |
| Tumors of the pericardium |

**Table 23.2** Incidence of different subtypes of primary malignant cardiac tumors [1–7].

| Primary cardiac tumors | Incidence |
|---|---|
| **Benign** | 70%–75% |
| **Malignant** | 25%–30% |
|   Angiosarcoma | 9% |
|   Rhabdomyosarcoma | 6% |
|   Mesothelioma | 4% |
|   Fibrosarcoma | 3% |
|   Lymphoma | 2% |
|   Other sarcomas | 3% |
|   Teratoma | <1% |
|   Other | <1% |

**Table 23.3** Incidence of cardiac metastasis in several malignancies [1–7].

| Secondary cardiac tumors | Rate of heart metastasis % |
|---|---|
| Pleural mesothelioma | 48.4% |
| Melanoma | 27.8% |
| Lung adenocarcinoma | 21% |
| Undifferentiated carcinoma | 19.5% |
| Lung squamous cell carcinoma | 18.2% |
| Breast carcinoma | 15.5% |
| Ovarian carcinoma | 10.3% |
| Lymphoproliferative neoplasms | 9.4% |
| Bronchoalveolar carcinoma | 9.8% |
| Gastric carcinoma | 8% |
| Renal cell carcinoma | 7.3% |
| Pancreatic carcinoma | 6.4% |

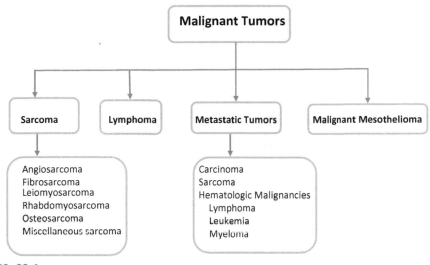

**FIG. 23.4**

Outlines of malignant cardiac tumors.

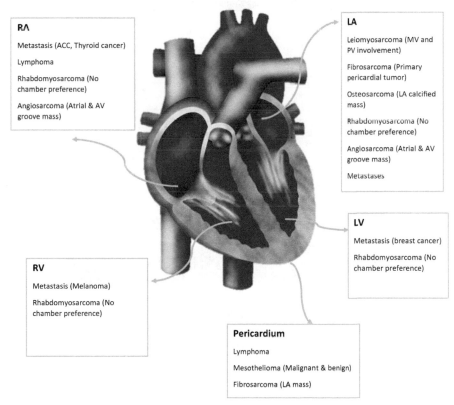

**FIG. 23.5**

Location of different cardiac malignant tumors in heart.

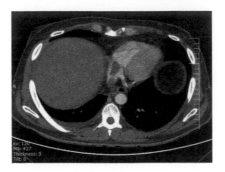

**FIG. 23.6**

A 44-year-old man with new onset hypertension and abdominal mass extended to IVC and RA. He was diagnosed with metastatic adrenocortical carcinoma.

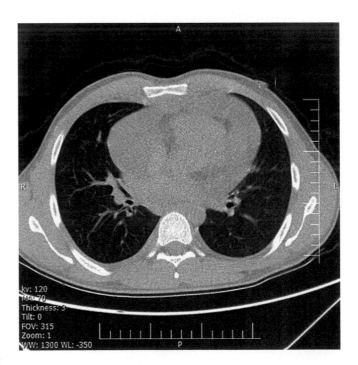

**FIG. 23.7**

A 27-year-old man admitted to emergency department because of progressive functional NYHA class 3 dyspnea. Malignant involvement of the pericardium with leukemic cells was detected. He was diagnosed with pre-B-cell ALL.

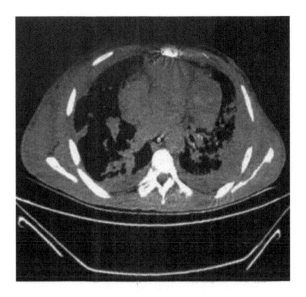

**FIG. 23.8**

A 31-year-old man with metastatic primary cardiac rhabdomyosarcoma.

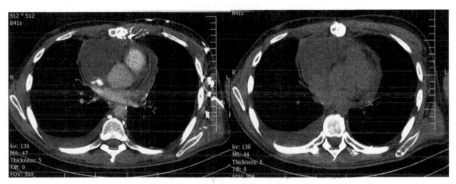

**FIG. 23.9**

A 33-year-old man with metastatic malignant mesothelioma (postthoracotomy).

## Approach and diagnostic workup

The clinical history and physical examination are critical to decide what types of laboratory tests and imaging studies are optimal for an individual. A cardiac mass in a patient with atrial fibrillation or heart failure most probably is intracardiac thrombi; instead in prosthetic valvular disease or endocavitary catheters, vegetation, calcifications, thrombus, and tumors should be taken into account. In most cases, multimodality noninvasive imaging is used. Usual imaging studies consist of TTE, CMR, and contrast TTE that provide useful information before histopathologic procedures [6–13].

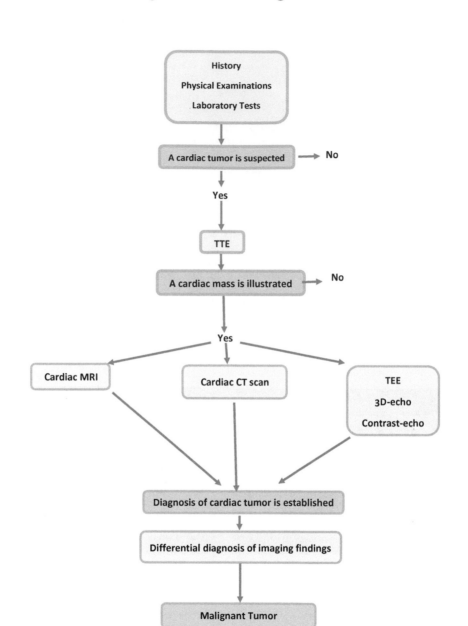

**FIG. 23.10**

Schema of approach to a suspected cardiac mass.

*Continued*

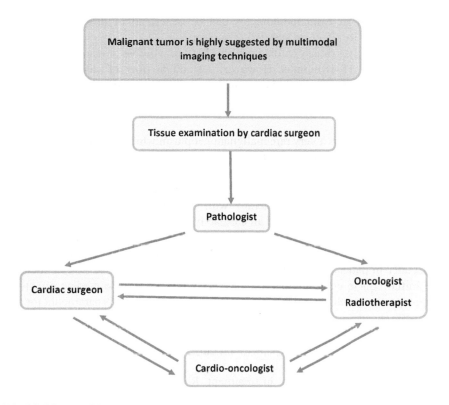

**FIG. 23.10—cont'd**

# Treatment and prognosis
## Primary cardiac tumors
### *Sarcoma*

Generally, sarcomas proliferate locally and cause obstruction of blood flow. In more advance cases, widespread metastasis may happen.

The standard treatment of malignant sarcoma is complete resection, yet most patients experience tumor recurrence.

In patients with low-grade cardiac sarcoma and limited disease, complete resection with valve reconstruction when indicated should be carried out.

In those with unresectable or metastatic tumors, surgery can improve hemodynamic status and prevent or ameliorate heart failure symptoms. Pericardiotomy and pericardial window are also useful palliative options.

Neoadjuvant or adjuvant chemotherapy has not been studied in a randomized clinical trial yet. However, it has been employed to improve the poor outcome with surgery alone and the benefit remained unknown.

Postsurgical adjuvant radiotherapy can be beneficial in subsiding unpleasant symptoms, but its effect on survival is unclear.

Unfortunately, primary cardiac sarcoma has unfavorable prognosis with an overall survival of 11–18 months. However, a small number of case series showed improved survival to about 2–4 years with heart transplantation [12–14].

### Lymphoma

Cardiac lymphoma is a very rare malignant neoplasm which accounts for about 1%–2% of primary malignant cardiac tumors and 10% of metastatic tumors to the heart. It is typically non-Hodgkin type and can originate from pericardium or cardiac chambers. Involvement of the right side of the heart predominates.

A combination of immunotherapy with chemotherapy backbone remains the mainstay of treatment for almost all cardiac lymphoma. The most common chemotherapy regimen widely used is at least 6 cycles of R-CHOP (Rituximab, Cyclophosphamide, Doxorubicin, Vincristine, Prednisone), but this can be challenging especially in patients with left-sided heart failure. Anthracycline dose reduction in the initial course of chemotherapy may decrease the adverse cardiac effects and its prospective death. Addition of rituximab to CHOP regimen is paramount for overall treatment success in cardiac lymphoma patients and enhanced complete response and duration of remission. Massive pulmonary embolism or tissue necrosis and subsequent death may happen postchemotherapy, especially in extensive myocardial lymphomatous infiltration.

Surgery has a limited role in treatment. Radiotherapy has been used in some cases, but pros and cons are still vague.

Generally, prognosis of cardiac lymphoma is poor. In a retrospective study, median survival was 2.2 years [15,16].

## Malignant mesothelioma

Primary pericardial malignant mesothelioma is exceptionally rare. It accounts for 1% of all mesothelioma cases. Like pleural and peritoneal mesothelioma, pericardial type has also been linked to asbestosis, although its association is less significant.

Due to sparsity of the disease, no treatment guideline has been established. For localized tumor, complete resection is the treatment of choice. As most of patients present with advanced disease, surgery is usually used as a palliative approach. Radiation has been utilized in adjuvant setting; though in SMART trial (Surgery for Mesothelioma After Radiation Therapy) it has been employed before surgery and showed to be of use. Chemotherapy with platins (cisplatin or carboplatin) plus pemetrexed is also appraised as first-line therapy in some studies and increased survival in combination with surgery.

Pericardial mesothelioma has very poor prognosis, and 50%–60% of patients die before 6 months of diagnosis [17–20].

## Metastatic tumors

Metastases to the heart and pericardium are much more common than primary cardiac tumors and are generally associated with a poor prognosis. Treatment options are generally directed to symptom control, and long-term survival is rare. Metastasis to the heart is almost always a systemic disease and treatment basically depends on the underlying pathology [21].

## References

[1] Kun Y, Liu Y, Wang H, et al. Epidemiological and pathological characteristics of cardiac tumors: a clinical study of 242 cases. Interact Cardiovasc Thorac Surg 2007;6(5):636–9.

[2] Rahouma M, Arisha MJ, Elmously A, et al. Cardiac tumors prevalence and mortality: a systematic review and meta-analysis. Int J Surg 2020;76:178–89.

[3] Shinichi T. Comprehensive review of the epidemiology and treatments for malignant adult cardiac tumors. Gen Thorac Cardiovasc Surg 2018;66:257–62.

[4] Burke A, Tavora F. The 2015 WHO classification of tumors of the heart and pericardium. J Thorac Oncol 2016;11(4):441–52.

[5] Mankad R, Herrmann J. Cardiac tumors: echo assessment. Echo Res Pract 2016;3: R65–77.

[6] Bussani R, Castrichini M, Restivo L, et al. Cardiac tumors: diagnosis, prognosis, and treatment. Curr Cardiol Rep 2020;22.169.

[7] Bruce CJ. Cardiac tumours: diagnosis and management. Heart 2011;97:151–60.

[8] Hoffmeier A, Sindermann JR, Scheld HH, et al. Cardiac tumors—diagnosis and surgical treatment. Dtsch Arztebl Int 2014;111(12):205–11.

[9] Shapiro LM. Cardiac tumours: diagnosis and management. Heart 2001;85:218–22.

[10] Lestuzzi C, De Paoli A, Baresic T, et al. Malignant cardiac tumors: diagnosis and treatment. Future Cardiol 2015;11(4):3.

[11] Salcedo EE, Cohen GI, White RD, et al. Cardiac tumors: diagnosis and management. Curr Probl Cardiol 1992;17(2):77–137.

[12] Hamidi M, Moody JS, Weigel TL, et al. Primary cardiac sarcoma. Ann Thorac Surg 2010;90(1):176–81.

[13] Burke A, Jean Jeudy Jr RV. Cardiac tumours: an update. Heart 2008;94:117–23.

[14] Orlandi A, Ferlosi A, Roselli M, et al. Cardiac sarcomas: an update. J Thorac Oncol 2010;5(9):1483–9.

[15] Gowda RM, Khan IA. Clinical perspectives of primary cardiac lymphoma. Angiology 2003;54(5):599–604.

[16] Zhao Y, Huang S, Ma C, Zhu H, Bo J. Clinical features of cardiac lymphoma: an analysis of 37 cases. J Int Med Res 2021;49(3), 0300060521999558.

[17] Vigneswaran WT, Stefanacci PR. Pericardial mesothelioma. Curr Treat Options Oncol 2000;1(4):299–302.

[18] Eren NT, Akar AR. Primary pericardial mesothelioma. Curr Treat Options Oncol 2002;3(5):369–73.

[19] Levý M, Boublíková L, Büchler T, Šimša J. Treatment of malignant peritoneal mesothelioma. Klin Onkol 2019;32(5):333–7.

[20] Webb J, Yiu YW, Giastefani S, Carr-White G. Pericardial mesothelioma. QJM 2016; 109(9):631–2.

[21] Poterucha TJ, Kochav J, O'Connor DS, Rosner GF. Cardiac tumors: clinical presentation, diagnosis, and management. Curr Treat Options Oncol 2019;20(8):66.

# Primary cardiac lymphoma

# 24

**Vincenzo Caruso[a], Carlo Maria Cipolla[b], and Daniela Cardinale[a]**

[a]*Cardioncology Unit, European Institute of Oncology, Istituto di Ricovero e Cura a Carattere Scientifico, Milan, Italy* [b]*Cardiology Department, European Institute of Oncology, Istituto di Ricovero e Cura a Carattere Scientifico, Milan, Italy*

## Introduction

Primary cardiac lymphoma (PCL) is an extranodal lymphoma which involves the heart and pericardium. It is a very rare tumor, representing 0.5% of all extranodal lymphomas and 1%–2% of primary cardiac tumors [1]. PCL is most frequently detected in immune-compromised patients [2], predominantly in males (3:1 ratio) [3], with a median age of occurrence of 63 years [4] although it can develop at any age [5]. PCL is often an aggressive lymphoma, and the short-term prognosis is usually unfavorable with a high mortality rate, unless it is identified early and promptly treated [6]. Cardiac lymphomas are infiltrative, intramural, with a specific tropism for the pericardium and the right side of the heart. The pericardium is affected in approximately 33% of cases [7]. The right atrium is the most involved site followed by right ventricle, left atrium, atrial septum, and ventricular septum. However, multichamber involvement has been seen in up to 75% of cases [7].

PCL has no typical clinical presentation, and clinical characteristics are not distinctive, with variable symptoms depending on location, amount of cardiac structure infiltration, proliferation, and friability [8].

At present, diagnosis mainly relies on multiple imaging techniques that include echocardiography, cardiac computed tomography (CT), and cardiac magnetic resonance (CMR) [9].

## Case report 1

A 79-year-old man, with no immunodepression, was referred to our outpatient clinic for moderate dyspnea (New York Heart Association Class, NYHA II), without signs of acute or unstable heart failure. A surface electrocardiogram (ECG) showed sinus tachycardia (110 bpm), right bundle branch block, and left anterior hemiblock (Fig. 24.1). Blood pressure was 120/80 mmHg. Chest X-ray indicated obliteration of the right costophrenic sinus due to mild flap of pleural effusion (Fig. 24.2).

**349**

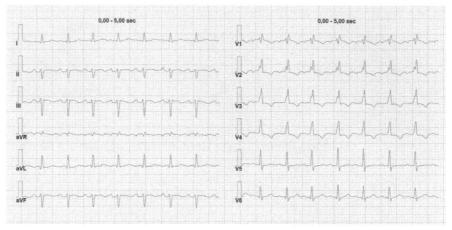

**FIG. 24.1**

Baseline electrocardiogram showing right bundle branch block and left anterior hemiblock.

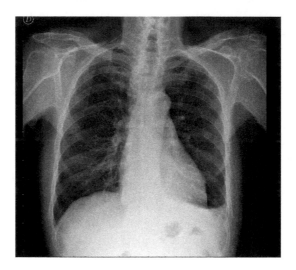

**FIG. 24.2**

Chest X-ray showing obliteration of the right costophrenic sinus due to mild flap of pleural effusion.

A complete transthoracic (TT) echocardiographic exam was then performed, revealing severe dilatation of the right chambers and the presence of a large (120 mm × 60 mm, in apical 4 chamber view) hyperechoic mass occupying two-thirds of the right heart, and including the anterior and posterior tricuspid valve

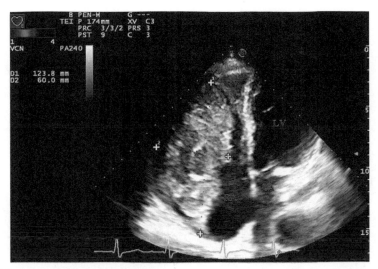

**FIG. 24.3**

Transthoracic echocardiographic exam revealed severe dilatation of the right chambers, the presence of a large (in apical 4 chamber view; 120 mm long × 60 mm transverse diameter) hyperechoic mass occupying two-thirds of the right heart, and including the anterior and posterior tricuspid valve leaflets. *RV*, right ventricle; *RA*, right atrium; *, lymphoid mass; *LV*, left ventricle; *LA*, left atrium.

leaflets. Further findings included paradoxical septal motion (with no evidence of pulmonary hypertension) and mild pericardial effusion, without significant tricuspid obstruction at Doppler analysis (Figs. 24.3 and 24.4A and B and Movies 24.S1–24.S4 in the online version at https://doi.org/10.1016/B978-0-323-84906-7.00023-6).

The patient underwent CMR and CT imaging that confirmed the size of the mass and excluded additional extracardiac masses (Figs. 24.5 and 24.6A and B).

The endomyocardial biopsy, performed by cardiac right catheterization, was consistent with the diagnosis of non-Hodgkin high-cell positive B-cell lymphoma, with positive immunophenotype for CD45, CD20; negative for cytokeratin pool, S-100 protein, synaptophysin, CD3, CD10, BCL-6, BCL-2, CD138, and for HHV-8; absence of rearrangement of the 8q24 (MYC) locus assessed by FISH.

After onco-hematologic evaluation, the patient started high-dose chemotherapy, according to the R-CHOP regimen (rituximab, cyclophosphamide, doxorubicin, vincristine, and prednisone) for 8 cycles.

Further, serial echocardiographic controls were performed that showed an impressive mass reduction soon after the 1st chemotherapy cycle (Movie 24.S5 in the online version at https://doi.org/10.1016/B978-0-323-84906-7.00023-6) with a complete resolution after three months (Movie 24.S6 in the online version at https://doi.org/10.1016/B978-0-323-84906-7.00023-6). At present, after 5 years, at the age of 84, the patient is in complete remission, with good performance status.

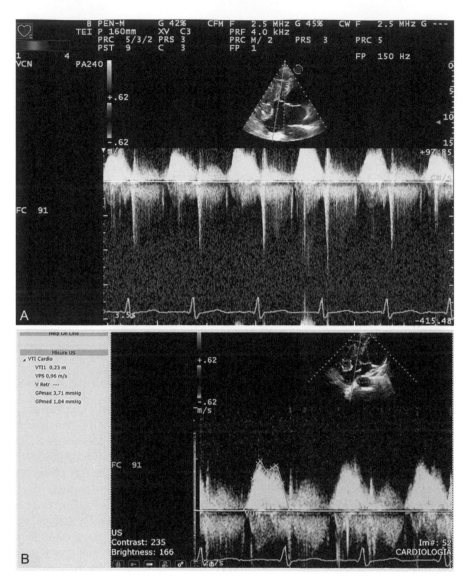

**FIG. 24.4**

(A) and (B) Continuous Doppler. Mild tricuspid regurgitation and no doppler velocities indicating valvular stenosis.

## Case report 2

A sixty-one-year-old woman presented at the Emergency Department for heart palpitation and worsening dyspnea. She was assuming antiarrhythmic therapy with flecainide for complex supraventricular arrhythmias.

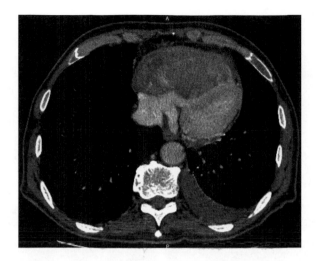

**FIG. 24.5**

Computed tomography imaging confirmed the presence of a voluminous mass in the right heart of about 105 × 71 mm with dishomogeneous contrastographic impregnation, which determines pericardial infiltration in the right antero-lateral site, where it is possible to recognize a modest layer of effusion, infiltration probably of the right atrium and right auricle and medially slight compression of the interventricular septum; this tissue anteriorly reaches the anterior thoracic wall where it is however recognizable in a plane of cleavage with the sternal body. Suspicious lymph nodes in the pericardial-phrenic fat and along the internal mammary chains bilaterally. Minimal flap of left pleural effusion.

ECG showed sinus rhythm, vertical axis, signs of right atrial overload, atrioventricular (AV) block grade I (Fig. 24.7).

Chest X-ray did not report any major pathological findings (Fig. 24.8).

The TT echocardiogram showed a large mass at the right cavities (78.9 mm × 43 mm) with mixed echographic pattern and characteristic "hammer" movement between the interatrial and interventricular septa. Hemodynamically, the mass occupying most of the right cardiac sector obstructed the tricuspid valve, creating an increased mean gradient (11 mmHg). The mass encompassed the septal flap of the tricuspid valve and the interatrial septum, with suspected infiltration of the AV ventricular plane as well. Mild pericardial effusion and thickening of pericardial leaflets, that appeared hyperechogenic, were observed (Figs. 24.9 and 24.10 and Movies 24.S7 and 24.S8 in the online version at https://doi.org/10.1016/B978-0-323-84906-7.00023-6).

Computed tomography imaging confirmed the presence of the mass in the right cardiac cavities (transverse diameter of about 7.5–8 cm) and evidenced presence of bilateral pulmonary pleural effusion more represented on the right side, causing atelectasis of the lower lung lobe (Fig. 24.11).

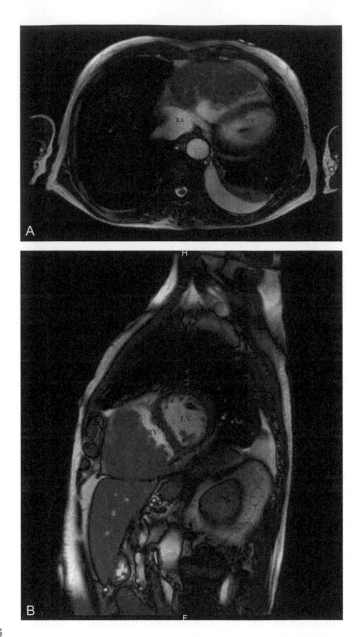

**FIG. 24.6**

(A) and (B) Cardiac magnetic resonance imaging documented a mass of size 7.6 × 12 × 5.5 cm extended along the free wall of the right ventricle infiltrating the ventricular wall at full thickness. *LV*, left ventricle; *RV*, right ventricle; *LA*, left atrium; *RA*, right atrium; *, lymphoid lesion.

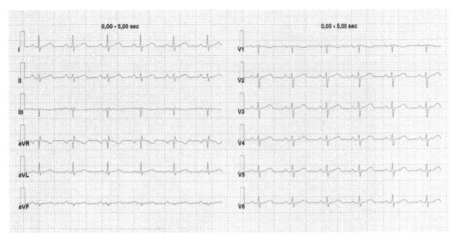

**FIG. 24.7**

Baseline electrocardiogram showing sinus rhythm, vertical axis, signs of right atrial involvement, atrioventricular block grade I.

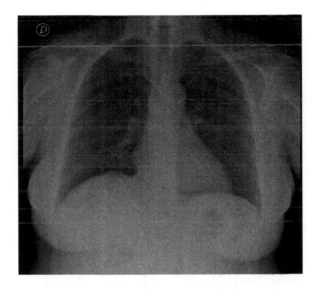

**FIG. 24.8**

Chest X-ray did not report major pathological findings.

Coronary CT scan excluded the presence of significant stenosis of the coronary tree, or direct infiltration or compression of coronary arteries.

An intracardiac biopsy was performed under transfemoral ultrasound guidance and the histopathological examination confirmed the diagnosis of diffuse large

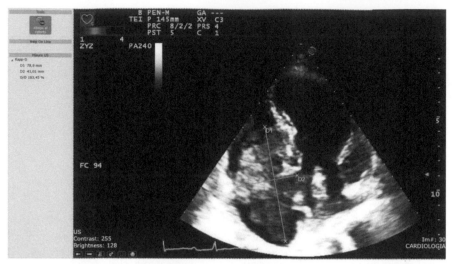

**FIG. 24.9**

Apical 4 chamber view. Dimensions of primary cardiac lymphoma mass.

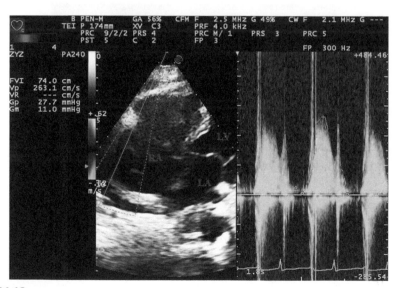

**FIG. 24.10**

Continuous Doppler waves showing severe tricuspid stenosis (mean gradient 11.0 mmHg).

B-cell lymphoma. The immunophenotype of the neoplastic cells was positive for cardiac lymphoma and negative for AE1-AE3 cytokeratins. The proliferating index was 80%. Immunoreactivity was positive for CD79a and, focally, for CD20.

After onco-hematologic evaluation, the patient was assigned to high-dose chemotherapy, according to the R-CHOP regimen (rituximab, cyclophosphamide, doxorubicin, vincristine, and prednisone) for 6 cycles.

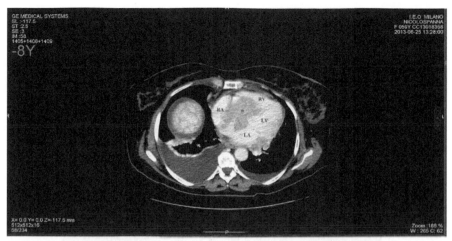

**FIG. 24.11**

CT imaging. Mediastinum view showing bilateral pleural effusion. *RV*, right ventricle. *RA*, right atrium. *LV*, left ventricle; *LA*, left atrium; *, primary cardiac lymphoma mass.

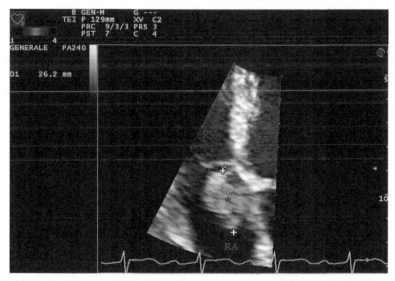

**FIG. 24.12**

Zoom acquisition of the right atrium. After 3 cycles of treatment with R-CHOP, the dimensions of the mass are reduced. Longitudinal axis of the mass is 26.2 mm. *RV*, right ventricle; *LV*, left ventricle; *RA*, right atrium; *, primary cardiac lymphoma mass.

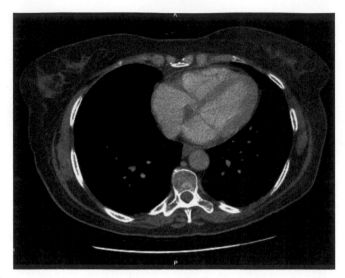

**FIG. 24.13**

CT lung after 3 cycles of R-CHOP regimen showed reduced mass with pedicle at the level of the interatrial septum.

Subsequent echocardiographic and tomographic reevaluations showed clear reduction in the size of the intracardiac mass already after 3 cycles of chemotherapy (Figs. 24.12 and 24.13 and Movie 24.S9 in the online version at https://doi.org/10.1016/B978-0-323-84906-7.00023-6). Reevaluation after 6 cycles of R-CHOP chemotherapy with positron emission tomography (PET) and TT echocardiogram showed complete remission (Movie 24.S10 in the online version at https://doi.org/10.1016/B978-0-323-84906-7.00023-6).

At present, after 5 years, at the age of 56, the patient is in complete remission, with good performance status.

## Discussion

The first observation of primary cardiac lymphoma dates back to the 1930s [10].

Due to the rarity of the disease, only isolated cases and limited reviews are published in the literature to date. Data refer to cases collected over a large period of time and managed very variably [5].

### Clinical presentation

Cardiac lymphomas often have mixed symptomatology, or, as other cardiac masses, may remain asymptomatic for a long time. Consequently, diagnosis may result to be challenging and delayed.

**Table 24.14** Clinical feature/manifestation more frequently reported in PCL patients [6,7,15].

| Sign/symptom | Incidence |
|---|---|
| Arrhythmia | 23% |
| Atrioventricular blocks 2–3 | 15%–27% |
| B-symptoms | 16% |
| Chest pain | 13%–24% |
| Cough | 8% |
| Dyspnea | 64% |
| Heart failure | 53%–64% |
| Pericardial effusion | Up to 58% |
| Pericardial mass | 30% |
| Peripheral edema | 13% |
| Pleural effusion | 62% |
| Superior vena cava syndrome | 5%–15% |
| Cardiac tamponade | 8%–34% |

Dyspnea is the most common presenting symptom, but also chest pain, palpitations, syncope, and dry cough are often reported as an onset symptom. Most frequent clinical pictures are heart failure and pericardial and pleural effusion (Table 24.14).

Extracardiac symptoms may hide cardiac ones as in case of paraneoplastic syndrome, superior vena cava syndrome, cardioembolic stroke, pulmonary embolism, and adrenal involvement. In some patients, general symptoms such as weight loss, fever, night sweat, and generalized pruritus, the so-called B symptoms, may also occur (Table 24.14).

Diagnosis may be deferred due to heterogeneous clinical presentation and limited availability of diagnostic tools. Diagnostic delay results in a poor prognosis; therefore, careful and thorough investigation of the clinical picture is required to make the correct diagnosis quickly and improve outcome. In this regard, a multidiagnostic technique approach is strongly recommended [6].

## 12-Lead ECG

The lymphomatous cells can infiltrate the electrical conduction system of the heart resulting in several ECG abnormalities, but none can be considered diagnostic. The ECG reported findings are summarized in Table 24.15.

Complete atrioventricular block is the most frequently observed ECG abnormality in patients with PCL. Many of these abnormalities often disappear during or following systemic oncologic therapy and radiotherapy [6,8].

**Table 24.15** Electrocardiographic findings in patients with PCL.

| |
|---|
| Any grade of atrioventricular block |
| Atrial fibrillation |
| Atrial flutter |
| Bradycardia |
| Ectopic beats |
| Inverted T waves |
| Low voltage QRS complex |
| Right bundle branch block |
| Ventricular tachycardia |

## Chest X-ray

Chest X-ray has limited value for the detection of cardiac masses or suspect cardiac infiltration. In most cases cardiomegaly is seen, especially at the right atrium. Pleural effusions and pulmonary venous congestion can also be observed. Notably, the chest X-ray may be without pathological findings [6].

## Transthoracic echocardiography

TT echocardiography allows for an initial, noninvasive, quick assessment of PLC and it is generally considered the first imaging assessment choice to identify the cardiac mass, and evaluate its extent and hemodynamic burden [11]. TT echocardiogram provides information on tumor size and echo-structure, Doppler velocity for evaluation of functional stenosis, relationships with surrounding structures, presence of pericardial effusion and thickening, possible kinetic abnormalities related to hypo- or akinetic areas due to tumor infiltration. It is the imaging technique that offers the greatest advantages (including the lower cost) for carrying out serial checks during follow-up to document mass regression [8].

The use of trans-esophageal echocardiography (TEE) is more sensitive in the diagnosis of primary cardiac tumors but has the disadvantage of being less tolerated by the patient. Its use remains essential for assessment of the auricle and superior vena cava [6].

## Computed tomography

Computed tomography (CT) provides optimal anatomic assessment of involvement of cardiac structures by PLC, mostly due to its high isotropic spatial and temporal resolution. CT has the advantage of a fast acquisition time and is a first-choice alternative as an imaging technique in patients with known contraindications to MRI or in patients with poor-quality images from TT echocardiography. Thanks to its tissue resolution, CT can define morphology, location, and extension of the cardiac mass. In addition, CT provides a field of view that includes the whole thorax and thus maximizes evaluation of extracardiac localizations of disease [7].

## Cardiac magnetic resonance

Cardiac magnetic resonance (CMR) is the gold standard imaging technique for cardiac mass evaluation [5]. Despite the wider availability of other imaging modalities, CMR is the preferred imaging modality owing to its higher soft tissue characterization, high temporal resolution, multiplanar imaging power, and wide field of view [7]. CMR is superior to other imaging techniques in detecting tumor infiltration [12]. On MRI, PCL shows a variable signal intensity due to its cellularity: PCL tumor cells have a higher free-water content, so they usually look hypointense on T1-weighted MR sequences and hyperintense in T2. Conversely, late gadolinium enhancement does not present a specific pattern for cardiac lymphoma (commonly minimal or no enhancement) [8].

## 18F-Fluorodeoxyglucose positron emission tomography

PCL is a fluoro-deoxy-glucose (FDG)-avid tumor. The utility of FDG-PET for the specific diagnosis of cardiac lymphoma is still questionable because of the physiologic storage of radiotracer within the myocardium cells and the poor anatomic resolution of FDG-PET. However, when coupled with CT anatomic information, FDG-PET has enhanced diagnostic and staging accuracy and became a useful tool in the evaluation of PCL body-wide for early staging and response to treatment [7].

Very recently, Liu et al. reported that the intensity and volume-based PET indexes of PLC are significantly greater than those of primary cardiac angiosarcoma, which is the most common primary tumor of the heart, and the most challenging differential diagnosis. The enhancement pattern and tumor morphology were also different. Based on these features, using FGD-PET-CT the two types of primary cardiac malignancies can be distinguished [13].

## Multimodality imaging approach

A multimodality imaging approach is pivotal in the characterization of a cardiac tumor, enabling clinicians to formulate a presumptive diagnosis and to distinguish PCL from other more prevalent cardiac malignancies, such as angiosarcoma [9]. Echocardiography is the first step examination to identify the mass and estimate its hemodynamic burden. However, complementary evaluations with cross-sectional imaging are crucial for additional characterization of the tumor and its extension. CT and CMR are helpful for additional mass details such as size, location, extent, and tissue characterization; 18-FDG PET-TC confirms cardiac isolation and is very useful in determining diagnosis and ascertaining treatment response [9].

## Intracardiac biopsy examination

Histological evaluation of the tumor is a pivotal step for definitive diagnosis and prompt treatment program. PCL and cardiac angiosarcoma are difficult to differentiate by imaging techniques in many patients and a biopsy examination may be crucial [14]. It can be performed by cardiac right catheterization with the help of fluoroscopy or TEE imaging [6]. In addition, transvenous biopsy guided by TT imaging is a novel optional technique. Both approaches were successfully used in our two patients with no side effects. Cytological examination can be a good alternative to or prior to endomyocardial biopsy in the presence of significant pericardial or pleural effusion [6].

## Differential diagnoses

As a very rare tumor, PCL is of course not the first diagnostic hypothesis for a cardiac mass, in particular in patients presenting with nonspecific symptoms. Most common differential diagnoses include cardiac benign tumors, primary cardiac sarcomas, and thrombus [15].

Most primary cardiac tumors are benign and cardiac myxoma, mainly located at left side of the heart in 75% of cases, is the most frequent in adults [2], generally presenting as an intracavitary, mobile mass of the left atrium, adhered to the endocardial surface by a pedicle, and potentially associated with thromboembolism events [2,15]. Differently from left side predominance of atrial myxoma, PCL is more often located at the right heart. More challenging is the differential diagnosis with primary cardiac sarcomas, which are more frequent than PCL, but usually develop from the left heart cavities (46% of cases), generally without being paired with pericarditis (3% of cases) or extracardiac lesion (7% of cases) [2]. Notably, a tumor situated on the right side of the heart points to a malignant primary cardiac tumor in nearly 50% of cases [9]. Angiosarcoma is the most important differential diagnosis. It is typically more aggressive than lymphomas, and, conversely, often infiltrates the vessels and valves. However, previous studies report a remarkable overlap of imaging findings between cardiac lymphomas and angiosarcomas, which brings great difficulties to the diagnosis of PCLs based on morphologic characteristics [16].

Other frequent differential diagnoses include intracardiac thrombus, which usually develops in the left atrium often in presence of hypokinetic-dilated cardiomyopathy [15].

## Treatment

As no clinical and/or prospective studies have ever been conducted, there are currently no clear guidelines on the treatment of PCL, and cancer therapy is mostly based on data from other extranodal lymphomas or on physicians' personal opinion.

There is no evidence of improved survival with surgery. Cardiac surgery in PCL is not only technically challenging but may also be associated with many damaging complications [17,18]. Therefore a curative surgical approach should be avoided and surgery should be performed only in patients with PCL who are hemodynamically unstable, unable to tolerate chemotherapy, or needing a palliative resection to control symptoms [18].

Conversely, video-assisted thoracoscopic surgery (VATS) has been successfully carried out in patients with PCL. VATS is a useful option in draining pericardial effusion, especially if recurrent [19].

Chemotherapy appears to have the best impact on survival and should be started as soon as possible [6,15,18,20]. Since 2010, the chemotherapy regimens are similar to that used for other subtypes of non-Hodgkin lymphoma, such as CHOP (cyclophosphamide, doxorubicin, vincristine, and prednisone) or CHOP regimen associated to rituximab. In a study by Carras et al., the overall response rate to these regimens was as high as 85%, with 62% complete response [15]. For refractory cases, autologous hematopoietic stem cell transplantation is also performed [21]. Recurrence after first-line chemotherapy mostly occurs at extracardiac sites and is burdened by poor survival [15].

The role of radiotherapy is controversial. It seems to add no benefit to systemic chemotherapy in terms of overall survival [22]. Usually cardiac infiltration is sensitive to radiotherapy [8]. However, the direct toxic effect caused by radiotherapy on cardiac tissues and structures may outweigh its positive antitumor effects. Therefore radiotherapy should be indicated only in patients with PLC which progresses despite chemotherapy [23].

## Outcome

Currently, PCL prognosis remains poor, mainly due to late diagnosis and the aggressiveness of the tumor. Immunocompromise, presence of extracardiac disease, and left ventricular involvement have been described as poor prognostic factors [2]. If not treated, PCL has a reported survival of about one month. However, with appropriate and prompt treatment, as in our two patients, survival can be prolonged for up to 5 years [24,25].

## Conclusion

Primary cardiac lymphoma is a very rare disease with nonspecific onset symptoms and associated with a poor prognosis. Early diagnosis and prompt treatment are of pivotal importance, significantly impacting on prognosis and survival rate. The presumptive diagnosis relies greatly on the use of multiple imaging techniques, including TT and TE echocardiography, CT scan, and CMR. At present, the most effective treatment is anthracycline-containing chemotherapy. As no well-defined guidelines on the management of PCL exist so far, future prospective studies for better defining the optimal approach of patients with this rare disease are strongly required.

## Appendix: Supplementary material

Supplementary material related to this chapter can be found on the accompanying CD or online at https://doi.org/10.1016/B978-0-323-84906-7.00023-6.

# References

[1] Burke A, Tavora F. The 2015 WHO classification of tumors of the heart and pericardium. J Thoracic Oncol 2016;11:441–52.

[2] Miyawaki M, Aoyama R, Ishikawa J, et al. BMJ Case Rep 2021;14, e243068.

[3] Travis W, Brambilla E, Nicholson A, et al. The 2015 World Health Organization classification of lung tumors: impact of genetic, clinical and radiologic advances since the 2004 classification. J Thorac Oncol 2015;10(9):1243–60.

[4] Jonavicius K, Salcius K, Meskauskas R, et al. Primary cardiac lymphoma: two cases and a review of literature. J Cardiothorac Surg 2015;10:138.

[5] Lucchini E, Merlo M, Ballerini M, et al. Case report: cardiac involvement by lymphoma: rare but heterogeneous condition with challenging Behaviors. Front Oncol 2021;11, 665736.

[6] Miguel C, Bestetti R. Primary cardiac lymphoma. Int J Cardiol 2011;149:358–63.

[7] Jeudy J, Burke A, Frazier A. Cardiac lymphoma. Radiol Clinics North America 2016;54:689–710.

[8] Bonelli A, Paris S, Bisegna S, et al. Cardiac lymphoma with early response to chemotherapy: a case report and review of the literature. J Nucl Cardiol 2021. https://doi.org/10.1007/s12350-021-02570-5.

[9] Serra V, De Luca F, Savino K, et al. Syncope and cardiac tamponade: multimodality imaging of primary cardiac lymphoma. J Cardiovasc Echogr 2021;31:42–4.

[10] Yu J, Zhao X, Liu Y, et al. The diagnosis of a giant cardiac malignant lymphoma in the right ventricle: a case report. ESC Heart Fail 2021;8:1620–6.

[11] Scheggi V, Mazzoni C, Mariani T, et al. Left-sided primary cardiac lymphoma: a case report. Egypt J Int Med 2020;32:27.

[12] Nijjar P, Msri S, Tamene A, et al. Benefits and limitations of multimodality imaging. Tex Heart Inst J 2014;41:657–9.

[13] Liu E, Huang J, Dong H, et al. Diagnostic challenges in primary cardiac lymphoma, the opportunity of 18F-FDG PET/CT integrated with contrast-enhanced CT. J Nucl Cardiol 2021. https://doi.org/10.1007/s12350-021-02723-6.

[14] Tanking C, Ratanapo S. Diagnostic challenge in primary cardiac lymphoma: a case report. Eur Heart J Case Rep 2020;4:1–5.

[15] Carras S, Berger F, Chalabreysse L, et al. Primary cardiac lymphoma: diagnosis, treatment and outcome in a modern series. Hematol Oncol 2017;35:510–9.

[16] Colin G, Symons R, Dymarkowski S, et al. Value of CMR to differentiate cardiac angiosarcoma from cardiac lymphoma. JACC Cardiovasc Imaging 2015;8:744–6.

[17] Ceresoli G, Ferreri A, Bucci E, et al. Primary cardiac lymphoma in immunocompetent patients. Diagn Ther Manage Cancer 1997;80:1497–506.

[18] Yin K, Brydges H, Lawrence K, et al. Primary cardiac lymphoma. J Thorac Cardiovasc Surg 2020. https://doi.org/10.1016/j.jtcvs.2020.09.102.

[19] Stoica C, Ferguson T, Monaghan H, et al. Video-thoracoscopic management of primary pericardial Hodgkin's lymphoma. EJSO 2001;27:325–31.

[20] Petrich A, Cho S, Billett E, et al. Primary cardiac lymphoma: an analysis of presentation, treatment, and outcome patterns. Cancer 2011;117:581–9.

[21] Usry C, Wilson A, Bush K. Primary cardiac lymphoma manifesting as complete heart block. Case Rep Cardiol 2020;2020, 3825312.

[22] Xiao M, Lin J, Xiao T, et al. The incidence and survival outcomes of patients with primary cardiac lymphoma: a SEER-based analysis. Hematol Oncol 2020;38:334–43.

[23] O'Mahomy D, Piekarz R, Bandettini P, et al. Cardiac involment with lymphoma: a
review of the literature. Clin Lymphoma Myeloma 2008;8:249–52.

[24] Sultan I, Aranda-Michel E, Kilic A, et al. Long-term outcome of primary cardiac lymphoma. Circulation 2020;142:2194–5.

[25] Chen X, Lin Y, Wang Z. Primary cardiac lymphoma: a case report and review of literature. Int J Clin Exp Pathol 2020;13:1745–9.

# Pericardial masses

**Hamidreza Pouraliakbar[a], Saifollah Abdi[b], Azin Alizadehasl[c],
and Niloufar Akbari Parsa[d]**

[a]*Department of Radiology, CardioOncology Research Center, Iran University of Medical Sciences,
Rajaie Cardiovascular Medical and Research Center, Tehran, Iran* [b]*Cardiovascular Intervention
Research Center, Rajaie Cardiovascular Medical and Research Center, Iran University of Medical
Sciences, Tehran, Iran* [c]*Cardio-Oncology Research Center, Rajaie Cardiovascular Medical and
Research Center, Iran University of Medical Sciences, Tehran, Iran* [d]*Echocardiography Depart-
ment, Guilan University of Medical Sciences, Rasht, Iran*

## Key points

- Pericardial tumors can be benign or malignant. Of the benign pericardial tumors,
  pericardial cysts are the most common. Other benign pericardial tumors include
  angiomas, lymphangiomas, fibromas, teratomas, and lipomas.
- Primary malignant pericardial tumors include mesotheliomas, lymphomas,
  thymomas (may be benign or malignant), sarcomas, and liposarcomas.
- Metastatic pericardial tumors occur 20 to 40 times more common than primary
  pericardial tumors and mostly result from the direct extension of tumors,
  principally the lung and the breast, producing a pericardial effusion that can
  progress to cardiac tamponade.
- Echocardiography, computed tomography, and magnetic resonance imaging are
  diagnostic modalities for detecting pericardial masses (Box 25.1).

**Multimodal Imaging Atlas of Cardiac Masses.** https://doi.org/10.1016/B978-0-323-84906-7.00011-X

**Box 25.1**

Primary pericardial tumors are rare and may be classified as benign or malignant. The most common benign lesions are pericardial cysts and lipomas. Mesothelioma is the most common primary malignant pericardial neoplasm. Other malignant tumors include a wide variety of sarcomas, lymphoma, and primitive neuroectodermal tumor. When present, signs, and symptoms are generally nonspecific. Patients often present with dyspnea, chest pain, palpitations, fever, or weight loss.

The diagnostic workup often starts with transthoracic echocardiography (TTE), which usually identifies the mass. Further evaluation using transesophageal echocardiography (TEE) may be indicated to complement the TTE assessment. Often, investigation with other imaging modalities such as CT, CMR, or PET is warranted for more detailed assessment by visualization of the entire pericardium, tissue characterization, and evaluation of surrounding structures. Although imaging may help in the identification and characterization of the mass, a biopsy is often needed for definitive tissue diagnosis [1,2].

Information on whether a mass is malignant or benign is important to direct surgical versus medical management. In addition, the extent of cardiac and extracardiac involvement is also important to determine the potential for complications such as pericardial effusion with or without cardiac tamponade, constrictive pericarditis [1]. Large masses deemed to be benign based on imaging can often be completely surgically excised to not only provide tissue for pathologic analysis, which remains the gold standard for definitive identification but also to provide symptom relief [2].

Small masses may be best assessed using CT given its high spatial resolution while larger masses may be better assessed using CMR due to its superior tissue characterization abilities [3]. Progression of the disease can be assessed using TTE if there are optimal acoustic windows or using CT or CMR if not easily visualized by TTE while the metabolic response to treatment can be evaluated using PET [1,4].

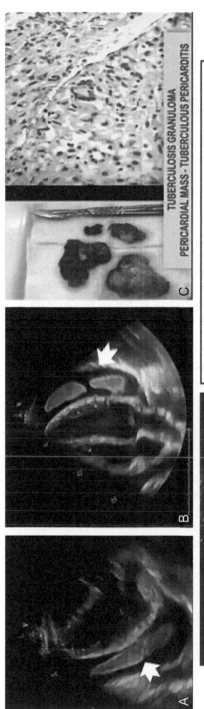

TUBERCULOSIS GRANULOMA
PERICARDIAL MASS - TUBERCULOUS PERICARDITIS

## Tuberculous Pericarditis

- Four pathological stages
  - DRY
    - Isolated granulomas
  - EFFUSIVE
    - Serosanginous effusion with lymphocytic exudate
  - ABSORPTIVE
    - Absorption of effusion and resolution of symptoms without treatment
  - CONSTRICTIVE
    - Fibrosis of visceral and parietal pericardium
    - +/- effusion

E

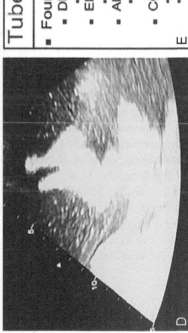

**FIG. 25.2**

The images depict tuberculous pericarditis. (A and B) TTE in a 29-year-old man presenting with orthopnea, peripheral edema, and progressive dyspnea over the preceding 2 weeks after protracted low fever, arthralgia, and weight loss (16 kg) over the preceding 5 months shows a large pericardial effusion, thickened pericardium with surface irregularities, and 2 large intrapericardial masses with regular contours (*white arrows*) (5.5 cm × 2.0 cm and 4.3 cm × 2.3 cm). The masses are interconnected with a bridge of tissue and are attached to the visceral and parietal layers of the pericardium with fibrinous strands. The masses float inside the pericardial fluid and have not invaded the surrounding tissues. (C) The patient underwent urgent pericardiotomy, and the masses were completely excised. The masses were disk-shaped and macroscopically composed of a lobulated, *yellowish* soft tissue. The histopathology results revealed a pattern of chronic granulomatous inflammation with necrosis, consistent with tuberculosis. (D) Another patient is presented herein with tuberculous pericarditis with a thick fibrin strand in the pericardial space, mimicking an intrapericardial mass (Supplementary Video 25.1 in the online version at https://doi.org/10.1016/B978-0-323-84906-7.00011-X). (E) The 4 stages of tuberculous pericarditis are presented herein.

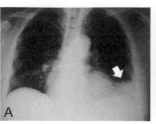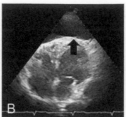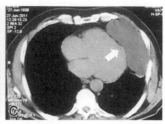

**FIG. 25.3**

The images illustrate a pericardial cyst. (A) The chest X-ray shows a large density adjacent to the cardiac apex *(white arrow)*. (B) TTE reveals a large echo-free space (14 cm × 5.2 cm) anterior to the left and right ventricles without compressive effects *(black arrow)*. (C) Thoracic CT scan shows a large cystic lesion in the left hemithorax adjacent to the cardiac apex *(white arrow)*. The final diagnosis was a pericardial cyst.

Pericardial masses are relatively rare and are mostly caused by malignancies. The metastatic involvement of the pericardium is more frequent than that by primary tumors and often carries a poor prognosis. Inflammatory and infectious diseases are very rarely reported as causes of pericardial masses in the literature, with a few reports of cardiac echinococcosis, rheumatoid arthritis, inflammatory pseudotumors, and tuberculous pericarditis. The presentation varies, and patients are often asymptomatic, with pericardial involvement detected only at the autopsy or as an incidental finding during thoracic imaging tests. Some patients, however, may develop progressive symptoms of venous congestion due to the evolution of pericardial effusion (diastolic restriction) or constriction, presenting with dyspnea, orthopnea, and peripheral edema [5].

Pericardial cysts are rare congenital anomalies located in the mediastinum. They are usually asymptomatic; nonetheless, they rarely produce symptoms based on their location and size. Commonly, they are located in the right cardiophrenic angle, followed by the left, anterosuperior, and posterior mediastinum. They are usually unilocular, well-marginated, spherical-shaped cysts lined with a single layer of mesothelial cells histologically. Most cysts are asymptomatic, but occasional complications include the obstruction of the right ventricular outflow tract, the obstruction of the main bronchi and atelectasis, cardiac tamponade, and sudden death. Imaging modalities include echocardiography, CT, and MRI. Usually, close follow-ups are sufficient in asymptomatic patients. Percutaneous drainage and surgical resection are the usual treatment modalities for symptomatic individuals [6].

**Table 25.4** Differential diagnoses of isolated cystic shadows adjacent to the heart.

| Lesions | Differentiating features |
|---|---|
| Bronchial cysts | Lined with the bronchial epithelium |
| Localized pericardial effusions | Fluid between the visceral and parietal pericardium |
| Teratomas | Usually associated with some solid components along with cystic components |
| Neurenteric cysts | Located in the right posterior chest and associated with vertebral anomalies |
| Lymphangiomas | Multilocular or multiple cysts |
| Congenital cysts of primitive foregut origins (e.g., bronchogenic cysts, gastroenteric cysts, and esophageal duplication cysts) | Usually located in the posterior mediastinum and lined by the epithelium |

**Table 25.5** Etiologies of pericardial cysts.

1. Congenital
2. Inflammatory (e.g., rheumatic pericarditis, bacterial infection, particularly tuberculosis, and echinococcosis)
3. Traumatic
4. Postcardiac surgery
5. Patients on chronic hemodialysis

**Table 25.6** Echocardiography in pericardial cysts.

| | |
|---|---|
| Characteristics | A homogeneous echolucent mass with minor attenuation of the ultrasound through a low-density fluid-filled structure<br>An echo-free space, indicating its separation from the cardiac chambers |
| Advantages | Safe<br>Low cost<br>May be performed on unstable patients<br>Diagnostic modality for follow-ups and image-guided percutaneous aspiration |
| Disadvantages | Limited windows and narrow fields of view<br>Technical difficulties in patients with obesity or obstructive lung disease, as well as in patients immediately post cardiothoracic surgery<br>Difficulty in the localization of cysts at uncommon locations<br>Operator dependent |

*Reproduced with permission form Kumar Kar S, Ganguly T. Current concepts of diagnosis and management of pericardial cysts. Indian Heart J 2017; 69:364–70. https://doi.org/10.1016/j.ihj.2017.02.021.*

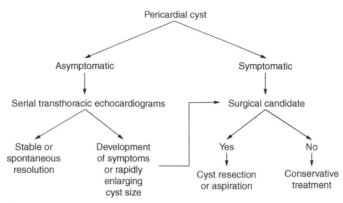

**ALGORITHM 25.7**

The image depicts the approach to pericardial cysts.

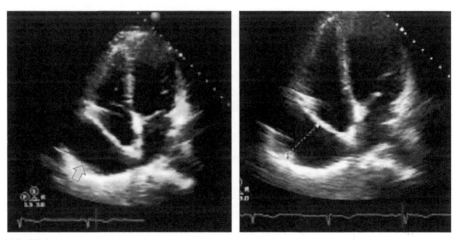

**FIG. 25.8**

The images illustrate a pericardial simple cyst in transthoracic echocardiography. The apical 4-chamber view of transthoracic echocardiography in a patient presenting with atypical chest pain shows an echolucent space adjacent to the right atrium without compressive effects *(yellow arrow)*. This finding is compatible with a pericardial simple cyst.

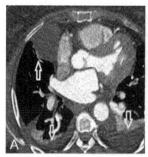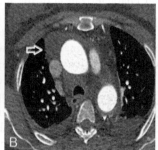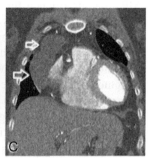

**FIG. 25.9**

Pericardial cyst on computed tomography (CT). High pitch prospective ECG-triggered CT angiography was performed for a patient suspicious of acute aortic dissection. Hypodense (densitometry: 10 HU) oval shape mass *(white arrow)* at right cardiophrenic angle and pericardial base. Intramural hematoma *(red arrow)* in descending aorta and bilateral pleural effusion *(yellow arrows)*.

Typically, pericardial cysts appear on CT images as well-defined, nonenhancing, homogeneous fluid-attenuation lesions that contain no internal septa. On CT, these thin-walled, homogeneous structures are nonenhancing with iodinated contrast and have an attenuation between −10 and 20 HU. Occasionally, the cyst may contain proteinaceous fluid, in which case the lesion will demonstrate intermediate attenuation at CT. Pericardial cysts with hemorrhagic contents appear with hyperattenuation at CT [7].

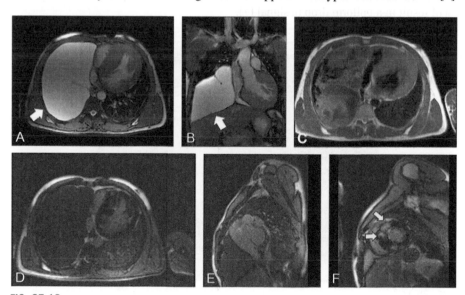

**FIG. 25.10**

Pericardial cyst on CMR. (A and B): Large cystic lesion *(white arrow)* in right hemithorax and pericardial based has shown high T2 signal cystic lesion in SSFP sequences in axial and coronal view in order. (C) Iso to hyposignal T1 lesion in HASTE sequence. (D and E) Late gadolinium enhancement (LGE) sequence revealed no enhancement. (F) Asymmetric hypertrophy of septum *(yellow arrows)* and patchy LGE due to concomitant hypertrophic.

MR imaging offers a further characterization of the internal contents of the cysts. Usually, pericardial cysts demonstrate intermediate to low signal intensity on T1-weighted images and high signal intensity on T2-weighted images. Pericardial cysts with proteinaceous content show high signal intensity with T1-weighted sequences and intermediate to the low signal intensity with T2-weighted sequences. Diffusion-weighted imaging may be useful in these cases, as pericardial cysts do not demonstrate restricted diffusion and show high signal on apparent diffusion coefficient (ADC) maps. Hemorrhagic cysts are hyperintense with T1-weighted sequences and demonstrate susceptibility with gradient recalled echo sequences. Surgical resection or percutaneous drainage is reserved for symptomatic individuals, when complications are present, or when the diagnosis is uncertain and pathologic analysis is needed [7].

Pericardial lipomas are benign lesions that most commonly grow insidiously, therefore resulting in few symptoms. As with subcutaneous lipomas, pericardial lipomas are encapsulated; however, unlike their subcutaneous counterparts, lipomas in the pericardium tend to be less circumscribed: Their contours are determined by the space they occupy. Symptoms, when present, are usually related to compression of adjacent structures. CT findings are usually diagnostic, as these lesions demonstrate homogeneously low attenuation (<0 HU) without enhancing components. A capsule may or may not be identified. MR imaging may be useful because of its superior contrast resolution. Lipomas appear as nonenhancing lesions that are hyperintense on T1-weighted MR images and intermediate to high signal intensity on T2-weighted MR images. Use of fat-saturated sequences to confirm the fatty nature of the lesion is helpful, as these sequences will result in a uniform drop in signal [7].

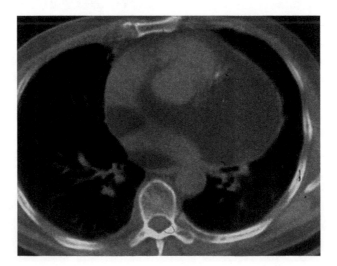

**FIG. 25.11**

Pericardial lipoma. A noncontrast CT image of the chest demonstrates a large, low-attenuation intrapericardial lesion that insinuates into the pericardial recesses and conforms to the pericardial space.

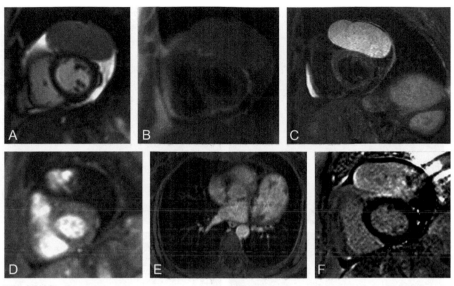

**FIG. 25.12**

Pericardial hemangioma. A 65-year-old female patient was admitted to the emergency department due to palpitation and atypical chest pain. In echocardiography, a large tumor was defined. CMR displays a large, well-defined pericardial tumor. In short-axis view, the cine SSFP sequence demonstrates hypersignal mass (A), the intermediate signal in the T1-W sequence (B), and a very high signal in the STIR sequence (C). In short-axis view, early perfusion sequence shows avid early enhancement at some part of the mass (D) and displays marked enhancement at early gradient-echo T1-W sequence in axial view (E). LGE sequence (F) demonstrates intense homogeneous enhancement of the mass lesion [Movie Online].

Pericardial hemangiomas can occur in any age group and are commonly found incidentally at autopsy. When arising from the pericardium, hemangiomas are most often of the cavernous type and they usually arise from the visceral pericardium. As with hemangiomas that occur elsewhere in the body, pericardial hemangiomas appear as heterogeneous lesions on noncontrast-enhanced CT images and may contain foci of calcification. When a contrast material is administered, it avidly enhance. At MR imaging, the hemangioma appears as a mass with intermediate T1-weighted signal intensity and high T2-weighted signal intensity. Upon contrast material administration, hemangiomas demonstrate nodular areas of enhancement with progressive filling on delayed images [7,8]. Hemangiomas show benign features, such as well-circumscribed borders and no evidence of invasion of neighboring structures. These features help differentiate these lesions from angiosarcoma.

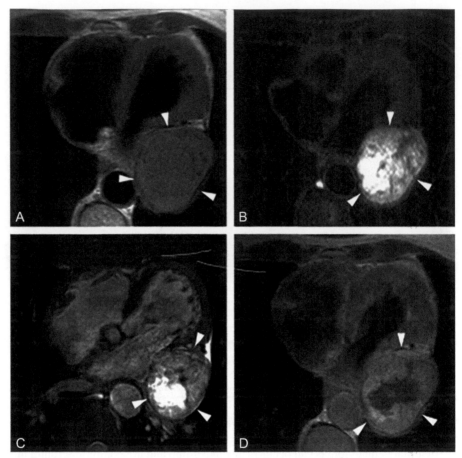

**FIG. 25.13**

Cardiac paraganglioma (or pheochromocytoma) in a 68-year-old man. T1w-imaging (A), T2w-imaging (B), 3D bright-blood imaging with high-spatial resolution (C), postcontrast T1wimaging (D). All images are obtained in the axial plane. A large well-circumscribed mass is shown at the lateral and upper border of the left atrium *(arrowheads)*. The appearance is fairly homogeneous on T1w imaging but is strongly heterogeneous on T2w imaging and cine imaging, and the mass shows a strong peripheral enhancement with a central nonenhancing zone. The adjacent cardiac structures are compressed by the large mass.

Intrapericardial paragangliomas are slow-growing tumors derived from neural crest cells and most often are nonfunctioning [9,10]. Their functioning counterpart is exceedingly rare [11]. Although most paragangliomas are benign, a minority of these neoplasms may exhibit locally invasive behavior or distant metastatic disease. Intrapericardial paragangliomas most commonly arise adjacent to the left atrium or anterior to the aortic root near the origin of the coronary arteries [4]. CT and MR imaging

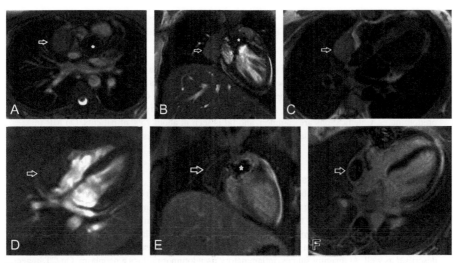

**FIG. 25.14**

The figure demonstrates subacute intrapericardial hematoma. The patient had a history of prosthetic aortic valve replacement (asterisk). Cardiac MRI demonstrates mass (arrow) in pericardial space. (A, B) Cine SSFP sequences display high signal oval shape mass, T1-W sequence (C) shows iso-high signal mass. (D) Early perfusion sequence reveals a nonenhancing mass. Early gadolinium (E) and late gadolinium (F) sequences display low signal mass and hyperenhancement of surrounding pericardium. These findings suggest the diagnosis of subacute intrapericardial hematoma.

are useful in localizing and characterizing the lesion and play important roles in surgical planning. On contrast-enhanced CT images, the paraganglioma appears as a hyperenhancing vascular mass. In approximately one-half of the patients, a central area of low attenuation that most likely represents necrosis or degeneration is seen. The characteristic MR imaging feature is a hyperintense signal with T2-weighted sequences. Contrast-enhanced T1-weighted images demonstrate findings similar to those seen on CT images. Cross-sectional imaging is useful for assessing the relationship of the tumor to adjacent structures, in a particular invasion of the adjacent atrium [10]. Patients may undergo imaging with indium 111 pentreotide, 131I MIBG, or 123I MIBG scintigraphy as part of their workup. Scintigraphy demonstrates an intrathoracic focus of increased tracer activity and is especially useful when the lesion remains occult with other imaging modalities. Indium 111 pentreotide is the nuclear medicine agent of choice, with a sensitivity of 94%. The sensitivity of MIBG scintigraphy is lower, as it accumulates in only functioning paragangliomas [12].

Pericardial hematomas are a common mimic of tumors, making differentiation between the two entities essential. Hematomas usually form after surgery or trauma, and although can be initially diagnosed by echocardiography, CT or CMR is often performed for confirmation and delineation of the extent of involvement. In an acute hematoma, CT will detect the high attenuation of initial blood, which decreases as

---

### Box 25.15

#### Germ cell tumors

Germ cell tumors may arise from the pericardium. These tumors are composed of tissue from at least two of the three germ cell layers. The majority of germ cell tumors are located anteriorly and to the right. Most of them manifest in the newborn period or infancy. On CT images, germ cell tumors are usually well-defined, heterogeneous, multilocular masses. Typically, the cystic component predominates. Calcifications are common, and fat is seen in about 75% of patients. On MR images, teratomas are heterogeneous masses with signal intensity characteristics that correspond to those of their components.

#### Inflammatory pseudotumors

Inflammatory pseudotumor is a benign process most commonly seen in the lung and orbit, but it can arise anywhere in the body, including the pericardium. The cause of inflammatory pseudotumor is unknown. Some cases develop secondary to surgery or trauma; some have been associated with IgG4-related sclerosing disease. Some authors argue in favor of a low-grade neoplastic process. Inflammatory pseudotumor is most often seen in children and young adults, but cases in older patients have been described as well. At imaging studies, inflammatory pseudotumor mimics a neoplasm. On CT images, these lesions have a variable appearance. Typically, a mass of heterogeneous attenuation and enhancement is seen [16]. An associated pericardial effusion may be present. On T1- and T2-weighted MR images, inflammatory pseudotumor usually has low signal intensity due to the fibrotic nature of the lesion. After administration of gadolinium contrast material, these lesions may show homogeneous or heterogeneous enhancement. On PET/CT images, these lesions show increased FDG uptake [7,16].

---

time progresses. As the hematoma matures, CT will detect fibrosis and calcification with high sensitivity. Further, hematomas do not enhance with iodinated contrast [1]. CMR has been shown to have excellent accuracy in the differentiation of cardiac thrombi or hematoma from tumors [13,14].

Acute phase hematomas display high intensity on T1- and T2-weighted sequences; subacute-phase hematomas appear as a fluid collection with heterogeneous intermediate to high signal on T1- and T2-weighted sequences; and chronic-phase hematomas display low signal with a dark rim due to its lower water content [15] (Box 25.15).

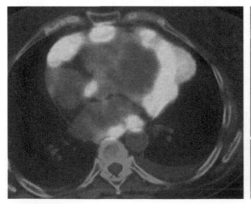 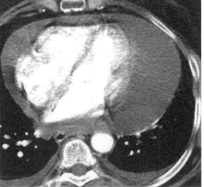

**FIG. 25.16**

Primary pericardial mesothelioma in a 65-year-old woman. *Left panel*: PET/CT image demonstrates a pericardial mass with avid FDG uptake that encases the heart. *Right panel*: Contrast-enhanced CT image obtained at a later date demonstrates interval development of an associated large pericardial effusion. The solid component is less conspicuous at CT.

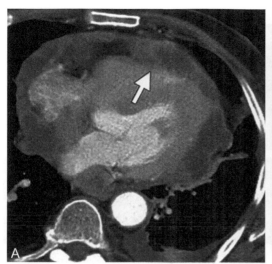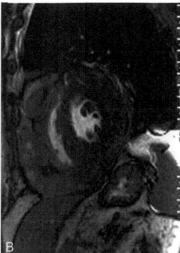

**FIG. 25.17**

Pericardial mesothelioma. (A) Contrast-enhanced CT image demonstrates a heterogeneously enhancing mass that involves the pericardium and completely encases the heart. There is loss of the epicardial fat plane along most of the ventricular walls *(arrow)*, a finding consistent with epicardial and possibly myocardial invasion. (B) Balanced steady-state free precession MR image obtained during diastole shows the heterogeneous mass confined to the pericardium and encasing the heart. Cine loop (not shown) demonstrated marked diastolic impairment.

Primary malignant pericardial mesothelioma is extremely rare, with a reported prevalence of 0.0022% at autopsy series. It is, however, the most common primary malignancy of the pericardium. Symptoms are vague and similar to those of other pericardial malignancies. Manifestations include constrictive pericarditis, pericardial effusion, tamponade physiology, and myocardial infiltration, which may result in conduction abnormalities [4]. Pericardiocentesis commonly reveals a hemorrhagic fluid, with malignant cells seen in only 20% of the cases. The sensitivity of echocardiography in the detection of pericardial mesothelioma is low [15]. CT and MR imaging offer an advantage, as these modalities better depict the extent of disease. On both CT and MR images, pericardial mesothelioma appears as a heterogeneously enhancing mass that involves both the parietal and visceral layers of the pericardium, with possible invasion of the adjacent vascular and anatomic structures. MR imaging helps provide information regarding the degree of constriction and diastolic impairment. At FDG/PET, these neoplasms demonstrate hypermetabolic activity. Metastatic disease is found in approximately 50% of the cases, most commonly in local mediastinal lymph nodes and the lungs [17].

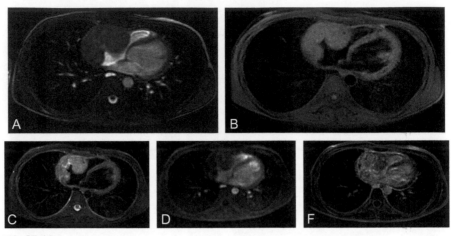

**FIG. 25.18**

The figure shows pericardial angiosarcoma. CMR from a young male patient with fever and malaise reveals infiltrative mass from the pericardium and right atrium. (A) Cine SSFP sequence image shows heterogeneous hypersignal mass. (B) T1-W fat saturation sequence image reveals iso-signal mass. (C) STIR sequence image displays high signal mass. (D) The early perfusion sequence image shows early enhancement of the mass. (E) LGE sequence demonstrates heterogeneous enhancement of the mass [Movie Online].

Pericardial angiosarcomas are vascular, highly aggressive neoplasms that frequently manifest with associated hemopericardium [18–20]. Echocardiography commonly demonstrates a pericardial effusion, but it may fail to show a mass because the depiction depends on a good acoustic window. Pericardiocentesis will often yield bloody fluid that may not contain malignant cells [18,19].

CT reveals the vascular and aggressive nature of angiosarcomas. These lesions are usually lobulated, vegetated masses that heterogeneously enhance at CT with areas of necrosis [19]. On T1-weighted MR images, the signal intensity of angiosarcoma is heterogeneous and variable, depending on the degree of hemorrhage and necrosis in the tumor; however, angiosarcoma is predominantly isointense relative to the myocardium. On T2-weighted and steady-state free precession images, these masses appear heterogeneous and hyperintense relative to the myocardium. Angiosarcoma is usually associated with the right atrioventricular groove, parasitizing blood flow from the right coronary artery. Large vascular channels may be seen as intralesional flow voids [18]. On contrast-enhanced images, angiosarcomas may show avid enhancement with a "sun ray" appearance. Both CT and MR imaging play an important role in depicting the degree of tumor invasion of adjacent structures. MR imaging may demonstrate constrictive physiology with diffuse thickening of the pericardium [20].

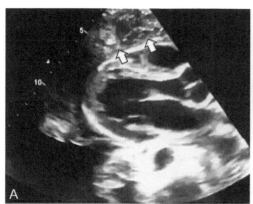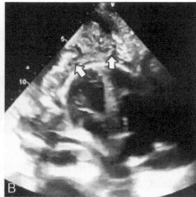

**FIG. 25.19**

The images illustrate a primary pericardial lymphoma. Transthoracic echocardiography shows pericardial and pleural effusions. There is notable pericardial thickness with a large, nonhomogeneous mass surrounding the heart *(white arrows)*. The anterior and inferior aspects of the pericardial space are filled with the mass, causing constriction physiology. The pathology results confirmed the diagnosis of a T-cell lymphoblastic lymphoma.

Most primary pericardial lymphomas are diffuse, large B-cell lymphomas [21]. Pericardial lymphoma most frequently manifests as an ill-defined, infiltrative soft tissue mass with an associated pericardial effusion.

On CT images, the soft tissue component of pericardial lymphoma may appear iso- to hypoattenuating with heterogeneous enhancement. Pericardial lymphoma is hypermetabolic at PET/CT. At MR imaging, it appears hypointense with T1-weighted sequences and iso  to hyperintense with T2-weighted sequences with variable heterogeneous enhancement. On occasion, a discrete mass is not seen, and the sole imaging finding may be diffuse pericardial thickening or effusion, which is commonly hemorrhagic [4] (Box 25.20).

### Box 25.20

Cardiac metastases are 20 to 40 times more frequent than primary tumors [22]. The pericardium is the most frequently involved site of cardiac metastasis, comprising 64% to 69% of all cardiac metastases in 2 recent large case series [23]. Tumor metastasis to the pericardium may initially result in pericarditis, with subsequent development of serosanguineous or hemorrhagic malignant pericardial effusions [24]. Spread to the heart occurs through direct extension from adjacent tumors, hematogenously spread, transvenous invasion, or lymphatic spread. Metastatic tumors display different characterization depending on the route; however, generally metastatic tumors show hypodense in CT and heterogeneous enhancement after IV contrast administration. Most pericardial metastases are of low signal intensity on T1-weighted images and are brighter on T2-weighted images. Most malignant disease enhances after administration of contrast material [25].

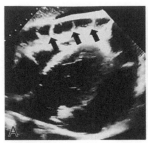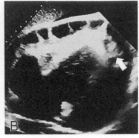

| Potential Clinical Manifestations of Pericardial Metastasis |
| --- |
| Pericarditis |
| Pericardial effusions |
| Cardiac tamponade |
| Pericardial adhesions |
| Constrictive pericarditis |

**FIG. 25.21**

The images demonstrate pericardial metastasis. Bedside transthoracic echocardiography in a patient, a known case of renal adenocarcinoma with a large pericardial effusion, shows notable pericardial thickening with multiple pericardial adhesion bands *(black arrows)*. Additionally, a large, semimobile, irregular echodensity is detectable. It is attached to the outer aspect of the apicolateral segment *(white arrow)*, suggestive of metastasis. Potential clinical manifestations of pericardial metastases.

*From Goldberg AD, Blankstein R, Padera RF. Tumors metastatic to the heart. Circulation 2013;128 (16):1790–94. https://doi.org/10.1161/CIRCULATIONAHA.112.000790; Maleki M, Alizadehasl A, Haghjoo M. Practical cardiology. 2nd ed. Elsevier; 2021.*

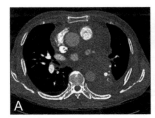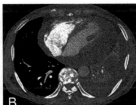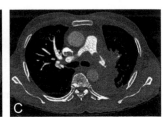

**FIG. 25.22**

Bronchogenic carcinoma. Thorax multislice CT with IV contrast demonstrates infiltrative bronchogenic carcinoma of the left lung with direct invasion to the pericardium, left atrium, and left pulmonary artery and encasement of descending aorta. Large pericardial effusion and left pleural effusion are noted.

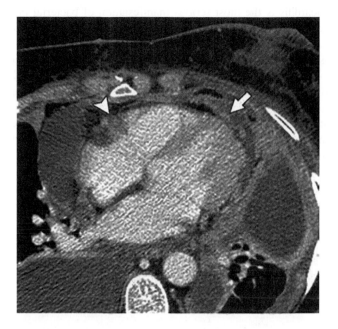

**FIG. 25.23**

A 45-year-old woman with metastatic breast cancer. Axial contrast-enhanced CT image shows large circumferential pericardial effusion, enhancing nodular visceral pericardium *(arrow)*, and soft tissue mass in right atrioventricular groove *(arrowhead)*. Lymphatic spread is common in patients with epithelial cancers such as breast carcinomas, and visceral pericardium and epicardial surface contain the largest distribution of heart lymphatics. Note left breast mass and skin thickening. Loculated pleural effusions and enhancing pleural nodules are also suspicious for metastatic disease, and incidence of cardiac metastasis increases with increasing overall metastatic burden.

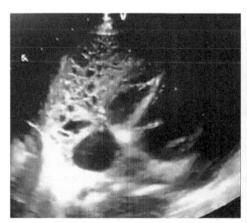 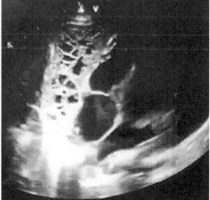

**FIG. 25.24**

The images depict bacterial pericarditis. Transthoracic echocardiography in a very ill patient shows large amounts of pus collected anteriorly to the heart, indicative of purulent bacterial pericarditis. Loculated, echogenic, septated collection can mimic masses like hydatid cysts.

Purulent pericarditis is the most serious manifestation of bacterial pericarditis. It is characterized by gross pus in the pericardium or a microscopically purulent effusion. Purulent pericarditis is an acute, fulminant illness with fever in virtually all patients. Chest pain is uncommon. Purulent pericarditis is always fatal if untreated. Sometimes, a localized pericardial effusion can extrinsically compress the heart, and its high echogenicity can make it appear as a solid mass on echocardiographic imaging [26].

All chronic pericardial effusions like tuberculosis pericarditis, infectious pericardial effusions, malignant pericardial effusions, and even chronic idiopathic pericardial effusions could have the above appearance.

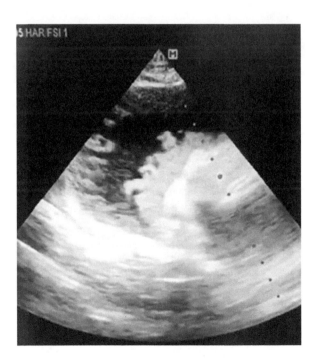

**FIG. 25.25**

The figure presents uremic pericarditis. Transthoracic echocardiography in an 18-year-old girl with lupus nephropathy presenting with dyspnea shows a massive pericardial effusion with large amounts of fibrin deposition as well as the shaggy appearance of the pericardium. The differential diagnosis of this finding is uremic pericarditis, and an infectious etiology should be borne in mind. These large fibrin strands and debris can mimic pericardial masses (Supplementary Video 25.2 in the online version at https://doi.org/10.1016/B978-0-323-84906-7.00011-X).

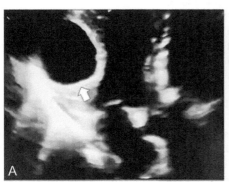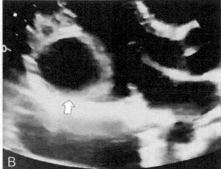

**FIG. 25.26**

The images depict pericardial hydatid cysts. Incidental finding in a patient during transthoracic echocardiography shows a large, echolucent mass with thick borders in the posterior aspect of the left ventricle *(white arrows)*. The concomitant liver cysts in this patient led to the diagnosis of a hydatid cyst.

## References

[1] Zhou W, Srichai MB. Multi-modality imaging assessment of pericardial masses. Curr Cardiol Rep 2017;19:32.

[2] Klein AL, Abbara S, Agler DA, et al. American society of echocardiography clinical recommendations for multimodality cardiovascular imaging of patients with pericardial disease: endorsed by the society for cardiovascular magnetic resonance and society of cardiovascular computed tomography. J Am Soc Echocardiogr 2013;26(9):965–1012.e15.

[3] Kassop D, Donovan MS, Cheezum MK, et al. Cardiac masses on cardiac CT: a review. Curr Cardiovasc Imaging Rep 2014;7(8):1–13.

[4] Restrepo CD, Vargas D, Ocazionez D, et al. Primary pericardial tumors. Radiographics 2013;33:1613–30.

[5] Santos Felix AD, Pinheiro da FonsecaRodrigo VB, Segalote C, et al. Arq Bras Cardiol 2021;116(2 Suppl. 1):12–6. https://doi.org/10.36660/abc.20190876.

[6] Nayak K, Shetty RK, Vivek G, et al. Pericardial cyst: a benign anomaly. BMJ Case Rep 2012. https://doi.org/10.1136/bcr-03-2012-5984.

[7] Narla LD, Newman B, Spottswood SS, et al. Inflammatory pseudotumor. Radiographics 2003;23(3):719–29.

[8] Shojaeifard M, Saedi S, Alizadeh Ghavidel A, et al. Concomitant cardiac and hepatic hemangiomas. Echocardiography 2020;37(3):462–4. https://doi.org/10.1111/echo.14614.

[9] Hamilton BH, Francis IR, Gross BH, et al. Intrapericardial paragangliomas (pheochromocytomas): imaging features. AJR Am J Roentgenol 1997;168(1):109–13.

[10] Hawari M, Yousri T, Hawari R, et al. Intrapericardial paraganglioma directly irrigated by the right coronary artery. J Card Surg 2008;23(6):780–2.

[11] Shimoyama Y, Kawada K, Imamura H. A functioning intrapericardial paraganglioma (pheochromocytoma). Br Heart J 1987;57(4):380–3.

[12] Intenzo CM, Jabbour S, Lin HC, et al. Scintigraphic imaging of body neuroendocrine tumors. Radiographics 2007;27(5):1355–69.

[13] Pazos-López P, Pozo E, Siqueira ME, et al. Value of CMR for the differential diagnosis of cardiac masses. JACC Cardiovasc Imaging 2014;7(9):896–905.

[14] Sparrow PJ, Kurian JB, Jones TR, Sivananthan MU. MR imaging of cardiac tumors. Radiographics 2005;25(5):1255–76.

[15] Lamba G, Frishman WH. Cardiac and pericardial tumors. Cardiol Rev 2012;20(5): 237–52.

[16] Patel R, Lim RP, Saric M, et al. Diagnostic performance of cardiac magnetic resonance imaging and echocardiography in evaluation of cardiac and paracardiacmasses. Am J Cardiol 2016;117(1):135–40.

[17] Fazekas T, Tiszlavicz L, Ungi I. Primary malignant pericardial mesothelioma. Orv Hetil 1991;132(48):2677–80.

[18] Holtan SG, Allen RD, Henkel DM, et al. Angiosarcoma of the pericardium presenting as hemorrhagic pleuropericarditis, cardiac tamponade, and thromboembolic phenomena. Int J Cardiol 2007;115(1):e8–9.

[19] Park SM, Kang WC, Park CH, et al. Rapidly growing angiosarcoma of the pericardium presenting as hemorrhagic pericardial effusion. Int J Cardiol 2008;130(1):109–12.

[20] Timóteo AT, Branco LM, Bravio I, et al. Primary angiosarcoma of the pericardium: case report and review of the literature. Kardiol Pol 2010;68(7):802–5.

[21] Miguel CE, Bestetti RB. Primary cardiac lymphoma. Int J Cardiol 2011;149(3):358–63.

[22] Motwani M, Kidambi A, Herzog BA, et al. MR imaging of cardiac tumors and masses: a review of methods and clinical applications. Radiology 2013;268:26–43.

[23] Bussani R, De-Giorgio F, Abbate A, et al. Cardiac metastases. J Clin Pathol 2007;60:27–34.

[24] Goldberg AD, Blankstein R, Padera RF. Tumors metastatic to the heart. Circulation 2013;128(16):1790–4. https://doi.org/10.1161/CIRCULATIONAHA.112.000790.

[25] Chiles C, Woodard PK, Gutierrez FR, et al. Metastatic involvement of the heart and pericardium: CT and MR imaging. Radiographics 2001;21:439–49.

[26] Kiavar M, Azarfarin R, Totonchi Z, et al. Comparison of two pain assessment tools, "Facial Expression" and "Critical Care Pain Observation Tool" in intubated patients after cardiac surgery. Anesth Pain Med 2016;6(1):e33434. https://doi.org/10.5812/aapm. 33434. 27110536. PMC4834529.

# Anesthetic considerations in cardiac mass

## 26

**Rasoul Azarfarin**

*Cardio-Oncology Research Center, Rajaie Cardiovascular Medical and Research Center, Iran University of Medical Sciences, Tehran, Iran*

## Key points

- Hemodynamic instability or even collapse, hypotension, and arrhythmias caused by a large right/left atrial or atrioventricular valve mass, limiting venous return and obstruction/restriction of intracardiac blood flow.

    (Anesthetic implications: Careful positioning of patient, preparation for major volume replacement, large bore IV and central venous access, vasoactive drug ready for immediate use, surgeon present in operating room during anesthesia induction, cardiopulmonary bypass primed and prepared for immediate use)

- Possibility of myocardial depression (intramural mass), reduction in coronary perfusion pressure, and systemic vascular resistance (SVR).

    (Anesthetic implications: Minimize dose of preoperative sedatives, titration of anesthesia induction drugs)

- Mass particle embolization.

    (Anesthetic implications: IOTEE for intraoperative monitoring, placing central venous catheter at femoral site is preferred)

- Atrial fibrillation or ventricular arrhythmias are not uncommon.

    (Anesthetic implications: Placing defibrillator pads before anesthesia induction for instantaneous cardioversion/defibrillation as needed)

Anesthetic management for resection of cardiac mass (including tumor, large clot, or vegetation) begins with an inclusive review of the preoperative imaging modalities by the cardiac anesthesiologist [1]. This evidence will enable the anesthesiologist to anticipate the possible intraoperative pathophysiologic considerations of the mass, based on size, mobility, and location [2]. For example, if a large mass (tumor or clot) is present in the right atrium (RA) [3], restriction or obstruction of venous return could potentially cause severe hypotension or arrhythmias (Fig. 26.1). The anesthetic implications in the approach to such an event should include careful positioning of the patient on the operating table to reduce the risk of impaired venous return [1–3].

   The anesthesiologist also needs to be ready for rapid volume replacement and resuscitation and immediate administration of a vasopressor if the patient becomes

Multimodal Imaging Atlas of Cardiac Masses. https://doi.org/10.1016/B978-0-323-84906-7.00021-2

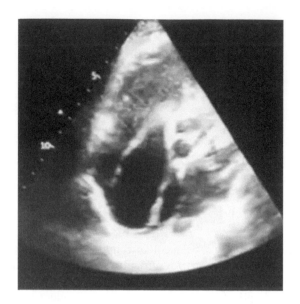

**FIG. 26.1**

Huge tricuspid valve blood cyst.

hemodynamically unstable due to decreased venous return or blood flow obstruction because of a large mass effect in the RA restricting blood flow through the tricuspid valve [4]. Because of the probability of hemodynamic collapse in such situations, the surgeon should be present in the operating room and ready for cardiopulmonary bypass (CPB) at all times, including during anesthesia induction. The anesthesiologist should minimize the use of sedative drugs in the preoperative period, and the dosage of induction agents must be titrated and administered cautiously in such patients. The aim of this practice is to avoid myocardial depression and to maintain adequate systemic vascular resistance (SVR) and coronary perfusion pressure. Maintaining adequate right ventricular filling pressure and volume and maintaining normal sinus rhythm reduces hemodynamic instability during anesthesia induction [1,5].

If the patient presents with a large intracardiac mass located in the atria or the tricuspid (or mitral) valves (Fig. 26.2), although administration of inotropes may be necessary to increase myocardial contractility, it is crucial to know that enhanced contractility can increase outflow tract obstruction (mimic valve stenosis) and may cause a dramatic decrease in intracardiac blood flow (Fig. 26.3). In addition, chronic mass effects could result in valvular stenosis or incompetence. Because of possible hepatic metastasis (Fig. 26.4), the anesthesiologist must assess liver function tests preoperatively in patients presenting with a malignant tumor so that drug dosage may be adjusted if indicated (Supplementary Videos 26.1–26.4 in the online version at https://doi.org/10.1016/B978-0-323-84906-7.00021-2).

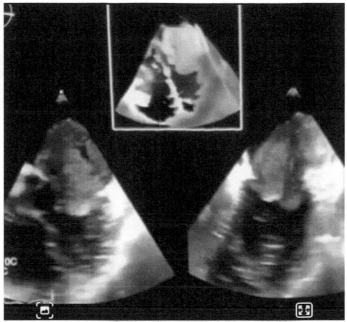

**FIG. 26.2**

Cardiac mixofibrosarcoma; a large and obstructive mass.

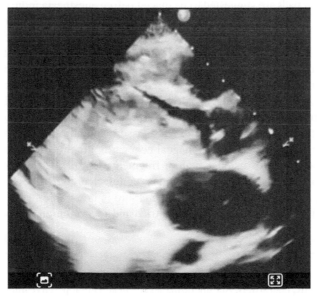

**FIG. 26.3**

Large life threatening outflow tract obstructing left ventricular mass (metastatic melanoma).

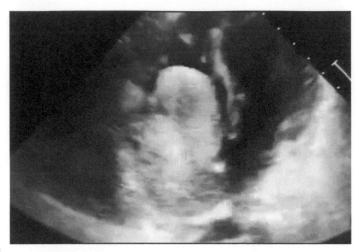

**FIG. 26.4**

Large and obstructive metastatic lesion (liver cancer).

In right side cardiac masses, particle embolization can lead to acute pulmonary hypertension with or without hemodynamic instability or even collapse [3]. The anesthesiologist might consider placement of a central venous catheter at the femoral vein instead of the internal jugular (or subclavian) vein, as a safer alternative to avoid atrial fibrillation or contact with the right side cardiac mass (especially fresh clots). Defibrillation pads are suggested to be placed before anesthesia induction so that the patient can be immediately cardioverted-defibrillated if needed. Atrioventricular block and ventricular arrhythmias are not uncommon in the perioperative period, particularly in patients who present with intramyocardial or intracavity masses that infiltrate to or cause inflammation of conduction fibers [6,7]. Arrhythmias can occur acutely after surgical resection, and may require a permanent pacemaker [3]. During anesthesia we must ensure that an adequate anesthesia depth is provided, especially in stimulating events such as laryngoscopy, surgical incision, and sternotomy, to prevent an acute hypertension or rise in RA pressure and atrial dysrhythmia [4].

Use of intraoperative transesophageal echocardiography (IOTEE) enables us to (1) detect cardiac mass dislodgement or fragmentation, (2) perform a postresection evaluation of the presence of a residual mass or defect, and (3) assess patient volume status, particularly if the central venous pressure is unreliable in the presence of a large mass in the RA that causes severe tricuspid regurgitation or obstruction [7].

## References

[1] Cushing MR, Leonardi B. Anesthetic management and intraoperative implications for surgical resection of a recurring primary cardiac rhabdomyosarcoma: a case report. AANA J 2017;85(1):36–41.

[2] Melnyk V, Hackett PJ, Subramaniam K, Badhwar V, Esper SA. Complex considerations and anesthetic management in patient with multiple intracardiac myxomas. J Cardiothorac Vasc Anesth 2018;32:1374–6.

[3] Essandoh M, Andritsos M, Kilic A, Crestanello J. Anesthetic management of a patient with a giant right atrial myxoma. Semin Cardiothorac Vasc Anesth 2016;20(1):104–9.

[4] Alizadehasl A, Saedi T, Saedi S. Huge right ventricular thrombus clot in renal cell carcinoma without inferior vena cava involvement. Iran Heart J 2021;22(4):135–7.

[5] Alexis A, Origer P, Hacquebard JP, Cannière DD, Germay O, Vandenbossche JL, Kapessidou Y. Anesthetic management of a voluminous left atrial myxoma resection in a 19 weeks pregnant with atypical clinical presentation. Case reports. Anesthesiology 2019. https://doi.org/10.1155/2019/4181502. 210139204.

[6] Saed D, Alizadehasl A. Challenging left ventricular apical mass: a case review. Iran Heart J 2018;19(4):62–5.

[7] Maleki M, Alizadehasl A, Behjati M, Youssef M. Metastatic cardiac mass: role of transthoracic echocardiography. Iran Heart J 2018;19(3):64–7.

# Other masses with the differential diagnosis of cardiac tumors

# 27

**Azin Alizadehasl[a], Hamidreza Pouraliakbar[b], and Sheikh Mohammed Shariful Islam[c]**

[a]*Cardio-Oncology Research Center, Rajaie Cardiovascular Medical and Research Center, Iran University of Medical Sciences, Tehran, Iran* [b]*Department of Radiology, CardioOncology Research Center, Iran University of Medical Sciences, Rajaie Cardiovascular Medical and Research Center, Tehran, Iran* [c]*Institute for Physical Activity and Nutrition, School of Exercise and Nutrition Sciences, Deakin University, Melbourne, VIC, Australia*

## Key points

- Extracardiac cardiac masses are important to the cardiologist because they can sometimes compress the heart or the great vessels, which enter or emerge from the heart, and, thus, simulate tamponade, constrictive pericarditis, or congestive heart failure.
- They are important also to the echocardiographer because their presence may be unexpectedly revealed on routine echocardiography, or because by encroachment on the cardiac chambers such as the atria, they distort normal anatomic contours or mimic intraatrial neoplasms or thrombi.

**Table 27.1** Mechanisms of the involvement of echocardiographic views by mediastinal masses [1].

| | |
|---|---|
| Proximity | The abnormal mass is contiguous or adjacent to the heart and recognizable in 1 or more of the 2D echocardiographic views, but it does not deform or indent the cardiac chambers |
| Encroachment | The mediastinal mass encroaches on 1 or more heart chambers, narrowing or otherwise distorting them, but it does not cause adverse hemodynamic effects (However, the patient may be symptomatic from the pressure effects of the mass on the esophagus, the trachea, or the other noncardiac structures.) |
| Compression | The mediastinal mass is large and rigid or, if cystic, under high pressure, and can compress the heart. Thereby, it produces hemodynamic effects and symptoms like tamponade. This mechanism is mostly due to a large, firm, solid mass; a high-tension fluid accumulation; or an aortic aneurysm to seriously impair cardiac filling, in effect like tamponade |

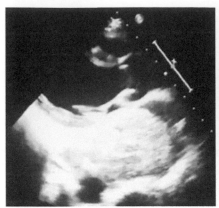 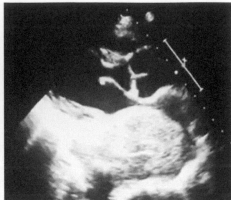

**FIG. 27.2**

The images illustrate an esophageal tumor. Transthoracic echocardiography shows the external compression of a large mass posterior to the left atrium with external compressive effects. The mass, however, does not exert obstructive effects on the left ventricular inflow. The mass is an esophageal tumor (Supplementary Video 27.1). The important point is that performing transesophageal echocardiography could be fatal in such a patient, and the external compression of esophageal masses should be in mind in all patients with left atrial masses before deciding to perform a transesophageal echocardiographic examination.

By transthoracic echocardiography, it is hard to distinguish a left atrial mass as an intraatrial or extraatrial tumor, which makes clinical decision-making difficult. If a fluid accumulation is found over the pericardial space, a differentiation between the extracardiac and intracardiac tumor can be made more easily. If the tumor mass in the heart chamber is without clear margins, it may be due to myocardial invasion by esophageal carcinomas or metastatic neoplasms (Supplementary Video 27.1 in the online version at https://doi.org/10.1016/B978-0-323-84906-7.00018-2).

The detection of an echodensity over the left atrium by echocardiography underscores the significance of skillful manipulations such as (1) the use of harmonic images that can improve the quality of the far gain image; (2) the employment of color flow images since there will be some blood flow around the mass if the mass, either primary or secondary in origin, is really inside the chamber; and (3) the adjustment of the probe angulation to see the tumor margin. If the convex margin of the tumor mass is found, extracardiac tumors should be considered. The probe angulation can see the correlation between the tumor motion and the chamber motion; nonetheless, moving the probe too fast can mimic the tumor moving

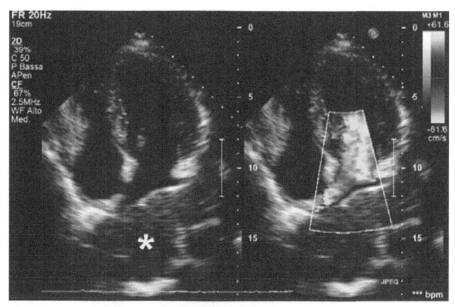

**FIG. 27.3**

The images demonstrate a lung tumor. Transthoracic echocardiography in the apical 4-chamber view shows an extracardiac, isoechoic mass compressing the left atrium. The mass is a pulmonary neoplasm.

*From L'Angiocola PD, Donati R. Cardiac masses in echocardiography: a pragmatic review. J Cardiovasc Echogr 2020;30(1):5–14. https://doi.org/10.4103/jcecho.jcecho_2_20.*

with the heartbeats. Additionally, if the mass lesion is found by echocardiography with a target characteristic, a tumor in the lower third of the esophagus with circumferential wall thickness compressing the left atrium could be another differential diagnosis [2].

It is well known that extracardiac structures such as hiatal hernias, pleural effusions, and ascites can be evaluated with transthoracic echocardiography. The reason that primary lung tumors can be visualized by transthoracic echocardiography is their proximity to the heart and, therefore, their placement in the field of view. It could be suggested that transthoracic echocardiography might be a method for the visualization of primary lung tumors. This case highlights the importance of the careful inspection of the extracardiac space when performing transthoracic echocardiography [3].

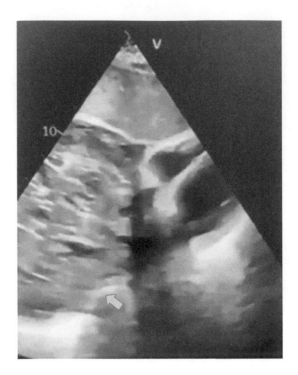

**FIG. 27.4**

The image illustrates a lung sarcoma. The subcostal view of transthoracic echocardiography shows a huge pulmonary mass with compressive effects on the heart and the inferior vena cava *(yellow arrow)*. The pathology results confirmed the presence of a right lung sarcoma.

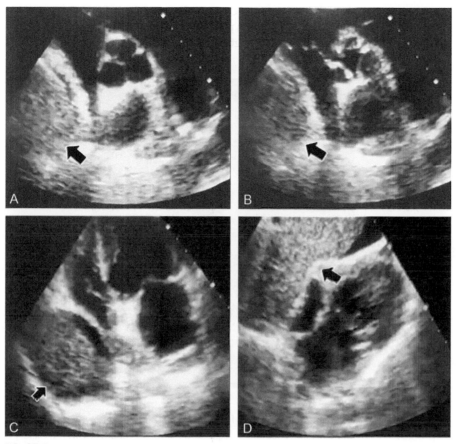

**FIG. 27.5**

The images demonstrate hepatomegaly. The parasternal short-axis view in the diastole (A) and the systole (B) and also the apical 4-chamber (C) and subcostal (D) views of transthoracic echocardiography in a 55-year-old woman with a history of common bile duct stenting 10 days earlier presenting with jaundice show ascites with huge hepatomegaly, compressing the right atrium *(black arrow)* (Supplementary Video 27.2).

Huge hepatomegaly, large hepatic cysts, or liver metastases can compress the right heart and even result in tamponade physiology in a few patients. Diaphragmatic hernia or eventration can also cause right heart compression by the liver.

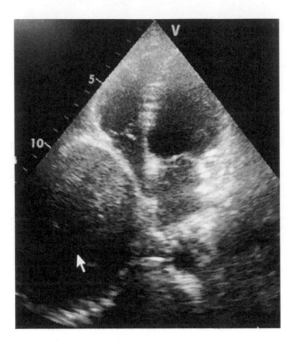

**FIG. 27.6**

The image depicts the compressive effect of liver metastasis in a patient with breast cancer. The apical 4-chamber view of transthoracic echocardiography in a patient with a history of metastatic breast cancer presenting with dyspnea shows a huge, round, well-defined extracardiac mass compressing the right atrium *(white arrow).*

The compression of the heart by liver metastases has been reported in the medical literature, most commonly presenting as right-sided heart failure or rarely tamponade. They can also result in atrial fibrillation, atrial flutter, or even variable atrioventricular conduction (Supplementary Video 27.2 in the online version at https://doi.org/10.1016/B978-0-323-84906-7.00018-2).

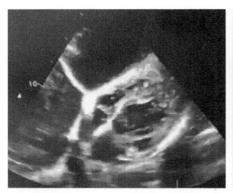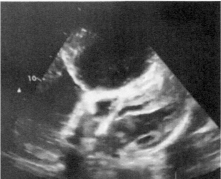

**FIG. 27.7**

The images illustrate the compressive effect of tense ascites. The subcostal view of transthoracic echocardiography in a patient with a history of chronic liver disease presenting with dyspnea, hypotension, and abdominal distention shows massive ascites with compressive effects on the right heart (left panel). Progression of the ascites resulted in tamponade hemodynamic effect and diastolic collapse of right ventricle (right panel).

Cardiac tamponade is a common and often life-threatening presentation. Classically, cardiac tamponade is associated with a pericardial effusion in most cases, but it is rarely seen in association with external cardiac compression.

Ascites is a common finding in patients with chronic liver disease and cirrhosis. It is frequently associated with dyspnea due to abdominal distension and less frequently with the development of a right-sided pleural effusion. Additionally, cirrhosis patients are often noted to be hypotensive and have tachycardia during hospitalization.

Performing an echocardiogram to look for a cardiac etiology for breathing distress and hemodynamic compromise is not a routine practice. It requires a high index of suspicion with thorough history taking and physical examination to suspect cardiac tamponade and to carefully select a patient who may be suitable for further cardiac testing. Tamponade in cirrhotic patients is usually caused by pericardial or large pleural effusions, but ascites can rarely be the reason. Given the high mortality among patients with cardiac tamponade, an early diagnosis and treatment of the underlying etiology can improve the clinical outcome significantly among patients suffering from liver disease [4,5].

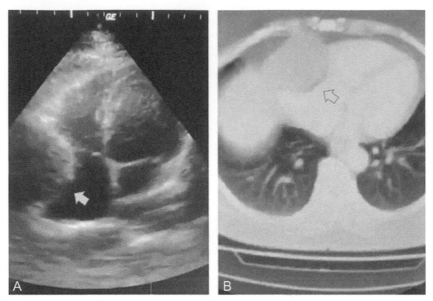

**FIG. 27.8**

The images demonstrate a thymoma. (A) The apical 4-chamber view of transthoracic echocardiography shows a large, well-defined mass compressing the right atrium *(yellow arrow)*. (B) Thoracic computed tomography scan shows a large, anterior mediastinal mass with compressive effects on the right heart *(yellow arrow)*. The differential diagnoses of this mass encompass thymomas, lymphomas, lipomas, and teratomas. The pathology results confirmed the presence of a large thymoma.

Typically, thymomas cause few symptoms unless they reach large dimensions. Thus these lesions may be occasionally discovered during imaging examinations in completely asymptomatic patients.

The symptoms of chest pain and dyspnea occur typically because of the compressive characteristic of the tumor, which, in significant volume, can compress the right atrium and cause hemodynamic alterations. These hemodynamic alterations not only change the venous flows at the entrance of the right atrium and the tricuspid valve but also may cause changes in the coronary reserve flow, which may certainly contribute to the symptoms of chest pain and dyspnea. These symptoms may also be aggravated by the degree of heart compression by the tumor and might worsen with certain positions adopted by the patient. Therefore mediastinal tumors as a differential diagnosis of patients with chest pain should be in mind [6,7].

# References

[1] Dcruz I, Feghali N, Gross CM. Echocardiographic manifestations of mediastinal masses compressing or encroaching on the heart. Echocardiography 1994;11(5):523–33.

[2] Huang SH, Tzeng BH, Tsai TN, et al. An image pitfall of esophageal carcinoma imitating left atrial tumor detected by transthoracic echocardiography. Acta Cardiol Sin 2006;22: 244–8.

[3] Dencker M, Cronberg C, Damm S, et al. Primary lung tumour visualised by transthoracic echocardiography. Cardiovasc Ultrasound 2008;6. https://doi.org/10.1186/1476-7120-6-60.

[4] Ahmad S, Jamali HJ, Waqar F, et al. Cardiac tamponade physiology secondary to tense ascites. Cardiology 2016;134:423–5. https://doi.org/10.1159/000445048.

[5] Maleki M, Alizadehasl A, Haghjoo M. Practical cardiology. 2nd ed. Elsevier; 2021.

[6] Filho JR, Melo RF, Macedo MD, et al. Chest pain due to right atrial compression caused by a thymolipoma. Arq Bras Cardiol 2004;82(5). https://doi.org/10.1590/S0066-782X2004000500011.

[7] Sadeghpour A, Alizacasl A. The right ventricle: a comprehensive review from anatomy, physiology, and mechanics to hemodynamic, functional, and imaging evaluation. Arch Cardiovasc Imaging 2015;3:4. https://doi.org/10.5812/acvi.35717.

# Fossa ovalis, patent foramen ovale, and cardiac masses

# 28

**Afsheen Nasir[a], Mohammad A. Zafar[b], and John A. Elefteriades[b]**

[a]Yale University School of Medicine, New Haven, CT, United States [b]Aortic Institute at Yale-New Haven Hospital, Yale University School of Medicine, New Haven, CT, United States

## Key points

- Fossa ovalis is a depression on the right atrial side of interatrial septum. It is an embryonic remnant of a once patent channel between the right and left atria of the fetal heart, serving fetal circulatory system. In adults, this landmark is often used surgically for accessing the left atrium from right atrium for various surgical procedures.

- In about a quarter of the population, this channel fails to close leading to patent foramen ovale. This foramen is implicated in various pathologies like paradoxical thromboembolism leading to conditions like cryptogenic stroke. This patency may also be associated with atrial septal aneurysm, that increases the risk for associated pathologies. Patent foramen ovale can be diagnosed using transesophageal echocardiography with bubble study, and transthoracic echocardiography, among other radiological techniques. Management involves percutaneous closure of the foramen ovale using occluder devices.

- Cardiac masses can range from simple cardiac growths to benign cardiac tumors and malignant neoplasms. Management involves resection of most tumors depending on their size and severity of the associated symptoms.

## Morphology

The fossa ovalis is a three-dimensional structure consisting of the septum itself and the annulus or limbus fossa ovalis, the raised edge around the perimeter of the fossa [1]. The annulus gives the margins of the fossa a crater-like appearance. Although there is a wide variation in the location and geometry of the fossa ovalis, structurally, the fossa can vary from being smooth to a net-like formation. The fossa can also be patent or form a right-sided pouch (RSP) [2]. The RSP may imitate a PFO channel. The shape of the fossa is oval in most people [3].

**403**

Multimodal Imaging Atlas of Cardiac Masses. https://doi.org/10.1016/B978-0-323-84906-7.00013-3

## Anatomical relations

The septum that separates the right atrium from the left atrium has an oval thumbprint size depression called the fossa ovalis on the lower portion of its right atrial side. It has a prominent margin, the limbus fossa ovalis (border of the oval fossa). The fossa lies cephalad and left of the inferior vena cava, and the coronary sinus lies caudal and anterior to the fossa, whereas His bundle shares the same horizontal plane with the fossa ovalis (Fig. 28.2). The depression in the fossa represents the residuum of the embryonic oval foramen and its valve—important components of the fetal circulation. The interatrial septum faces forward and to the right, corresponding to the location of left atrium that lies posteriorly and to the left of right atrium. The interatrial septum forms the anterior wall of the left atrium.

Surgically, the fossa ovalis, along with the midseptal region, represents the true interatrial septum and comprises only 20% of the entire interatrial septum. The fossa ovalis and this midseptal region are the only places where one can penetrate and create an interconnection between the two atria without exiting the heart [2,5].

## Embryology

In the primitive atrium of the fetal heart, two partially muscular embryonic structures called septum primum and septum secundum fuse to form the interatrial septum (Fig. 28.3).

The ostium primum in the septum primum serves the purpose of shunting oxygenated blood from the umbilical vein through inferior vena cava and right atrium directly to the left atrium, bypassing the pulmonary system and the nonfunctional fetal lungs. Oxygen-rich blood hence shunts directly into the systemic circulation, a process necessary for the normal expansion of left atrium and left ventricle.

During the 4th week of fetal life, as the septum primum grows, the evolving atrioventricular mesenchymal complex begins to fill the gap in the interatrial connection of ostium primum (Fig. 28.3A and B). At the same time, as the ostium primum is gradually disappearing, new tiny perforations are created in the central region of septum primum by programmed cell death; those coalesce to form a new foramen called the ostium secundum (Fig. 28.3C), which is purposed for continued right to left shunting of blood before ostium primum finally closes.

Around 5–6 weeks, a second ridge called septum secundum begins to grow craniocaudally and dorsoventrally, overlapping the ostium secundum (Fig. 28.3D and E). This muscular ridge leaves an opening near the floor of the right atrium, forming the foramen ovale.

The cranial part of the septum primum, initially attached to the roof of the left atrium, gradually disappears (Fig. 28.3E). The remaining part of the septum, attached to the fused endocardial cushions, forms the flap-like valve of the foramen ovale. This valve prevents the backflow of blood away from the left atrium by collapsing

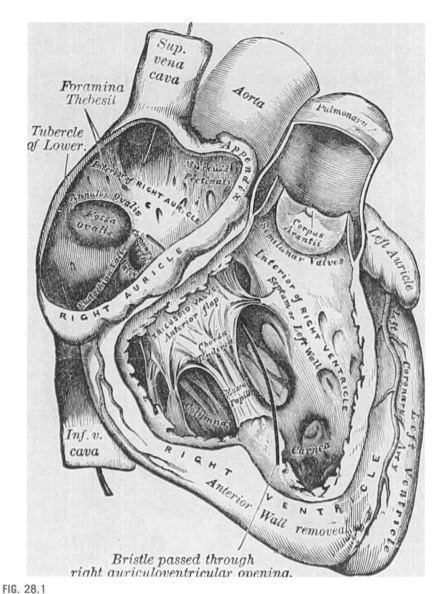

**FIG. 28.1**

Fossa ovalis on the interatrial septum as seen through the right atrium.

*Reproduced with the permission of Alamy, alamy.com (Public domain).*

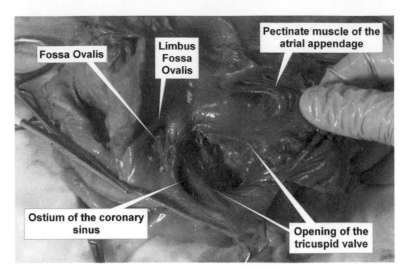

**FIG. 28.2**

Anatomic relations of fossa ovalis.

*Reproduced with permission from Clinical Anatomy Associates, Inc.*

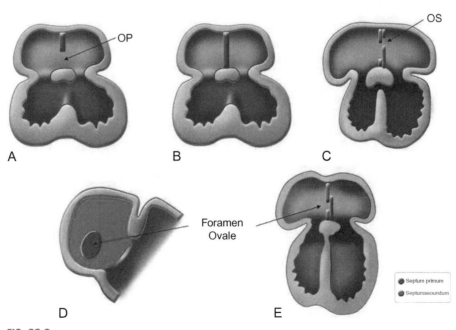

**FIG. 28.3**

Embryonic formation of fossa ovalis. (A) Ostium primum in septum primum. (B) Septum primum growing caudally toward the atrioventricular mesenchymal complex. (C) Formation of ostium secundum in septum primum, and formation of septum secundum. (D and E) Formation of foramen ovale.

*Reproduced with permission from Cruz-González I, Solis J, Inglessis-Azuaje I, Palacios IF. Patent foramen ovale: current state of the art. Rev Esp Cardiol. 2008;61(7):738–751.*

against the stiff septum secundum. This shunt continues for the rest of the fetal development during the intrauterine life.

## Functional closure of the foramen ovale

After birth, as the lungs become functional with neonatal breathing, the pulmonary vasculature abruptly dilates. This, combined with the cessation of umbilical flow, reverses the pressure difference, significantly decreasing the pressure in right atrium compared to the left. Increased pressures in the left atrium push the flexible septum primum (valve of the foramen ovale) against the more rigid septum secundum, even during atrial diastole, thus leading to functional closure of the foramen ovale.

## Anatomical closure of the foramen ovale

Anatomical closure is achieved at around 3rd month when tissue proliferation and adhesion of the septum primum to the left margin of the septum secundum are complete, obliterating the foramen ovale.

As a result, the interatrial septum becomes a complete partition between the atria in about 75% of humans, carrying the memory of fetal foramen ovale as a depression, called the fossa ovalis. The septum primum forms floor of the oval fossa. The inferior edge of the septum secundum forms a rounded fold, the border of the oval fossa (limbus fossa ovalis), which marks former boundary of the foramen ovale, giving it a crater-like appearance.

## Vascular supply

Right and left coronary arteries give off right and left anterior and posterior atrial branches, which anastomose to form Kugel's artery or the arteria anastomotica auricularis magna [6,7] (Fig. 28.4) which supplies the interatrial septum.

The midportion of the interatrial septum, together with the fossa ovalis, receives the least amount of vascular supply. The number and density of these vessel networks also decreases with age. In the antero-inferior part of the septum, a comparatively dense vascular network exists [8].

## Nerve supply

Angiotensinergic (renin–angiotensin–aldosterone dependent) innervation dominates the right atrium, which might also be a source of angiotensin II. It modulates autonomic nervous function in the heart thereby facilitating presynaptic noradrenaline

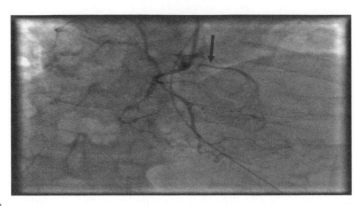

**FIG. 28.4**

Coronary angiogram of the right coronary system in the right anterior oblique view showing anomalous vessel connection (Kugel's artery) between the proximal RCA and distal RCA (*red arrow*), also demonstrating CTO of mid-RCA. *CTO*, complete total occlusion; *RCA*, right coronary artery.

*Reproduced with permission from Narh JT, Choudhary KV, Okunade A, et al. Kugel's artery: silent bystander or savior? Cureus 2021;13(8):e17039. https://doi.org/10.7759/cureus.17039.*

release. Vagal efferents and noncatecholaminergic afferents comprise the peripheral nerve fibers, a small amount of whose impact is sympathetic.

## Use of fossa ovalis as a surgical plane

For most surgical procedures that require access from the right atrium to the left heart chambers, the (limbus) fossa ovalis represents the most direct anatomical landmark and avenue of access [2] (Fig. 28.5). Situations requiring such access include hemodynamic assessment of the mitral valve, catheter-based mitral valve repair, paravalvular leak closure, and percutaneous balloon valvuloplasty. Left atrial appendix closure, pulmonary vein isolation, and radiofrequency catheter ablation also make use of the true interatrial septum formed by the fossa ovalis for transseptal puncture. In the presence of a prosthetic aortic valve, the fossa ovalis provides an alternate access to the left ventricle besides the retrograde route through the aortic valve. PFO and ASD repair also makes use of the same fossa landmark for access.

## Change of morphology of fossa ovalis in certain conditions
### Rheumatic heart disease

An increase in the surface area of fossa ovalis is observed and it tends to assume a more horizontal orientation in rheumatic heart disease that scars the valves [9] and other structures within the heart [10].

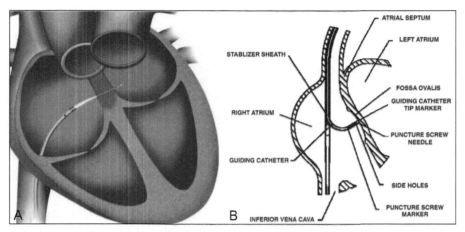

**FIG. 28.5**

Right heart catheter traversing through fossa ovalis to enter the left heart.

*Reproduced with permission from Babaliaros VC, Green JT, Lerakis S, Lloyd M, Block PC. Emerging applications for transseptal left heart catheterization: old techniques for new procedures. J Am Coll Cardiol. 2008; 51(22):2116–2122.*

## Amyloidosis

While amyloidosis causes diffuse thickening of the heart valves, it also thickens the interatrial septum including fossa ovalis, which is 100% specific for disease [11].

## Patent foramen ovale
### Incidence and morphology

In about 25%–35% [4] of the population, the fetal foramen ovale fails to close, leaving a patency between the right and left atria known as the "patent foramen ovale." It is not a true defect of the interatrial septum like the atrial septal defects, rather a variant of fossa ovalis occurring due to the failure of successful fusion of the septum primum and secundum [4]. There is variation in the location and size of the fossa ovalis from heart to heart [12]; therefore, a corresponding variation is seen in the corresponding characteristics of the patent foramen ovale. In most cases, the height of the curvilinear, oblong tunnel-like patent foramen ovale ranges anywhere between 1 and 6 mm and width between 5 and 13 mm [13] along the curve of the muscular rim formed by septum secundum, with a diameter of 1–10 mm. The size tends to increase with increasing age [4].

Antero-superiorly, the right atrial entrance of patent foramen ovale is bordered by the muscular rim of the fossa, whereas the thin flap valve forms the posterior border. A crescentic free edge of the embryonic septum primum forms the left atrial entrance [13]. This entrance is in proximity to the left atrial antero-superior wall and

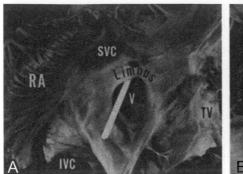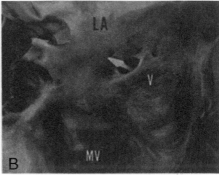

**FIG. 28.6**

Patent foramen ovale shown in autopsy specimen from a 85-year-old man. (A) Right atrial (RA) view shows a probe in foramen ovale, between limbus and valve (V) of fossa ovalis. (B) Left atrial (LA) view shows same probe as in (A) exiting through ostium secundum, the prominent fenestration in the valve. Normally, when left atrial pressure exceeds right atrial pressure, the valve of the fossa ovalis is pressed against the limbus and thereby closes the foramen ovale. *IVC*, inferior vena cava; *MV*, mitral valve; *SVC*, superior vena cava; *TV*, tricuspid valve [4].

*Reproduced with permission from Hagen PT, Scholz DG, Edwards WD. Incidence and size of patent foramen ovale during the first 10 decades of life: an autopsy study of 965 normal hearts. Mayo Clin Proc. 1984;59(1):17-20.*

is of surgical importance while advancing a catheter due to the risk of exiting the heart as this part of the left atrial wall is exceptionally thin (Fig. 28.6).

## Clinical pathology
### Patent foramen ovale, atrial septal aneurysm, paradoxical embolism, and cryptogenic stroke
#### Paradoxical embolism
Patent foramen ovale (PFO), although benign on its own, is usually too small to be hemodynamically significant. However, even a small patent foramen can provide a channel for thrombi, fat particles, and gas bubbles to enter the systemic circulation, bypassing the pulmonary arterial circuit. This right to left shunting of the embolus via PFO, called "paradoxical embolism" (Figs. 28.7 and 28.8), has been long associated with cryptogenic stroke, especially in a younger population without risk factors for ischemic stroke. In fact, out of all individuals who suffer cryptogenic stroke, nearly half harbor a PFO [14].

#### Atrial septal aneurysm
Atrial septal aneurysm (ASA), although rarely an isolated abnormality, is frequently associated (50%–89%) with PFO [15,16]. Presenting on echocardiography as a focal bulge of the IAS with displacement toward the left or right atrium [17–19], atrial septal aneurysm has been implicated as a source of cardiogenic emboli from thrombi

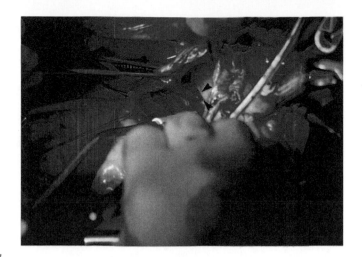

**FIG. 28.7**

Paradoxical embolism, intraoperative demonstration of the large thrombus traversing the patent foramen ovale (*arrows*). View is taken through the open right atrium, while on cardiopulmonary bypass. The patient is a young male graduate student who was working for 9 weeks on his PhD thesis dissertation, essentially never leaving his desk during that time. He developed chest pain and severe shortness of breath, prompting his presentation to the emergency room. Despite the massive venous thrombus (see also Fig. 28.7), he recovered completely postoperatively and achieved his PhD degree shortly thereafter.

*Published with permission from Koullias G, Elefteriades JA, Wu I, Jovin I, Jadbabaie F, McNamara R., Massive paradoxical embolism caught in the act. Circulation 2004;109:3056–3057.*

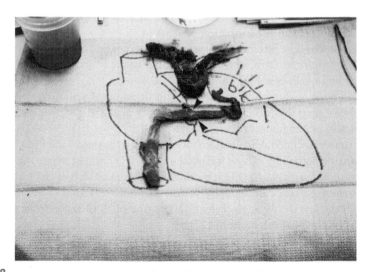

**FIG. 28.8**

Paradoxical embolism, intraoperative schematic reconstruction of the location of the massive volume of thrombotic material "caught in the act" of traversing the patent foramen ovale (*arrows*) into both the right and left pulmonary arteries.

*Reproduced with the permission from Koullias G, Elefteriades JA, Wu I, Jovin I, Jadbabaie F, McNamara R., Massive paradoxical embolism, caught in the act, Circulation 2004;109:3056–3057.*

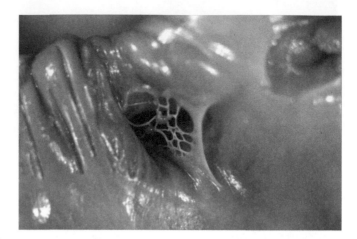

**FIG. 28.9**

The Chiari network.

*Reproduced with permission from Wikipedia (www.wikidoc.org/index.php/Chiari_network).*

formed by the stagnation of blood in the depth of its recess [20]. Atrial septal aneurysm has also been known to develop fibrosis of its wall. An associated preexisting ASD can provide the patent connection permitting left atrial to right atrial intracardiac shunting, with all of its associated consequences. Elevated intracardiac pressures secondary to cardiac pathologies (and increased left atrial pressures) are likely to be involved in the formation of ASA [17].

A Chiari network, a fine, net-like latticework of residual atrial tissue, can serve as a nidus for thrombi to form, potentially leading to paradoxical embolization via a patent foramen ovale (see Fig. 28.9).

One can easily picture how an ASA full of thrombus, oscillating (hypermobile) right and left during the cardiac cycle, could easily displace systemic emboli, resulting in initially cryptogenic stroke [3,21] (Fig. 28.10).

Other than associated ASA, certain morphologic features of the PFO confer high risk for causing pathology. These include large size ($\geq 2$ mm in height) and long tunnel ($\geq 10$ mm in length) of the PFO, prominent Eustachian valve, and large right-to-left shunt seen on echocardiography at rest and during Valsalva maneuver. Also included in the list is low-angle PFO ($\leq 10$ degree of PFO angle from the inferior vena cava longitudinal orientation) [22].

It is absolutely essential that individuals with otherwise unexplained embolic stroke undergo an echocardiogram with bubble study. The origin of the embolic material may often be ascertained by this simple, noninvasive study.

### Decompression sickness and gas embolism
Decompression sickness (DCS) is caused by the supersaturation of blood and tissues with dissolved gases caused by breathing under high pressure, with subsequent evolution of gas bubbles as the pressure decreases when a diver rises toward the surface.

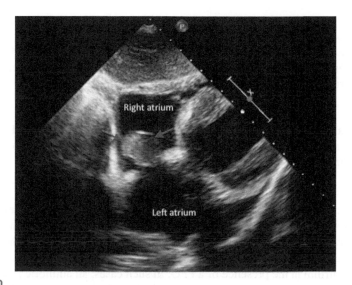

**FIG. 28.10**

Transthoracic echocardiogram (subcostal view) showing the atrial septal aneurysm (*red arrows*) bulging from the left atrium into the right atrium. Note the hyperechoic area within the atrial septal aneurysm suggestive of thrombus.

*Reproduced with permission from Aryal MR, Pradhan R, Pandit AA, Polinsky R. A "Teapot" atrial septal aneurysm with spontaneous thrombus in an asymptomatic patient, 2013. Circulation 2013;128:e409–e410.*

These gas bubbles embolize from a pulmonary or intravascular origin into the arterial circulation, causing occlusion of a distal systemic arterial locus, leading to symptomology of cutis marmorata and vestibular and neurological DCS [23]. PFO has been implicated to provide a channel for gas embolism to move from venous to arterial circulation via paradoxical embolism, especially in unprovoked [24] and "undeserved" decompression sickness, where diving has been done within accepted safety limits [25].

### Migraine

About half of the population suffering the symptoms of migraine headache with or without aura have a demonstrable concomitant PFO. A causal relation has so far not been established, but it is hypothesized that hypoxemia (via right to left shunting) or shunting of vasoactive chemicals (e.g., serotonin) which are ordinarily metabolized during their passage through the lungs, may be the cause of migraine headaches in patients with the right to left atrial shunt [26].

### Platypnea–orthodeoxia syndrome

Patent foramen ovale is also known to cause platypnea–orthodeoxia syndrome (POS), a rare condition presenting itself as orthostatic arterial desaturation and hypoxia. As such, a drop in $PaO_2 > 4\,mmHg$ or $Sao_2 > 5\%$ from supine to an upright position characterizes the syndrome. This positional change in oxygen saturation has been attributed to the mixing of the deoxygenated venous blood with the oxygenated arterial blood via a shunt in the heart chambers or an arteriovenous malformation in the pulmonary circuit. Interatrial shunt via PFO is the most common cause of platypnea–orthodeoxia [27].

### Fat embolism syndrome

PFO has also been implicated in paradoxical fat embolism syndrome (FES) [28] in cases of traumatic bone fractures [29]. This is of special consideration for orthopedic trauma surgeons [30].

### Miscellaneous pathologies

PFO, especially with high-risk morphology, coupled with multiple gestation and hypercoagulability, poses increased risk of stroke, pulmonary emboli, and myocardial infarction in pregnant women [31]. It is also hypothesized that the increased intrathoracic pressure during labor may lead to shunting of the blood from right to the left atrium in the presence of a PFO. In such cases, an amniotic fluid embolus may cause multiple cerebral infarcts using this channel to enter the systemic circulation [32].

It is also implicated in a minute number of acute myocardial infarctions by way of paradoxical embolism via interatrial communication [33]. The presence of a PFO has been implicated in both air embolism and thromboembolism in the setting of liver transplant surgery [34,35].

## Diagnosis
### Right heart catheterization

The most accurate method for confirming the presence of a PFO is through the demonstration of a guidewire crossing the septum during right heart catheterization [14]. However, due to the invasiveness of this procedure, it is not utilized in routine assessment for the presence of interatrial communication.

### Transesophageal echocardiography

Transesophageal echocardiography (TEE) with bubble study offers the benefit of relative lack of invasiveness while providing high accuracy for determining the presence and anatomic characteristics of a PFO, including size, all the while differentiating PFO from other atrial septal defects and intrapulmonary vascular shunts (e.g., pulmonary arteriovenous malformations). For this reason, TEE is the standard for diagnosing a PFO [36]. The significance of the shunt through a PFO is often estimated as a function of the degree of bubbles directly visualized passing from right to left atrium (Fig. 28.11). This is best assessed using the bicaval view.

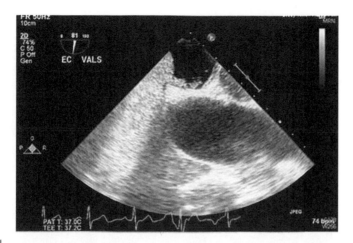

**FIG. 28.11**

Transesophageal echocardiogram with positive bubble study through a patent foramen ovale. *Reproduced with permission from Mojadidi MK, Gevorgyan R, Tobis JM. A comparison of methods to detect and quantitate PFO: TCD, TTE, ICE and TEE. In: Amin Z, Tobis J, Sievert H, Carroll J, editors. Patent foramen ovale. London: Springer; 2015. https://doi.org/10.1007/978-1-4471-4987-3_7.*

Furthermore, the sensitivity and specificity of TEE can be increased using:

- A provocation maneuver, with Valsalva or inferior vena cava (IVC) compression [37].
- Unloading the left ventricle with nitroglycerin, thus dropping left-sided pressure and promoting leftward bulging of the interatrial septum, by reversing the interatrial pressure gradient, thereby reducing the number of false negative TEEs [38] and eliminating the need for Valsalva in sedated patients.
- Use of at least five contrast injections for enhanced visualization of dense right atrial contrast filling along with the leftward bulging of the interatrial septum [39].
- Use of harmonic imaging mode for bubble studies performed with echocardiography, resulting in a higher yield for the detection of a PFO [40] compared to fundamental imaging [41].
- Addition of the patient's blood to agitated saline mixture to enhance sensitivity of bubble studies without compromising specificity when compared to agitated saline alone and other contrast agents [40].

## Transthoracic echocardiography

Transthoracic echocardiography (TTE) has a fairly low sensitivity (about 46%), with drastic improvement (of up to 90%) when performed with harmonic imaging [40–42] (Fig. 28.12).

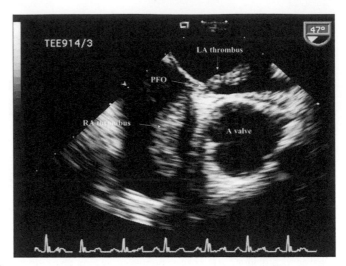

**FIG. 28.12**

Transthoracic echocardiographic imaging of a large waving tubular right atrial and left atrial thrombus through a patent foramen ovale (PFO).

*Reproduced with permission from Koullias G, Elefteriades JA, Wu I, Jovin I, Jadbabaie F, McNamara R, Massive paradoxical embolism caught in the act. Circulation. 2004;109:3056–3057.*

## Transcranial Doppler

Transcranial Doppler (TCD) is an excellent modality for detecting bubbles in the arterial circulation; however, this does not differentiate between cardiac and pulmonary shunting or directly implicate a PFO. Combined with TCD, a bubble study has a higher sensitivity for the detection of intracardiac right-to-left shunt, including the anatomic details of PFO, compared to TEE alone [41,43,44].

## Computed tomography angiography

PFO can be a frequent finding in routine coronary CTA done for other purposes. CT technology has enabled convenient assessment of the interatrial septum owing to high spatial and temporal resolution [45–47]. While CTA is capable of providing a detailed description of structure, assessment of flow through the shunt is limited [48].

## Cardiovascular magnetic resonance

Another method that can detect a PFO and an ASA is cardiac magnetic resonance imaging (CMR). Gadolinium-based contrast is injected (repeated 2–3 times, if necessary) to improve the sensitivity of the test. Appearance of the contrast in the right atrium is imaged in real time. Detection of the contrast signal can be plotted on a signal–time curve for both the right atrium and the left atrium [49]. Demonstration of the signal in the left atrium and the right atrium simultaneously is conclusive of the presence of PFO. CMR eliminates the need for sedation, hence improving patient cooperation while performing the Valsalva maneuver [49].

## Current application

In cases of a suspected cryptogenic stroke, most healthcare centers prefer initial screening with TCD followed by echocardiography for the diagnosis of PFO [14]. An isolated PFO for any suspected pathology is generally followed up initially with a TTE due to lack of invasiveness, although a TEE may be required for a definitive diagnosis. A PFO can be differentiated from an ASD as a PFO takes a tunneled intraseptal course. Presence of a flap valve on the left atrial side of the foramen is another indicator of PFO. Echocardiography also represents the best method of visualizing fossa ovalis membrane aneurysms in patients suspected to have cardiogenic emboli, although the emboli may arise from a different source [50,51].

## Management

Most patients with an isolated finding of a PFO without associated pathology require no special treatment. When a PFO manifests pathology (embolization), a choice must be made between medical and surgical management.

### Medical management

Traditional treatment of a PFO with associated pathology (such as a neurologic event) consists of antiplatelet therapy (i.e., aspirin) alone in low-risk patients or combined with warfarin (or other novel anticoagulants) in high-risk individuals to prevent a cryptogenic stroke. This reduces the risk of formation of clots that may later traverse the PFO to cause harm. Warfarin administration requires maintenance of the INR between 2 and 3.

### Interventional management

Percutaneous closure of the patent foramen ovale with occluder devices (Fig. 28.13) has been the mainstay of interventional management of PFO-related embolization as well as their prevention. Traditionally, PFO closure used to be done with open heart surgery. Over the past 4 decades, percutaneous catheter-based closure of the PFO has offered efficacy while sparing the invasiveness of open heart surgery.

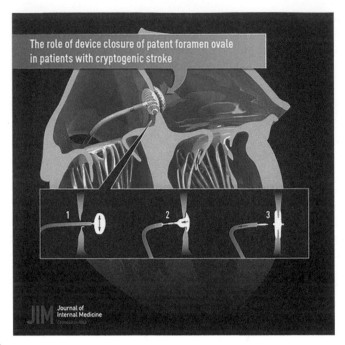

**FIG. 28.13**

Use of occluder device for closure of the patent foramen ovale (PFO).

*Reproduced with permission from: Fukutomi M, Wilkins B, Søndergaard L (Rigshospitalet, Copenhagen, Denmark). The role of device closure of patent foramen ovale in patients with cryptogenic stroke (Review-Symposium). J Intern Med 2020;288:400–409.*

### *Indications for percutaneous management*

PFO has long been closed surgically or by percutaneous means due to its implication in serious pathologies including cryptogenic stroke, migraine with or without aura, decompression syndrome, platypnea–orthodeoxia, and patients about to undergo liver surgery. Regarding the techniques for management of PFO, differing conclusions have been offered by the several meta-analysis of three randomized controlled trials for PFO treatment; some studies show a benefit from device closure, while others show no benefit [52–55]. Nonetheless, percutaneous closure is the preferred procedure for the following indications.

### Cryptogenic stroke

When all other causes of ischemic stroke have been eliminated, a presumptive diagnosis of cryptogenic stroke can be made. Evidence supporting PFO-mediated paradoxical embolic stroke includes cortical location of infarcts, strokes in multiple vascular distributions, and infarcts of different ages in the same vascular territory [56]. Knowing that 20%–30% of strokes are cryptogenic in etiology, a RoPE (Risk of Paradoxical Embolism) score has been developed which takes into account the age and smoking status of the patient as well as any history of hypertension, diabetes mellitus, transient ischemic attack (TIA), or stroke, along with the presence of cortical infarct on imaging [57]. The RoPE score determines the probability of a PFO being responsible for a cryptogenic stroke in a specific patient [58] with preexisting PFO. A high score correlates with increased likelihood that a PFO is responsible for the stroke. A RoPE score greater than or equal to 7 provides good reason for percutaneous surgical closure. The risk–benefit ratio of performing PFO closure in patients with a RoPE score less than 7 should be carefully weighed [58].

### Decompression sickness

Decompression sickness (DCS) is another potential application of PFO closure. Divers with diagnosed PFO and a history of DCS are recommended either to cease or limit diving, or, if they do not accept limitations, to undergo PFO closure. The benefit of PFO closure in this patient population has yet to be evaluated with randomized clinical trials for conclusive indication.

### Migraine

Several retrospective observational studies have noted improvement in migraine headaches in patients who have undergone PFO closure for nonmigraine indications [59,60]. A causal relationship between right-to-left shunting across a PFO and migraine headache is yet to be proven; hence, there is no consensus regarding the application of closure devices as a standard therapy for migraine.

### Platypnea–orthodeoxia syndrome

Although there is a paucity of data regarding the potential benefit of PFO closure for POS, improvement of symptoms has been noted after PFO closure in some studies [61]. In cases of severe hypoxia where pulmonary disease has been excluded, PFO closure could be considered.

### Liver transplant surgery

Routine PFO closure is not yet recommended for patients undergoing liver transplant surgery, despite the potential severity of massive intraoperative systemic air embolization obstructing either the pulmonary arteries, or, tragically, the coronary arteries [34,62].

### *Devices for PFO closure*

Among many commercially available devices for PFO closure, the Amplatzer PFO Occluder and the Gore Cardioform Septal Occluder are among the most studied and most commonly used (Fig. 28.14).

### *Imaging guidance during percutaneous closure*
### Imaging modality during surgery

Imaging modality during the procedure: Fluoroscopy, of course, is essential. Simultaneous echocardiographic imaging is desirable as well. While TEE provides excellent image quality of the entire interatrial septum as well as the adjacent structures,

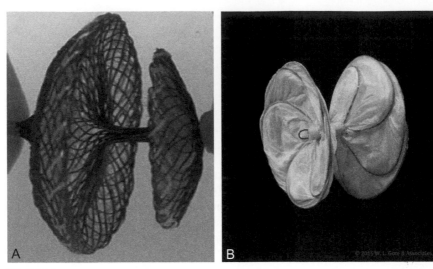

**FIG. 28.14**

(A) The Amplatzer patent foramen ovale (PFO) Occluder. (B) the Gore Cardioform Septal Occluder.

*Reproduced with permission from Collado FMS, Poulin MF, Murphy JJ, Jneid H, Kavinsky CJ, Patent foramen ovale closure for stroke prevention and other disorders. J Am Heart Assoc. 2018;7:e007146.*

and is a well-established imaging modality for procedural guidance, this requires general anesthesia and the presence of an additional physician to manipulate the TEE probe and acquire necessary images. The use of intracardiac echocardiography (ICE) as an alternate obviates the need for general anesthesia or an additional physician for the procedure but requires supplemental venous access and may be associated with rare complications of vascular injury, cardiac perforation, and atrial arrhythmias [63].

## Focus of imaging

Regardless of imaging modality, a comprehensive echocardiographic evaluation should be done, with special attention to the fundamental characteristics of the PFO (tunnel length, presence of atrial septal aneurysm, thickness of the septum secundum, presence of additional defects, and presence of additional structures in the right atrium, such as a Eustachian valve or a Chiari network). PFO closure can be technically challenging in the presence of a long tunnel morphology. Special note is taken for the transverse pericardial sinus, the aorta, the superior vena cava, and the atrioventricular rim [64]. The absence of right and left atrial thrombi should also be confirmed before the procedure, as thrombi may contraindicate the procedure. Meticulous, complete, careful imaging is critical for the safe and effective placement of a PFO device.

Postprocedure

After the procedure, patient's condition is monitored overnight for possible complications. Postprocedure ECG or telemetry detects any new atrial arrhythmia or an atrioventricular block. Patients are carefully assessed for any bleeding complications (from access sites or into the pericardial space). Generally, a TEE is also performed on post procedure day 1 or before the discharge to assess for residual shunts, device instability, evidence of device erosion, deformation of surrounding structures, and any new or worsening pericardial effusion [63]. Strict asepsis is required intraoperatively. Infection of a PFO device postimplant may require either intravenous antibiotics and/or surgical management [65,66].

## Complications of the procedure

While inadequate disc apposition, residual shunts, and inability to deploy the device are possible difficulties encountered during the closure of a PFO with a long tunnel, new arrhythmias, hypersensitivity to nickel [67], and vascular injury at the site of access [68] represent additional complications that may occur in the follow-up period. New onset periprocedural atrial fibrillation [69] is associated with an increased risk of left atrial thrombi and hence should be managed promptly [70,71]. The occluder device itself can also be a nidus for thrombus formation [63] although (fortunately) the incidence remains low [72]. Device erosion leading to cardiac perforation is another potential complication. Absence of the aortic rim in multiple views, poor posterior rim consistency, and septal malalignment are the echocardiographic features that may portend device erosion [64]. Finally, residual shunts may remain after the PFO closure, but associated embolic events are quite rare [73]. Of note, presence of an atrial septal aneurysm is also associated with an increased risk of device embolization; use of larger devices may mitigate some of this risk by stabilizing the aneurysmal portion of the septum [72].

## Cardiac masses

Cardiac masses vary from benign tumors to malignant tumors [74] of the heart, the latter including primary tumors and metastases from a distant malignant focus. Seventy-five percent of the cardiac neoplasms are benign [75], the majority of which are myxomas. Primary malignant cardiac tumors comprise only the minority (25%) of all cardiac neoplasms. The heart can also be a locus for secondary malignancies from systemic metastasis (Table 28.15). Tumors usually vary in their clinical presentation and symptomology, which can involve a spectrum of obstructive, embolic, and systemic symptoms. Other than tumors, nonneoplastic masses also arise in the heart, comprising a small proportion of all cardiac masses.

**Table 28.15** Types of cardiac masses

| Types of cardiac masses | Examples |
| --- | --- |
| Benign tumors | Myxomas, lipomas, fibroelastomas, rhabdomyomas, fibromas, hemangiomas, teratomas, hamartomas of mature cardiac cells, cystic tumors of the atrioventricular node |
| Primary malignant tumors | Undifferentiated pleomorphic sarcomas which include angiosarcomas, rhabdomyosarcomas, leiomyosarcomas, liposarcomas, osteosarcomas, fibrosarcomas, malignant fibrous histiocytomas [75,76], primary cardiac lymphomas |
| Secondary metastases | Lymphomas, melanomas, and carcinomas of the thorax including breast, lung, and esophagus [76], renal cell carcinomas |
| Nonneoplastic masses | Thrombi, vegetations, calcific lesions of the heart, lipomatous hypertrophy of the atrial septum (LHAS), foreign bodies, Prichard's structures of the fossa ovalis, papillary fibroelastomas |

Two types of structures particularly local to the fossa ovalis are myxomas, the most common benign tumor of the heart, and Prichard's structures, also a benign accumulation of mature endothelial cells.

## Structures of the fossa ovalis

### Myxoma

Originating from the multipotent mesenchymal cells [77] and benign in nature, myxomas represent the most common primary tumors of the heart [78]. These usually present between the fourth and sixth decades of life, with a preponderance toward female sex [79,80]. The mitral annulus or fossa ovalis border on the left atrial side hosts the majority (~75%) of these tumors, whereas the right atrium is the second most common location (~20%) [81,82]. While the majority of these endocardial tumors are sporadic in origin, a small percentage of myxomas constitute part of the rare MEN (multiple endocrine neoplasia) syndrome of Carney's complex [83]. Atrial myxomas are often pedunculated, with a smooth, villous, or friable surface [84] (Fig. 28.16).

### Symptomatology

Myxomas can cause both the obstructive symptoms and the embolic events [85]. Depending on the location, they can lead to mitral valve obstruction or mitral regurgitation in the left heart, or tricuspid stenosis on the right side. What follows is a sequelae of symptoms including dyspnea, orthopnea, and paroxysmal nocturnal dyspnea, potentially leading right up to pulmonary edema [86] culminating in left heart failure and shock. Secondary pulmonary hypertension, pedal edema, hepatomegaly, and ascites culminating in right heart failure, respectively, may complicate right- or left-sided myxomas [87].

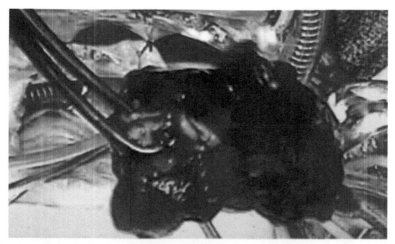

**FIG. 28.16**

Atrial myxoma after removal using transseptal approach.

*Reproduced with permission from Ziganshin BA, Anis O, Zafar MA, et al. Surgical correction of a giant left atrial myxoma producing critical mitral stenosis. June 2021. https://doi.org/10.25373/ctsnet.14749119.*

Myxomas of the left atrium also carry a high risk of systemic embolization, likely due to the high systolic pressures on the left side. These emboli can be catastrophic [88]. Presentation can vary from only dyspnea and chest pain to transient ischemic attack, hemiplegia, and vision loss [89]. Right atrial myxomas, on the other hand, can cause pulmonary embolism. In the presence of ASD or PFO, they are capable of systemic embolism paradoxically [90].

Of note is the productive capacity of the atrial myxoma: vascular endothelial growth factor production within the atrial myxoma can stimulate angiogenesis. Various cytokines like IL-6 and growth factors also result in constitutional symptoms, including fever, malaise, anorexia, weight loss, and high sedimentation rate [91,92].

### Diagnosis

Echocardiography (Fig. 28.17) and cardiac magnetic resonance (CMR) imaging are the modalities of choice for achieving diagnosis. While echocardiography can characterize the size, location, attachment, mobility, and extent of the tumor, CMR also gives details about the microenvironment of the myxomas (densities within the tumor) via T1- and T2-weighted sequences [93,94]. If the patient requires surgical resection, some authorities recommend assessment of the tumor's blood supply to be made with coronary angiography.

Cardiac computed tomography (cardiac CT) (Fig. 28.18) is a fair alternative to CMR if CMR is unavailable. PET scan can also be used to characterize atrial myxomas [95]. Transvenous biopsy is an invasive modality that carries the risk of dislodging emboli from the friable tumor; hence, it is not routinely performed.

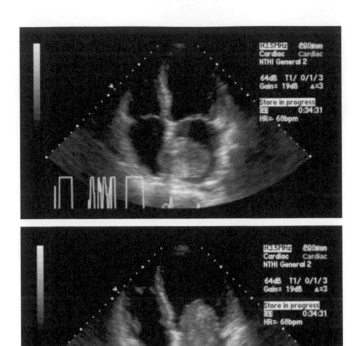

**FIG. 28.17**

Echocardiographic assessment of an atrial myxoma prolapsing into the mitral valve, causing severe mitral stenosis.

*Reproduced with permission from Ziganshin BA, Anis O, Zafar MA, et al. Surgical correction of a giant left atrial myxoma producing critical mitral stenosis. June 2021. https://doi.org/10.25373/ctsnet.14749119.*

## Management

After the characterization of cardiovascular complications and risk of embolization, the decision for surgical excision is made. Pericardial patch placement can help construct defects not amenable to primary closure after resection of the myxoma. Prognosis after resection is excellent. Pathologic examination of the resected tumor rules out other tumors in the differential diagnosis as well as metastases [96]. Despite resection, recurrence of atrial myxomas is common in patients with Carney's complex [85,97–99].

For left atrial myxoma, we prefer a right atrial, transseptal, "no touch" approach [100] (Fig. 28.19). After bicaval cannulation and institution of cardiopulmonary bypass, we excise the fossa ovalis in its entirety. We avoid touching the tumor at all, as myxomas are notoriously friable, and any dislodged pieces may disappear into

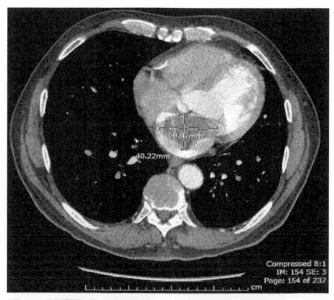

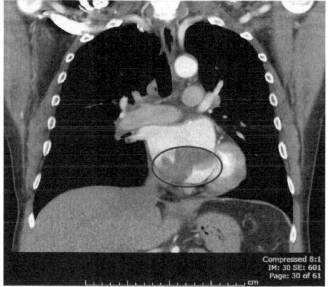

**FIG. 28.18**

CT scan demonstration of a large atrial myxoma filling left atrium (axial and coronal views).
*Reproduced with permission from Ziganshin BA, Anis O, Zafar MA, et al. Surgical correction of a giant left atrial myxoma producing critical mitral stenosis. June 2021. https://doi.org/10.25373/ctsnet.14749119.*

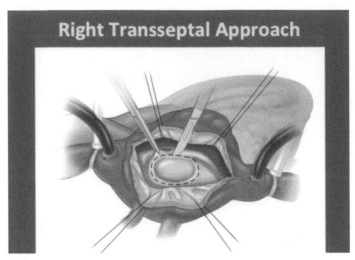

**FIG. 28.19**

Demonstration of the transseptal approach using fossa ovalis for removal of the left-sided atrial myxomas.

*Reproduced with permission from Ziganshin BA, Anis O, Zafar MA, et al. Surgical correction of a giant left atrial myxoma producing critical mitral stenosis. June 2021. https://doi.org/10.25373/ctsnet.14749119.*

atrial recesses or into the trabeculae of the left ventricle, never to be seen again until they cause stroke or other catastrophic embolization. After excising circumferentially around the fossa, we pick up the edge of the atrial tissue and lift it like a manhole cover. This allows light and vision into the left atrium. We then gently rock and tease the tumor out. Large myxomas may seem as if they cannot be removed through the fossa ovalis, but, as long as not touched by instruments, they will squeeze, deform mildly, and pass through the opening into the right atrium, being then removed as one piece with the tissue of the fossa ovalis. The cardiac chambers are exhaustively explored for any fragments.

### Prichard's structures

Commonly found on the left side of the fossa ovalis in individuals beyond 60 years of age, Prichard's structures are also benign growths derived from mature endothelial cells. Age-related formation of these small endocardial deformities is characterized by capillary sized lacunas lined by plump endothelial cells [101]. For long, they have been associated with cardiac myxomas; however, they have been proven to be unrelated to them [102]. These structures may be subendothelial or located within the atrial cavity (intracavitary) [101].

### Cardiac masses: Miscellaneous benign cardiac tumors

Table 28.20.

**Table 28.20** Benign cardiac tumors.

| Benign primary tumors | Features |
|---|---|
| Rhabdomyoma | • Congenital hamartoma [60]<br>• Most common benign cardiac neoplasm in the pediatric population [74,103]<br>• Multiple lesions, usually in the ventricles or the ventricular septum of the fetal heart [104]<br>• Presentation includes murmurs, cyanosis, respiratory distress, cardiac failure and cardiogenic shock, along with hydrops fetalis and ventricular inflow/outflow obstruction [75]<br>• Possible association with tuberous sclerosis [105]<br>• Known to regress spontaneously, so first-line management is conservative. For high-risk clinical presentations, surgery is considered [106,107] |
| Fibroma | • Connective tissue neoplasm<br>• Occurs mostly in childhood with a higher male predisposition<br>• Presents with ventricular arrhythmias, given that the most common tumor locations are the left ventricle and the interventricular septum<br>• Clinical manifestations include syncope, chest pain, and heart failure symptoms<br>• Associated with Gorlin syndrome or nevoid basal cell carcinoma |
| Lipoma | • Subendocardial, subpericardial, or endocardial encapsulated tumors<br>• Predisposition towards elderly women with increased body mass<br>• Monitored through active surveillance<br>• Surgical resection reserved for symptomatic patients |
| Hemangioma | • Rare neoplasms consisting of blood vessels (Fig. 28.23)<br>• Usually asymptomatic<br>• When symptomatic, clinical presentation depends on the location and size of the tumor. It can vary from pericardial effusion and arrhythmias to hemopericardium or cardiac tamponade and complete heart block or even sudden death<br>• Associated with Kasabach–Merritt syndrome<br>• Diagnosed with a combination of echocardiography, CCT, and CMR<br>• Surgical resection is recommended for symptomatic patients<br>• Prognosis is excellent |

*Malignant primary neoplasms*
Table 28.21.

*Nonneoplastic masses*
Table 28.22.

**Table 28.21** Primary malignant tumors of the heart.

| | | |
|---|---|---|
| Sarcoma | Angiosarcoma (Fig. 28.24) | • Originates from the vascular endothelial cells (endothelial cells lining the blood vessels)<br>• Most frequently occurring primary malignancy of the heart<br>• Higher predisposition in men<br>• Commonly affects the right atrium and invades adjacent structures<br>• Most common presenting symptoms include dyspnea, right-sided heart failure, cardiogenic shock and pericardial effusion, all of which occur very late in the course of the disease<br>• Poor prognosis, with high rates of recurrence<br>• Management is palliative rather than curative through partial or complete surgical resection and possible adjuvant chemotherapy |
| Sarcoma | Rhabdomyosarcoma | • Neoplasm of the striated cardiac musculature<br>• Second most common form of malignant cardiac tumors<br>• Most cases occur in children or adolescents<br>• They arise from any cardiac chamber but carry a predisposition for the ventricles<br>• Highly aggressive with frequent invasion and metastasis<br>• High rates of recurrence |
| Sarcoma | Undifferentiated pleomorphic sarcoma/malignant fibrous histiocytoma | • Account for 10% of all primary malignant cardiac tumors<br>• Present in the fifth decade of life<br>• More common in the left atrium<br>• Nonspecific symptoms such as dyspnea, chest pain and cough<br>• Surgical resection is the treatment of choice<br>• Adjuvant chemoradiotherapy offered to those undergoing partial resection |
| Lymphoma | | • Confined to the pericardium with no extracardiac involvement<br>• Twice as common in men as in women<br>• Most cases occur in patients over the age of 60 years |

**Table 28.21** Primary malignant tumors of the heart—*Cont'd*

| | | |
|---|---|---|
| | | • Associated with immunosuppression through organ transplantation, acquired immunodeficiency syndrome (AIDS), or infection with human herpes virus 8 (HHV-8) or Epstein–Barr virus |
| | | • Constitutional symptoms of lymphoma occur, including pyrexia, malaise, night sweats, weight loss, and specific cardiac conditions, such as atrial fibrillation, heart failure, and pericardial effusion |
| | | • Treatments are analogous to systemic lymphoma and include chemoradiotherapy and monoclonal antibody therapy |
| | | • Surgical treatments are typically palliative to relieve obstruction |
| Li–Fraumeni Syndrome | | • Rare, inherited autosomal dominant condition associated with germline mutations in the TP53 gene |
| | | • Younger patients present with recurrent cardiac tumor disease |

**Table 28.22** Nonneoplastic cardiac masses.

| Nonneoplastic masses | Features |
|---|---|
| Papillary fibroelastoma | • Benign endocardial papillary growths<br>• Most commonly found in the elderly population<br>• Equal prevalence in males and females<br>• Most commonly affect mural endocardium of the aortic and mitral valves<br>• High likelihood of embolization<br>• Clinical presentation may often be in the form of cerebral or coronary occlusive events<br>• Robotic or traditional surgical resection with valvular sparing should be offered to all patients |
| Lipomatous hypertrophy of the atrial septum | • Hypertrophy of the atrial septum (Fig. 28.25)<br>• Predominates in obese patients<br>• More commonly affects elderly female population<br>• Manifests as obstructive symptoms and arrhythmias<br>• Majority of the patients remain asymptomatic. This diagnosis is often made incidentally on imaging<br>• Characteristic "dumbbell-like appearance" seen on echocardiography |

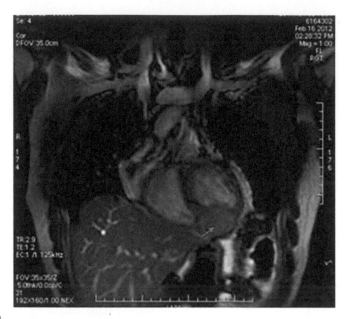

**FIG. 28.23**

Benign cardiac masses: cardiac hemangioma.

*Reproduced with permission from Columbia Heart Surgery (columbiasurgery.org).*

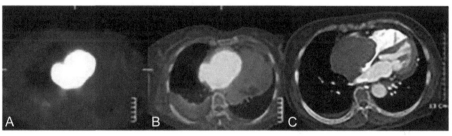

**FIG. 28.24**

Malignant primary cardiac tumors, angiosarcoma.

*Reproduced with permission from Columbia Heart Surgery (columbiasurgery.org).*

## Diagnosis of cardiac tumors

Clinical suspicion is of importance because initial workup, including blood work, electrocardiogram (ECG) and chest X-ray, usually offers only nondiagnostic findings [75]. Of note, a small proportion of these tumors are subclinical and are identified only incidentally during an investigation for other pathologies.

Echocardiography gives anatomical details of the tumor along with its attachments and any extension into the neighboring structures. It also confers information

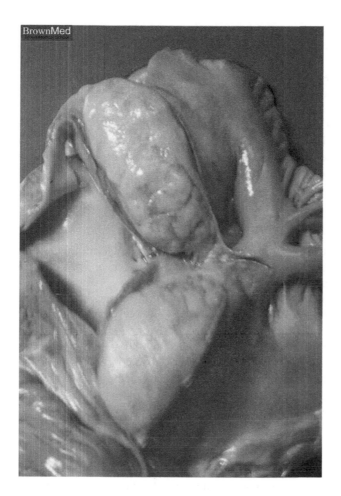

**FIG. 28.25**

Nonneoplastic cardiac masses: lipomatous hypertrophy of the interatrial septum.

*Reproduced with permission from Brown University (brown.edu).*

about the hemodynamic derangement caused by the tumor. Malignant cardiac tumors tend to show rich vascularity and enhancement of image upon contrast administration, and can be differentiated from thrombi by the use of contrast echocardiography [75,108,109].

Cardiac MRI provides excellent tissue characterization, and, when used with gadolinium contrast administration, can differentiate between cardiac tumors and thrombi.

Definitive diagnosis and grading can be done with histopathological evaluation of cardiac tumors after resection [75,110]. Care should be taken in order to prevent cancer seeding from a malignant tumor [75,76,110]. Cytological examination of pericardial or pleural fluid, echocardiographically guided cardiac biopsy and thoracoscopically guided biopsy are some of the methodologies employed for accurate diagnosis [75].

Fluorodeoxyglucose (FDG)-positron emission tomography (PET) (FDG-PET) is employed for the staging of disseminated disease and prognostication, which it accomplishes with great accuracy.

Contrast enhanced cardiac CT is capable of providing much more detailed imaging along with delineation of smaller tumors and evaluation of fat and calcification within studied structures by the use of multidetector CT, postprocessing algorithms, and ECG gating. CT is employed when C-MRI is unavailable.

## Management

Management of cardiac tumors involves a multidisciplinary team approach depending on histopathological classification, cancer invasion, and patient risk stratification [105].

Small, immobile masses, such as papillary fibroelastomas, lipomas, and lipomatous hypertrophy, which typically progress slowly, can be followed up by serial echocardiography to monitor tumor behavior. Benign growths in asymptomatic patients offer very good prognosis, which is not the case for malignant growths. Late presentation and difficult surgical management contribute to the poor prognosis of the malignant primary cardiac tumors. Management usually combines complete surgical resection and adjuvant chemoradiotherapy but varies depending on specific patient and tumor characteristics.

## References

[1] Barik R. The three-dimensional fossa ovalis. Indian Heart J 2016;68(2):211–2.
[2] Klimek-Piotrowska W, et al. Anatomy of the true interatrial septum for transseptal access to the left atrium. Ann Anat 2016;205:60–4.
[3] Joshi SD, Chawre HK, Joshi SS. Morphological study of fossa ovalis and its clinical relevance. Indian Heart J 2016;68(2):147–52.
[4] Hagen PT, Scholz DG, Edwards WD. Incidence and size of patent foramen ovale during the first 10 decades of life: an autopsy study of 965 normal hearts. Mayo Clin Proc 1984;59(1):17–20.
[5] Asirvatham SJ, Stevenson WG. Editor's perspective: the interatrial septum. Circ Arrhythm Electrophysiol 2013;6(5):e75–6.
[6] Boppana VS, et al. Atrial coronary arteries: anatomy and atrial perfusion territories. J Atr Fibrillation 2011;4(3):375.
[7] Krupa U. Arterial vascularization of the interatrial septum in the human heart in relation to the type of coronary ramification. Folia Morphol 1995;54(1):51–9.
[8] Sokolov VV, Brezhnev FF, Kharlamov EV. Sources of the vascularization of the human interatrial septum of the heart with different variants of the atrial blood supply. Arkh Anat Gistol Embriol 1986;91(7):29–34.

[9] Chaudhari RG, Shinde SV, Deshpande JR. Morphometric analysis of fossa ovalis in rheumatic heart disease. Indian Heart J 2005;57(6):662–5.

[10] Roberts WC, Ko JM. Some observations on mitral and aortic valve disease. Proc (Bayl Univ Med Cent) 2008;21(3):282–99.

[11] Munjewar C, Agrawal R, Sharma S. Cardiac amyloidosis: a report of two cases. Indian Heart J 2014;66(4):473–6.

[12] Hanaoka T, et al. Shifting of puncture site in the fossa ovalis during radiofrequency catheter ablation: intracardiac echocardiography-guided transseptal left heart catheterization. Jpn Heart J 2003;44(5):673–80.

[13] Rana BS, et al. Three-dimensional imaging of the atrial septum and patent foramen ovale anatomy: defining the morphological phenotypes of patent foramen ovale. Eur J Echocardiogr 2010;11(10):i19–25.

[14] Mojadidi MK, et al. Cryptogenic stroke and patent foramen ovale. J Am Coll Cardiol 2018;71(9):1035–43.

[15] Silver MD, Dorsey JS. Aneurysms of the septum primum in adults. Arch Pathol Lab Med 1978;102(2):62–5.

[16] Agmon Y, et al. Frequency of atrial septal aneurysms in patients with cerebral ischemic events. Circulation 1999;99(15):1942–4.

[17] Topaz O, et al. Aneurysm of fossa ovalis in adults: a pathologic study. Cardiovasc Pathol 2003;12(4):219–25.

[18] Katayama H, et al. Incidence of atrial septal aneurysm: echocardiographic and pathologic analysis. J Cardiol 1990;20(2):411–21.

[19] Ruiz de Larrea C, et al. Aneurysm of the atrial septum associated with interatrial communication: a study of 12 cases by 2-dimensional color echocardiography. Rev Esp Cardiol 1993;46(6):340–3.

[20] Schneider B, et al. Improved morphologic characterization of atrial septal aneurysm by transesophageal echocardiography: relation to cerebrovascular events. J Am Coll Cardiol 1990;16(4):1000–9.

[21] Turc G, et al. Atrial septal aneurysm, shunt size, and recurrent stroke risk in patients with patent foramen ovale. J Am Coll Cardiol 2020;75(18):2312–20.

[22] Nakayama R, et al. Low-angle patent foramen ovale (PFO): high-risk PFO morphology associated with paradoxical embolism. CASE (Philadelphia, PA) 2021;5(3):183–5.

[23] Loewenherz JW. Pathophysiology and treatment of decompression sickness and gas embolism. J Fla Med Assoc 1992;79(9):620–4.

[24] Honěk J, et al. High-grade patent foramen ovale is a risk factor of unprovoked decompression sickness in recreational divers. J Cardiol 2019;74(6):519–23.

[25] Koopsen R, et al. Persistent foramen ovale closure in divers with a history of decompression sickness. Neth Heart J 2018;26(11):535–9.

[26] Kumar P, et al. The connection between patent foramen ovale and migraine. Neuroimaging Clin N Am 2019;29(2):261–70.

[27] Agrawal A, Palkar A, Talwar A. The multiple dimensions of platypnea-orthodeoxia syndrome: a review. Respir Med 2017;129:31–8.

[28] Yang L, Wu J, Wang B. Fat embolism syndrome with cerebral fat embolism through a patent foramen ovale: a case report. Medicine (Baltimore) 2020;99(24), e20569.

[29] Vetrugno L, et al. Cerebral fat embolism after traumatic bone fractures: a structured literature review and analysis of published case reports. Scand J Trauma Resusc Emerg Med 2021;29(1):47.

[30] Piuzzi NS, et al. Paradoxical cerebral fat embolism in revision hip surgery. Case Rep Orthop 2014;2014, 140757.

[31] Chen L, et al. Patent foramen ovale (PFO), stroke and pregnancy. J Invest Med 2016; 64(5):992–1000.

[32] Woo YS, et al. Ischemic stroke related to an amniotic fluid embolism during labor. J Clin Neurosci 2015;22(4):767–8.

[33] Kleber FX, et al. Epidemiology of myocardial infarction caused by presumed paradoxical embolism via a patent foramen ovale. Circ J 2017;81(10):1484–9.

[34] Olmedilla L, et al. Fatal paradoxical air embolism during liver transplantation. Br J Anaesth 2000;84(1):112–4.

[35] Yerlioglu E, et al. Patent foramen ovale and intracardiac thrombus identified by transesophageal echocardiography during liver transplantation. J Cardiothorac Vasc Anesth 2012;26(6):1069–73.

[36] de Belder MA, et al. Transesophageal contrast echocardiography and color flow mapping: methods of choice for the detection of shunts at the atrial level? Am Heart J 1992;124(6):1545–50.

[37] Mojadidi MK, et al. Transesophageal echocardiography for the detection of patent foramen ovale. J Am Soc Echocardiogr 2017;30(9):933–4.

[38] Johansson MC, Guron CW. Leftward bulging of atrial septum is provoked by nitroglycerin and by sustained valsalva strain. J Am Soc Echocardiogr 2014;27(10):1120–7.

[39] Johansson MC, et al. Sensitivity for detection of patent foramen ovale increased with increasing number of contrast injections: a descriptive study with contrast transesophageal echocardiography. J Am Soc Echocardiogr 2008;21(5):419–24.

[40] Mojadidi MK, et al. Two-dimensional echocardiography using second harmonic imaging for the diagnosis of intracardiac right-to-left shunt: a meta-analysis of prospective studies. Int J Cardiovasc Imaging 2014;30(5):911–23.

[41] Mojadidi MK, et al. Accuracy of conventional transthoracic echocardiography for the diagnosis of intracardiac right-to-left shunt: a meta-analysis of prospective studies. Echocardiography 2014;31(9):1036–48.

[42] Madala D, et al. Harmonic imaging improves sensitivity at the expense of specificity in the detection of patent foramen ovale. Echocardiography 2004;21(1):33–6.

[43] Mojadidi MK, et al. Accuracy of transcranial doppler for the diagnosis of intracardiac right-to-left shunt: a bivariate meta-analysis of prospective studies. JACC Cardiovasc Imaging 2014;7(3):236–50.

[44] Spencer MP, et al. Power M-mode transcranial doppler for diagnosis of patent foramen ovale and assessing transcatheter closure. J Neuroimaging 2004;14(4):342–9.

[45] Incedayi M, et al. The incidence of left atrial diverticula in coronary CT angiography. Diagn Interv Radiol 2012;18(6):542–6. https://doi.org/10.4261/1305-3825.Dir.5388-11.1.

[46] Vural M, et al. Assessment of global left ventricular systolic function with multidetector CT and 2D echocardiography: a comparison between reconstructions of 1-mm and 2-mm slice thickness at multidetector CT. Diagn Interv Radiol 2010;16(3):236–40. https://doi.org/10.4261/1305-3825.Dir.2624-09.2.

[47] Kosehan D, et al. Interatrial shunt: diagnosis of patent foramen ovale and atrial septal defect with 64-row coronary computed tomography angiography. Jpn J Radiol 2011;29(8):576–82. https://doi.org/10.1007/s11604-011-0602-x.

[48] Rat N, et al. Cardiovascular imaging for guiding interventional therapy in structural heart diseases. Curr Med Imaging Rev 2020;16(2):111–22. https://doi.org/10.2174/1573405614666180612081736.

[49] Rustemli A, Bhatti TK, Wolff SD. Evaluating cardiac sources of embolic stroke with MRI. Echocardiography 2007;24(3):301–8.

[50] Mügge A, et al. Atrial septal aneurysm in adult patients. A multicenter study using transthoracic and transesophageal echocardiography. Circulation 1995;91(11):2785–92.

[51] Ilercil A, et al. Clinical significance of fossa ovalis membrane aneurysm in adults with cardioembolic cerebral ischemia. Am J Cardiol 1997;80(1):96–8.

[52] Udell JA, et al. Patent foramen ovale closure vs medical therapy for stroke prevention: meta-analysis of randomized trials and review of heterogeneity in meta-analyses. Can J Cardiol 2014;30(10):1216–24.

[53] Rengifo-Moreno P, et al. Patent foramen ovale transcatheter closure vs. medical therapy on recurrent vascular events: a systematic review and meta-analysis of randomized controlled trials. Eur Heart J 2013;34(43):3342–52.

[54] Khan AR, et al. Device closure of patent foramen ovale versus medical therapy in cryptogenic stroke: a systematic review and meta-analysis. JACC Cardiovasc Interv 2013; 6(12):1316–23.

[55] Stortecky S, et al. Percutaneous closure of patent foramen ovale in patients with cryptogenic embolism: a network meta-analysis. Eur Heart J 2015;36(2):120–8.

[56] Saver JL. Cryptogenic stroke. N Engl J Med 2016;375(11), e26.

[57] Kent DM, et al. An index to identify stroke-related vs incidental patent foramen ovale in cryptogenic stroke. Neurology 2013;81(7):619–25. https://doi.org/10.1212/WNL.0b013e3182a08d59.

[58] Prefasi D, et al. The utility of the RoPE score in cryptogenic stroke patients ≤50 years in predicting a stroke-related patent foramen ovale. Int J Stroke 2015;11(1), NP7-NP8.

[59] Tariq N, Tepper SJ, Kriegler JS. Patent foramen ovale and migraine: closing the debate—a review. Headache 2016;56(3):462–78.

[60] Rayhill M, Burch R. PFO and migraine: is there a role for closure? Curr Neurol Neurosci Rep 2017;17(3):20.

[61] Mojadidi MK, et al. The effect of patent foramen ovale closure in patients with platypnea-orthodeoxia syndrome. Catheter Cardiovasc Interv 2015;86(4):701–7.

[62] Collado FMS, Poulin MF, Murphy JJ, Jneid H, Kavinsky CJ. Patent foramen ovale closure for stroke prevention and other disorders. J Am Heart Assoc 2018;7, e007146.

[63] Silvestry FE, et al. Guidelines for the echocardiographic assessment of atrial septal defect and patent foramen ovale: from the American Society of Echocardiography and Society for Cardiac Angiography and Interventions. J Am Soc Echocardiogr 2015;28(8):910–58.

[64] Amin Z. Transcatheter closure of secundum atrial septal defects. Catheter Cardiovasc Interv 2006;68(5):778–87.

[65] Goldstein JA, et al. Infective endocarditis resulting from CardioSEAL closure of a patent foramen ovale. Catheter Cardiovasc Interv 2002;55(2):217–20 [discussion 221].

[66] Calachanis M, et al. Infective endocarditis after transcatheter closure of a patent foramen ovale. Catheter Cardiovasc Interv 2004;63(3):351–4.

[67] Wertman B, et al. Adverse events associated with nickel allergy in patients undergoing percutaneous atrial septal defect or patent foramen ovale closure. J Am Coll Cardiol 2006;47(6):1226–7. https://doi.org/10.1016/j.jacc.2005.12.017.

[68] Berdat PA, et al. Surgical management of complications after transcatheter closure of an atrial septal defect or patent foramen ovale. J Thorac Cardiovasc Surg 2000;120(6): 1034–9. https://doi.org/10.1067/mtc.2000.111054.

[69] Staubach S, et al. New onset atrial fibrillation after patent foramen ovale closure. Catheter Cardiovasc Interv 2009;74(6):889–95.

[70] Gevorgyan Fleming R, et al. Comparison of residual shunt rate and complications across 6 different closure devices for patent foramen ovale. Catheter Cardiovasc Interv 2020;95(3):365–72.

[71] Musto C, et al. Comparison between the new Gore septal and Amplatzer devices for transcatheter closure of patent foramen ovale. Short- and mid-term clinical and echocardiographic outcomes. Circ J 2013;77(12):2922–7.

[72] Goel SS, et al. Embolization of patent foramen ovale closure devices: incidence, role of imaging in identification, potential causes, and management. Tex Heart Inst J 2013; 40(4):439–44.

[73] Hammerstingl C, et al. Risk and fate of residual interatrial shunting after transcatheter closure of patent foramen ovale: a long term follow up study. Eur J Med Res 2011; 16(1):13–9.

[74] Burke A, Tavora F. The 2015 WHO classification of tumors of the heart and pericardium. J Thorac Oncol 2016;11(4):441–52.

[75] Paraskevaidis IA, et al. Cardiac tumors. ISRN Oncol 2011;2011, 208929.

[76] Maleszewski JJ, et al. Pathology, imaging, and treatment of cardiac tumours. Nat Rev Cardiol 2017;14(9):536–49.

[77] Pucci A, et al. Histopathologic and clinical characterization of cardiac myxoma: review of 53 cases from a single institution. Am Heart J 2000;140(1):134–8.

[78] Ha JW, et al. Echocardiographic and morphologic characteristics of left atrial myxoma and their relation to systemic embolism. Am J Cardiol 1999;83(11):1579–82. https://doi.org/10.1016/s0002-9149(99)00156-3.

[79] Wu HW, et al. [Clinical and pathological characteristics of cardiac tumors: analyses of 689 cases at a single medical center]. Zhonghua Bing Li Xue Za Zhi 2019; 48(4):293–7. https://doi.org/10.3760/cma.j.issn.0529-5807.2019.04.006.

[80] Yu K, et al. Epidemiological and pathological characteristics of cardiac tumors: a clinical study of 242 cases. Interact Cardiovasc Thorac Surg 2007;6(5):636–9. https://doi.org/10.1510/icvts.2007.156554.

[81] Jelic J, et al. Cardiac myxoma: diagnostic approach, surgical treatment and follow-up. A twenty years experience. J Cardiovasc Surg (Torino) 1996;37(6/1):113–7.

[82] Li H, et al. Clinical features and surgical results of right atrial myxoma. J Card Surg 2016;31(1):15–7. https://doi.org/10.1111/jocs.12663.

[83] Vidaillet Jr HJ, et al. "Syndrome myxoma": a subset of patients with cardiac myxoma associated with pigmented skin lesions and peripheral and endocrine neoplasms. Br Heart J 1987;57(3):247–55.

[84] Cohen R, et al. Atrial myxoma: a case presentation and review. Cardiol Res 2012; 3(1):41–4.

[85] Pinede L, Duhaut P, Loire R. Clinical presentation of left atrial cardiac myxoma. A series of 112 consecutive cases. Medicine (Baltimore) 2001;80(3):159–72.

[86] Goswami KC, et al. Cardiac myxomas: clinical and echocardiographic profile. Int J Cardiol 1998;63(3):251–9. https://doi.org/10.1016/s0167-5273(97)00316-1.

[87] Seol SH, et al. Left atrial myxoma presenting as paroxysmal supraventricular tachycardia. Heart Lung Circ 2014;23(2):e65–6.

[88] Wang Z, et al. Risk prediction for emboli and recurrence of primary cardiac myxomas after resection. J Cardiothorac Surg 2016;11:22.

[89] Lee VH, Connolly HM, Brown Jr RD. Central nervous system manifestations of cardiac myxoma. Arch Neurol 2007;64(8):1115–20.

[90] Ma G, et al. Pulmonary embolism as the initial manifestation of right atrial myxoma: a case report and review of the literature. Medicine (Baltimore) 2019;98(51), e18386.

[91] Amano J, et al. Cardiac myxoma: its origin and tumor characteristics. Ann Thorac Cardiovasc Surg 2003;9(4):215–21.

[92] Gavrielatos G, et al. Large left atrial myxoma presented as fever of unknown origin: a challenging diagnosis and a review of the literature. Cardiovasc Pathol 2007;16(6): 365–7.

[93] Kaminaga T, Takeshita T, Kimura I. Role of magnetic resonance imaging for evaluation of tumors in the cardiac region. Eur Radiol 2003;13(Suppl 6):L1–10.

[94] Gulati G, et al. Comparison of echo and MRI in the imaging evaluation of intracardiac masses. Cardiovasc Intervent Radiol 2004;27(5):459–69.

[95] Agostini D, et al. Detection of cardiac myxoma by F-18 FDG PET. Clin Nucl Med 1999;24(3):159–60.

[96] Loire R. Myxoma of the left atrium, clinical outcome of 100 operated patients. Arch Mal Coeur Vaiss 1996;89(9):1119–25.

[97] Shetty Roy AN, et al. Familial recurrent atrial myxoma: Carney's complex. Clin Cardiol 2011;34(2):83–6.

[98] Birla S, et al. Rare association of acromegaly with left atrial myxoma in Carney's complex due to novel PRKAR1A mutation. Endocrinol Diabetes Metab Case Rep 2014;2014, 140023.

[99] Okamoto T, et al. A familial case of multiple recurrent cardiac myxomas. J Cardiol Cases 2013;8(4):142–4.

[100] Ziganshin BA, Anis O, Zafar MA, et al. Surgical correction of a giant left atrial myxoma producing critical mitral stenosis; 2021. https://doi.org/10.25373/ctsnet. 14749119.

[101] Val-Bernal JF, et al. Prichard's structures of the fossa ovalis are age-related phenomena composed of nonreplicating endothelial cells: the cardiac equivalent of cutaneous senile angioma. Apmis 2007;115(11):1234–40.

[102] Acebo E, Val-Bernal JF, Gómez-Román JJ. Prichard's structures of the fossa ovalis are not histogenetically related to cardiac myxoma. Histopathology 2001;39(5):529–35.

[103] Bireta C, et al. Carney-complex: multiple resections of recurrent cardiac myxoma. J Cardiothorac Surg 2011;6:12.

[104] Amonkar GP, Kandalkar BM, Balasubramanian M. Cardiac rhabdomyoma. Cardiovasc Pathol 2009;18(5):313–4.

[105] Hoffmeier A, et al. Cardiac tumors—diagnosis and surgical treatment. Dtsch Arztebl Int 2014;111(12):205–11.

[106] Shapiro LM. Cardiac tumours: diagnosis and management. Heart 2001;85(2):218–22. https://doi.org/10.1136/heart.85.2.218.

[107] Goddard MJ. Cardiac tumours. Diagn Histopathol 2018;24(11):453–60. https://doi.org/10.1016/j.mpdhp.2018.10.003.

[108] Joshi M, et al. The current management of cardiac tumours: a comprehensive literature review. Braz J Cardiovasc Surg 2020;35(5):770–80.

[109] Mulvagh SL, et al. American Society of Echocardiography consensus statement on the clinical applications of ultrasonic contrast agents in echocardiography. J Am Soc Echocardiogr 2008;21(11):1179–201 [quiz 1281].

[110] Lampropoulos KM, Kotsas D, Iliopoulos T. Lipomatous hypertrophy of interatrial septum. BMJ Case Rep 2012;2012.

# Introduction to interventional radiology in cardiac mass

## 29

**Kiara Rezaei-Kalantari and Hamidreza Pouraliakbar**

*Department of Radiology, CardioOncology Research Center, Iran University of Medical Sciences, Rajaie Cardiovascular Medical and Research Center, Tehran, Iran*

## Key points

- Surgical removal is the mainstay of cardiac mass diagnosis and treatment.
- When complete tumor removal of the tumor is not possible or patient intention or condition does not allow proceeding toward the surgery, interventional radiology (IR) is a good option for the cardio-oncology team to consider.
- Interventional oncology (IO) is a rapidly developing branch of IR that encompass procedures to yield tissue sample for diagnosis, assist in treatment as neoadjuvant or palliation, and management of complications due to tumoral progression or treatment adverse effects.
- Accomplishment of the cardiac interventional procedures requires demanding skill, comprehensive knowledge, and specific preparation as well as appropriate setting (including available cardiac surgeon) for handling the occasional complications.

**Interventional radiology** (IR) is a specialized field, in which the physician not only interprets the medical images but also uses medical imaging to guide minimally invasive surgical procedures that diagnose, treat, and cure many kinds of conditions through small incisions in the body. The treatments IR can effectively perform are ever changing and expanding. Interventional Oncology (IO) is one of the fastest growing fields in interventional radiology, dedicated to the diagnosis, treatment, and palliation of cancer and cancer-related problems that had tremendous progress over the last decade, and has now successfully established as an essential and independent pillar within the firmament of multidisciplinary oncologic care. Cardiac mass interventions are one of the ignored interdisciplinary fields that have explored new encouraging horizons during past decade.

The appropriateness of minimally invasive interventions for any patient with cardiac tumor should be assessed individually by the multidisciplinary "cardio-oncology team."

## IR role in diagnosis

Minimally invasive diagnosis of the cardiac tumors can be performed either by percutaneous or endovascular approach obviating the need for open surgery.

- **Percutaneous transthoracic biopsy** of cardiac masses can be applied for pericardial, intramural, or even some cavitary lesions if trajectory access is appropriate. The procedure is mainly performed under CT scan or sometimes ultrasound guidance (Fig. 29.1) while the backup cardiac surgeon is available and informed. Interventionists try to choose tumoral regions with the lowest amount of vascularity in order to diminish the possible risk of hemopericardium [1] (Fig. 29.2). Filling the intralesional biopsy tract at the end of procedure with embolizing agents (e.g., gelfoam) will largely reduce the incidence.

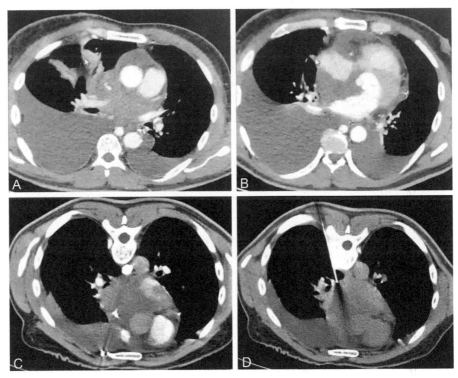

**FIG. 29.1**

(A) and (B) A 48-year-old man with an infiltrative pericardial mass which extensively encased the cardiac chambers and intrapericardial portion of the great vessels and has led to severe SVC stenosis. (C) and (D) After drainage of pleural effusion, percutaneous biopsy attempted by first delineating the vascular structure with contrast enhanced CT. Transthoracic biopsy result confirmed the diagnosis of lymphoma.

*Courtesy of Dr. Saleh Jafarpisheh, Isfahan University of Medical Science, Isfahan, Iran.*

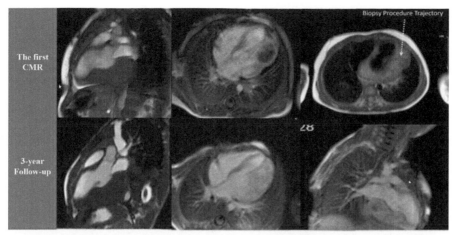

**FIG. 29.2**

A 1-year-old boy with a large incidental cardiac mass extending from inferior left atrium wall to involve inferior and lateral wall of the left ventricle. (A) Cardiac MRI was inconclusive for discriminating the neoplastic nature of the mass due to remarkable heterogeneous enhancement of the lesion. (B) Percutaneous ultrasound-guided biopsy of the mass (C) revealed hypercellular spindle cells with no atypia in favor of fibroma. (D), (E), and (F) Follow-up MRI three years later showed no significant change in extension of the fibroma with characteristic CMR features.

- **Endovascular biopsy** of the cardiac or central great vessel masses is a minimally invasive procedure that could be considered for right heart and septal tumor of adequate size in a manner commonly used for the blunt endomyocardial biopsy (Figs. 29.3–29.6). Cases of transseptal approach of the left atrial mass are also reported [2]. To guide the prompt site of target lesion for biopsy, concomitant echocardiography is crucial. TTE, although commonly used, gives less clear cardiac images than TEE, especially for the posterior wall mass and the patient with poor echo window, while the latter requires general anesthesia during the procedure. Intracardiac echocardiography (ICE) can provide better anatomical delineation of the lesion and targeting device without the need for general anesthesia, is more patient friendly, and will reduce radiation exposure for the echocardiographer during the procedure.

## IR role in tumoral treatment

Whenever possible, surgical removal is the main stay of management for cardiac tumors. But some masses are too large or extensively infiltrative that precludes curative excision or patient health condition is too poor to undergo surgery. IR therapies

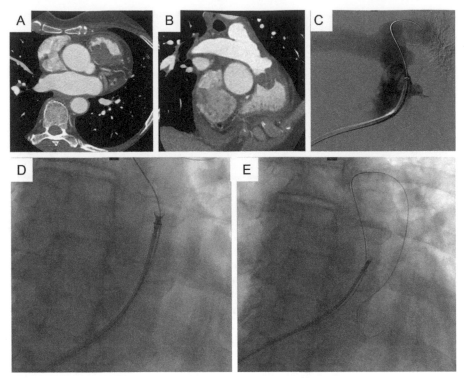

**FIG. 29.3**

A 70-year-old woman with a mass in the right ventricular outflow tract detected on echocardiography, during a routine workup for renal cancer. (A) and (B) Axial and oblique CT images demonstrate the exact location of the mass. (C) Pulmonary angiogram confirms the filling defect in subpulmonic region. (D) and (E) Due to the unstable position of the introducer sheath in the right ventricle, a 0.035 guide wire was positioned in the inferior left pulmonary lobar artery to stabilize the introducer in the target position. The biopsy device was advanced coaxially to the guide wire. Histopathological analysis revealed the lesion as coincidental myxoma.

*Courtesy of Prof. Salah D. Qanadli, Centre Hospitalier Universitaire Vaudois (CHUV), Laussane, CH.*

may be applied as neoadjuvant in order to reduce the diameters of the tumor and thus increase the chance of excision or palliative therapy to relieve the hemodynamic consequence of the mass—which obstructs the outflow tract or causes valvular annulus compression or insufficiency—and ultimately improve patient survival. Obviously, interventional techniques can also be used in combination with other treatments to help increase their efficacy.

- **Nonvascular techniques:** Successful application of radiofrequency (RF)-based techniques, microwaves, cryoablation, high-intensity focused ultrasound, and laser techniques for the treatment of neoplasms such as hepatic cancer [3,4], malignant lung tumors [5], and renal cancer [6] has led to considering these

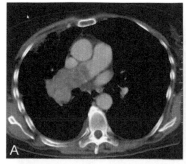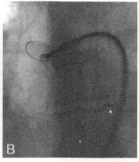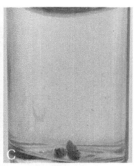

**FIG. 29.4**

A 62-year-old woman presented with dyspnea, pain, and weight loss for couple of months. (A) Axial CT images show heterogeneous enhancing intravascular mass in the right pulmonary artery extending to lobar branches. (B) Fluoroscopy view demonstrates the introducer placed in the pulmonary trunk as well as a 0.035 guide wire (Radiofocus Glidewire Advantage, Terumo) advanced to the right lobar pulmonary artery in order to stabilize the introducer in the target position. (C) The two obtained samples. Histopathological analysis revealed an intimal sarcoma of the pulmonary artery.

*Courtesy of Prof. Salah D. Qanadli, Centre Hospitalier Universitaire Vaudois (CHUV), Lausanne, CH.*

minimally invasive approaches as an alternative for patients with cardiac masses who cannot tolerate surgical procedures (Fig. 29.7).

- **Superselective embolization** of the feeding arteries is performed solely (for benign hypervascular masses) or in combination with chemotherapy. The procedure is done after at least 15 min of superselective balloon occlusion test of the feeder/s while monitoring patient for signs of myocardial ischemia. If no adverse effect is detected the feeder is occluded by coil or preferably dilute liquid agents, although the latter is technically more demanding and its nontarget embolization would be disastrous (Fig. 29.8).

- **Superselective chemotherapy** of the cardiac tumors is a promising option which can deliver intraarterial chemotherapy regimen to the lesion with very lower doses while increasing their potency, shortening the recovery times, and precluding the harsh systemic effects of the drugs. Further prospective multicenter clinical trials—like chemoembolization of other part of the body (e.g., liver, kidney)—are needed to confirm the compelling outcomes and change the therapeutic paradigms.

## IR role in complication management

Progression of the body neoplasms by direct invasion or metastatic dissemination can lead to cardiac or central vein involvement with disastrous consequences (Figs. 29.9 and 29.10). On the other hand, chemoradiation therapy and regimens for cardiac tumors could be accompanied by sometimes inevitable complications that may result in patient disability and demise (Figs. 29.11–29.13).

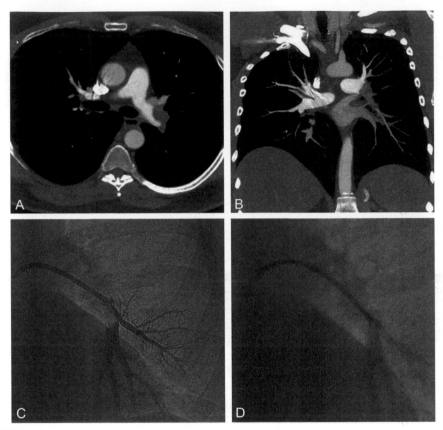

**FIG. 29.5**

A 56-year-old man past history of renal cell carcinoma. (A) and (B) Axial and coronal CT images demonstrate a "thrombus-like" heterogeneous enhancing mass of the left pulmonary artery. (C) Angiographic view demonstrates the endoluminal lesion of the left pulmonary artery. (D) Under fluoroscopic guidance the biopsy device was advanced within the left inferior lobar artery. Histopathological analysis revealed metastatic disease from the renal cell carcinoma.

*Courtesy of Dr. Salah D. Qanadli, Centre Hospitalier Universitaire Vaudois (CHUV), Laussane, CH.*

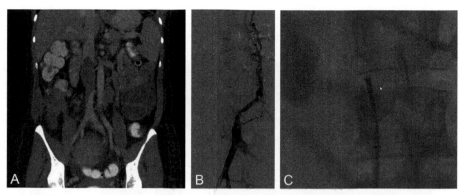

**FIG. 29.6**

A 51-year-old woman with abdominal pain without any specific relevant medical history. (A) Coronal CT images show an enhancing, heterogeneous endovascular mass of the inferior vena cava, a mass-like cecal wall thickening and a voluminous uterine mass. (B) Venography demonstrating an irregular occlusion 6 cm above the confluence of iliac veins with development of a collateral venous network. (C) Biopsy device with jaws opened just before the biopsy. Histopathological analysis revealed a tumor thrombus of a moderately differentiated adenocarcinoma originating from the cecum, confirmed by surgery.

*Courtesy of Dr. Salah D. Qanadli, Centre Hospitalier Universitaire Vaudois (CHUV), Lausanne, CH.*

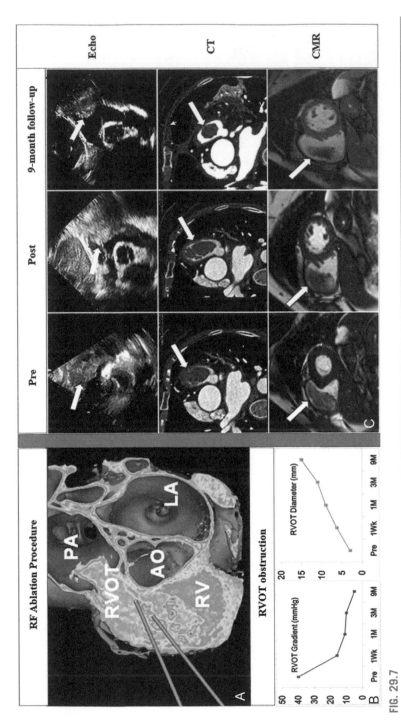

**FIG. 29.7**

A 70-year-old woman presented with chest pain, shortness of breath, and mild lower limb edema of more than 1 month (New York Heart Association [NYHA] classification IV). Imaging modalities (C) revealed a huge mass in the right ventricle causing right ventricular outflow tract (RVOT) obstruction. Because the mass was too huge to be completely resected by thoracotomy, and the patient was resistant to surgical treatment, a percutaneous ultrasound-guided biopsy and subsequent RF ablation were decided. Volume rendered image (A) to illustrate the needle positions in the tumor. RF ablation (Cool-tip System; Covidien/Medtronic, Minneapolis, MN) was performed at 120 W for 20 min until the concomitant contrast-enhanced echocardiograms showed no intratumor perfusion. Pathologic examination confirmed the tumor as myxoma. (B) and (C) Charts and images from different modalities display changes in the extent of right ventricular outflow tract (RVOT) obstruction over the 9-month follow-up period. *AO,* aorta; *LA,* left atrium; *PA,* pulmonary artery; *RV,* right ventricle.

*Adapted with permission from Zheng M-J, Yang J, He G-B, Zhou X-D, Li-Wen Liu L-W. Percutaneous radiofrequency ablation of obstructive right ventricular giant myxoma. Ann Thoracic Surg 2018;105(4):e159–e161.*

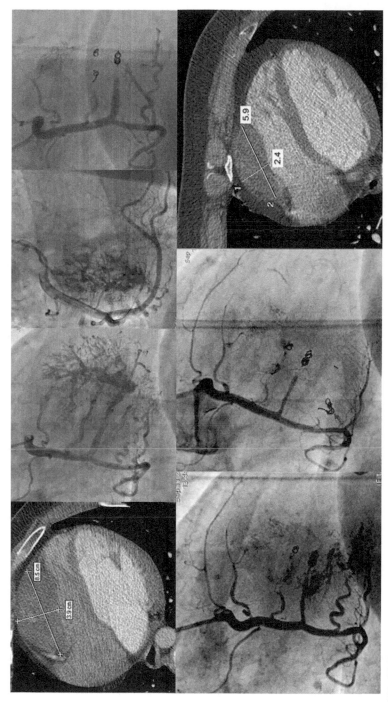

## FIG. 29.8

A 38-year-old male with atypical chest pain and gradually worsening shortness of breath on exertion for several months. (A) Computed tomography (CT) confirmed the presence of a vascularized 39 × 85 mm intramural RV mass that obstructed the RV outflow tract. (A) CT-guided percutaneous biopsy confirmed the tumor as fibrolipoma (not shown). (B) Coronary angiography showed a large area of hypervascular mass near the RV projection that was supplied by the acute marginal branches of the right coronary artery. (C) After 15-min balloon occlusion test of the 2nd and 3rd marginal branches, the two branches and distal segments of the 4th marginal branch were successfully embolized with Trufill pushable coils (Cordis Neurovascular, Inc., Miami Lakes, FL). Control coronary angiography showed recanalization of the 4th acute marginal branch (*red arrows*). Therefore, the branch was reembolized. (D) The size of the mass was reduced to 24 × 59 mm by contrast-enhanced computed tomography at 1-year follow-up. At short- and long-term follow-ups, the patient's clinical status dramatically improved: with significant reduction in chest pain, and near normal tolerance to general physical activity.

*Adapted with permission from Kipshidze N, Archvadze A, Kipiani V, Katsitadze Z, Matoshvili Z, Sigwart U. Endovascular treatment of right ventricular tumor. Circulation 2011;4(5):e33–e35.*

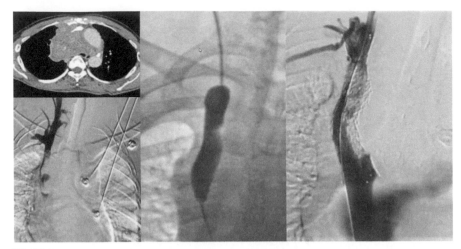

**FIG. 29.9**

Malignant SVC syndrome in a 56-year-old man. (A) Right lung adenocarcinoma invasion to cardiac and mediastinal great vessels has led to severe head and neck fullness and swelling. (B) Venography through right internal jugular vein shows complete occlusion of SVC. (C) and (D) Predilation of the obstructed region and subsequent stenting (wallstent 16*60mm, Boston Scientific, USA).

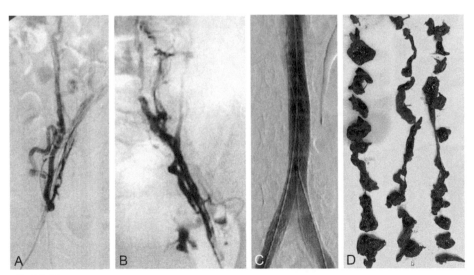

**FIG. 29.10**

A 71-year-old lady with metastatic rectosigmoid cancer with tumor thrombosis propagation to suprahepatic IVC. (A) and (B) Venography shows complete bilateral iliac vein occlusion. Cross-pelvic venous collaterals are seen. (C) Extensive mechanical thrombectomy (FlowTriever, T20, Inari Medical) was performed with subsequent iliocaval stent reconstruction (wallstent 16, 18, 22 mm). (D) extracted clots.

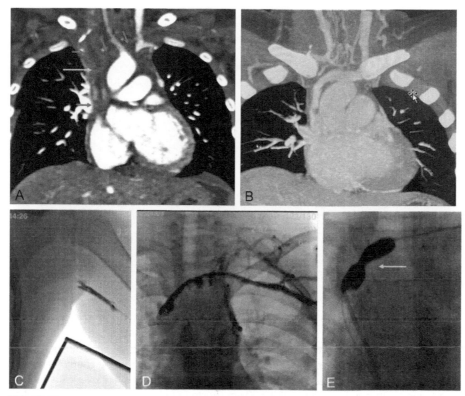

**FIG. 29.11**

A 5-year-old girl with history of recently cured acute lymphoblastic leukemia (ALL), referred for severe resistant SVC syndrome since 12 days. (A) CT angiography scan revealed complete right internal jugular and both brachiocephalic vein (BCV) thrombosis *(blue arrows)*, significant proximal SVC stenosis *(yellow arrow)* due to long-term chemotherapy port presence, and propagation of the partial thrombosis to the cavoatrial junction. (B) Venography from brachial vein shows the occlusion from left axillary vein. (C) Venography after more than 24 h of thrombolytic therapy with alteplase through infusion catheter (Cragg-McNamara Valved Infusion Catheter—Medtronic USA) shows partial recanalization. (D) Sequential venoplasty of the stenotic SVC (maximum 8 mm dimeter) as well as balloon maceration of the thrombus along the left brachiocephalic and subclavian veins. Swelling and symptoms started to subside from the day of thrombolysis. Follow-up CT (E) after 5 days demonstrated remarkable patency of the left BCV and SVC.

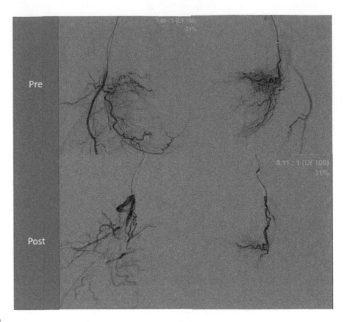

**FIG. 29.12**

A 60-year-old woman with cardiac lymphoma and chemotherapy-induced hemorrhagic cystitis from 3 weeks before, refractory to conservative treatments and continuous irrigations which led to several blood transfusion sessions and impeding chemotherapy continuation. Judicious bilateral embolization of the superior and inferior vesical arteries performed with polyvinyl alcohol 350–500 μm (Boston scientific) without any complication.

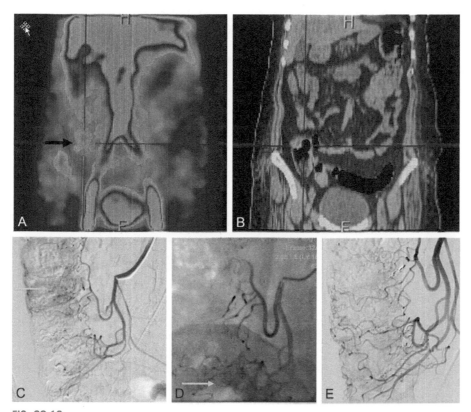

**FIG. 29.13**

An 80-year-old lady referred occult lower GI bleeding that resulted in severe anemia and several blood transfusion sessions. Endocolonoscopy was negative for abnormal finding. (A) and (B) Nuclear RBC scan demonstrated the cecum *(black arrow)* as the bleeding source. (C) and (D) Selective superior mesenteric angiography revealed two cecal and proximal ascending colon AV malformation. (E) Superselective embolization of the feeding arteries with detachable coils (Microvention, Terumo) resulted in cessation of bleeding.

# References

[1] Rezaei Kalantari K, et al. Transthoracic biopsy of the cardiac mass obviating open surgery. Iran Heart J 2019;20(3):91–4.

[2] Satya K, et al. Transseptal biopsy of a left atrial mass with 3-dimensional transesophageal echocardiographic guidance. Tex Heart Inst J 2012;39(5):707–10.

[3] Decadt B, Siriwardena AK. Radiofrequency ablation of liver tumours: systematic review. Lancet Oncol 2004;5(9):550–60.

[4] Poon D, et al. Management of hepatocellular carcinoma in Asia: consensus statement from the Asian Oncology Summit 2009. Lancet Oncol 2009;10(11):1111–8.

[5] Lencioni R, et al. Response to radiofrequency ablation of pulmonary tumours: a prospective, intention-to-treat, multicentre clinical trial (the RAPTURE study). Lancet Oncol 2008;9(7):621–8.

[6] Capitanio U, Montorsi F. Renal cancer. Lancet 2016;387(10021):894–906.

# Minimally invasive surgery in cardiac masses

# 30

**Alireza Alizadeh Ghavidel and Mahdi Daliri**

*Heart Valve Disease Research Center, Rajaie Cardiovascular Medical and Research Center, Iran University of Medical Sciences, Tehran, Iran*

## Key points

- Today minimally invasive cardiac surgery (MICS) is a good alternative for standard midsternotomy for many cardiac surgeries.
- Indications, technical issues, and the number of centers for MICS are improving.
- Less tissue damage and systemic inflammatory response syndrome (SIRS), less postoperative bleeding and pain, less need for transfusion, shorter hospital stay and early patient return to daily work and also the patients' satisfaction on small surgical scars are the main advantages of the MICS.
- Longer cardiopulmonary bypass and aortic cross-clamping time requires training courses and learning curves are the major drawbacks of MICS.
- Cardiac myxomas, as the most common heart tumor, are often easily resectable by minimally invasive approaches.
- The clinical outcome of the myxoma resection by MICS is comparable to the standard midsternotomy technique.
- Minimally invasive surgery can play a limited role in metastatic or primary malignant cardiac tumors because of tumor extension, surrounding tissue invasion, and requiring complex reconstructive procedures which is not feasible in most patients.
- Diagnostic tissue biopsy could be easily performed via minimally invasive approaches.
- Complete preoperative evaluation is crucial in selecting the best surgical approach.
- Secondary to the improvements in the cardio-oncology knowledge and minimally invasive approaches, the clinical results of the MICS for cardiac masses are encouraging.

## Principals of minimally invasive cardiac surgery (MICS)

The term "minimally invasive cardiac surgery" refers to a form of cardiac surgery performed using specialized surgical instruments through small incisions to minimize tissue damage and inflammation process and also patients' more satisfaction and quick recovery. Today minimally invasive cardiac surgery (MICS) is a good alternative for standard midsternotomy for many cardiac surgeries [1–3]. Although the smaller surgical incision scars seem to be the main advantage of this procedure among the general population, the main advantages of this surgical method are less tissue damage and systemic inflammatory response syndrome (SIRS), postoperative bleeding, less need for transfusion, and shorter hospital stay [1,2].

This procedure is technically rather more difficult for heart surgeons and requires training courses and learning curves; however, alleviating concerns about the mediastinitis nightmare and the need for reexploration to control bleeding and tamponade after heart surgery are good incentives for heart surgeons to use this minimally invasive method. Today, the use of this method is increasingly being used in different centers, and the results of surgery performed by cardiac surgeons with sufficient experience are comparable to the conventional method [1,2]. The need for peripheral cannulation and vascular complications with vascular access, limited vision, and lack of access to the entire field of cardiac surgery as well as the relatively long cardiopulmonary bypass (CBP) and cross-clamp time are the drawbacks of this surgical method. According to studies, adding a few minutes to the pump time and myocardial ischemia does not have a major negative impact on patients' prognosis [4].

The necessity for extracorporeal circulation and cardiopulmonary bypass (CPB) machine distinguishes minimally invasive cardiac surgery from other noncardiac minimally invasive operations. Upper J-shaped median sternotomy, right or left lateral thoracotomy, and right anterior thoracotomy are the main surgical approaches of MICS incisions that can be utilized based on operation type. For CPB establishment, peripheral femoral artery and venous cannulation are frequently utilized in minimally invasive procedures to diminish surgical incision, increase surgical view, and make surgery easier and safer [2,3]. Sometimes it is necessary to use percutaneous superior vena cava cannulation through the jugular vein in the neck for optimal venous drainage [3]. For minimally invasive aortic surgery such as aortic valve replacement or repair and aortic root reconstruction, some surgeons preferred to use the central aortocaval cannulation as standard fashion. Upper J-shaped ministernotomy is commonly used in such aorta surgeries in which only one-third of the sternum toward the third intercostal space is opened. This ministernotomy reduces the risk of dehiscence, mediastinitis, postoperative bleeding, and pain and results in a minimal surgical scar [4]. The main advantage of this surgical incision is that it can easily be converted to a full sternotomy in case of unexpected complications, technical challenges, or concomitant procedures without the need to change the patient's position or create another surgical incision. This procedure can be used for resection of thymoma or papillary fibroelastoma of the aortic valve [5].

Right anterior thoracotomy is the next common approach for minimally invasive aortic root and aortic valve surgeries. In this approach, a 4–5 cm incision is made in the second intercostal space, allowing the surgeon adequate access without the need for sternum incisions and providing better cosmetic results. Peripheral cannulation is the preferred method for this procedure; however, in some circumstances when there is good exposure, central cannulation can also be used [2,3]. Mitral valve surgery can also be performed using this approach by an atriotomy incision in the roof of the left atrium in highly selected patients. Two distinct surgical incisions for converting the approach to ministernotomy during intraoperative surgical complication and limitations in patients with a wide-angled ascending aorta are the main disadvantages of this minimal approach. This method can be very useful for the biopsy of middle and anterior mediastinal tumors.

A 4–5 cm incision of the right lateral minithoracotomy is the most common approach in MICS that is often used for different minimally invasive mitral and tricuspid operations, atrial septal defect (ASD), and PAPVC repair. This surgical approach is also very useful for the resection of masses from the right atrium, left atrium, IVC, or right and left ventricles. Peripheral arteriovenous cannulation must be used to establish the CPB. Two-stage femoral cannulas in which to separate lateral cannula holes inserted within both SVC and IVC can be utilized for complete venous system evacuation. Vacuum-assisted venous drainage (VAVD) can be used to facilitate optimal drain of the venous system on CPB machine. This allows the surgeon to use smaller venous cannulas to reduce the risk of vascular access complications. It is preferable to have the SVC vein independently and percutaneously from the right side of the neck through the right internal jugular vein if a total CBP pump is required, such as for surgery on the right heart including the tricuspid valve surgeries, resection of the right atrial tumor, and ASD closure [2,3]. Double lumen endotracheal tubes for single-lung ventilation are often used in this surgical approach to facilitate the procedures [6]. Special instruments are required to clamp the ascending aorta and induce cardiac arrest in this technique. This may be done either with a specialized surgical instrument named "Chitwood clamp" to occlude the ascending aorta externally or with an endoaortic clamp internally. The EndoClamp method, which passes through the femoral artery, can also be used to temporarily block the outflow of blood from the ascending aorta by filling the special balloon at the tip of EndoClamp, allowing the cardioplegia solution to perfuse the coronary arteries and induce cardiac arrest. Endoaortic clamp is less commonly used nowadays due to its high cost and vascular problems. Since the surgeon's finger cannot produce secure knots from a tiny thoracotomy incision, this surgical method requires a special instrument called "knot pusher" to securely tie the sutures. Today, the COR-KNOT device (LSI Solutions Victor NY) can be used to facilitate suture tying, which eliminates the need for normal suture tying by the surgeon [7].

This approach can also be used in selective patients with cardiac masses and preoperative evaluations have a major role in selecting the best surgical technique. Minimally invasive surgery can be a suitable option for patients with malignant tumors and patients with malignancy who are mostly frail with immune system deficiency;

however, optimal resection of the mass, patient's safety, and the outcome must be considered as the primary goals of surgical management. Although this procedure is technically rather more difficult for heart surgeons and requires training courses and learning curves, alleviating concerns about the mediastinitis nightmare and the need for reexploration to control postoperative bleeding and tamponade are good incentives for cardiac surgeons to use this minimally invasive method. Today, MICS is increasingly being used in different centers with comparable results with the conventional methods. Vascular complications secondary to the peripheral cannulation, lack of access to the entire field of cardiac surgery through a small incision, as well as the relatively longer cardiopulmonary bypass (CBP) and cross-clamp time are the drawbacks of this surgical method. However, adding a few minutes to the pump time and myocardial ischemia does not have a major negative impact on patients' prognosis [1,2,4].

## How to use MICS in cardiac tumors

Primary cardiac tumors are uncommon, with more than two-thirds of them being benign and the most prevalent type is atrial myxoma [8]. Primary malignant tumors are extremely rare and frequently presented in later stages of the disease, so in most cases the desired outcome of a cancer surgery cannot be obtained. Myxomas are the most common surgically treatable cardiac tumors, occurring most frequently in the left atrium, sometimes in the right atrium, and rarely in other heart chambers. As a result, excision of these tumors can be accomplished using minimally invasive techniques such as right minithoracotomy [8–10].

Fortunately, cardiac myxomas, as the most common heart tumor, are often easily resectable. Since echocardiographic or radiographic images of myxomas are usually typical and often single, and because they are well-defined mass attached with a short base on the atrial septum or adjacent tissues and do not invade adjacent tissues, the heart surgeon can confidently choose a minimally invasive surgical approach to resect these benign tumors [8,9]. In typical forms of atrial myxoma, the atrial septum adjacent to the tumor must be resected along with the mass and repaired with a patch, often from the patient's autologous pericardial tissue, which can be easily performed with a minimally invasive procedure using a small lateral thoracotomy incision. In myxoma resection, especially in the minimally invasive method, complete en bloc resection of the mass is very important because this tumor has a very fragile tissue that can be fragmented during resection and lead to embolism and cerebrovascular accident. Therefore it is critical to emphasize that surgeons with sufficient experience in routine MICS are eligible to perform minimally invasive surgery of the cardiac masses [10–13].

Minimally invasive surgery can play a limited role in metastatic or primary malignant cardiac tumors. It is usually not possible to perform safe and effective minimally invasive surgery for malignant tumor resection because complete resection of these malignant tumors often requires complex reconstructive procedures and good surgical access to whole parts of the heart and surrounding tissue that is impossible through small incisions. However, minimal approach video-assisted thoracoscopic surgery (VATS) is a well-known diagnostic tool for mediastinal masses and minimally invasive techniques could be very useful for tissue biopsy in mediastinal or cardiac masses when percutaneous methods failed [14,15]. With improving the cardio-oncology knowledge and minimally invasive cardiac surgery progressive development, we will see more and more good outcomes from minimally invasive approaches in the management of cardiac tumors in the future.

The main drawback of minimally invasive cardiac tumor surgery is the limited access to the whole heart and surrounding tissues. Cardiac tumor surgery might be unpredictable in terms of its extension and nature. Sometimes cardiac masses appear resectable according to the preoperative evaluations and cardiac imaging results but intraoperative findings are completely different and tumor resection is impossible or at least very challenging because of severe adhesions, tumor invasions, or potential coronary arteries involvement. These problems and possible surgical major complications or need for complex reconstructive operation after an invasive cardiac tumor resection may necessitate an unexpected procedure; and therefore, the operation may become so complicated that it is either impossible or at least unsafe to perform with a minimally invasive approach. Furthermore, relatively prolonged CBP pump and cross-clamp duration may affect the surgical result, and leaving a residual tumor worsens the patient's outcome during minimally invasive techniques [12,14]. Although reduced tissue damage, surgical bleeding, and inflammatory response might be highly beneficial to patients with malignancy and immune deficiency status, complete and safe excision of the tumor and proper reconstruction of cardiac cavities in excisable malignant tumors are much more critical whereas these objectives may not be feasible with a minimally invasive procedure.

Preoperative evaluations of patients with primary and secondary malignant tumors are very important. One of the major problems that can complicate minimally invasive surgery is the adhesions of lungs to the heart or thoracic wall, which may entirely exclude the possibility of performing minimally invasive surgery [14,15]. Peripheral cannulation through the femoral vessels can also be challenging due to the presence of pelvic and abdominal masses around the iliac and aortic arteries, as well as the IVC in patients with metastatic tumors.

## Case presentation

### Case 1

A 63-year-old female with chief complaints of palpitation and chest pain without important medical history. Coronary angiography showed stenosis in midportion of LAD. Echocardiography reported EF: 55%, mild mitral regurgitation and round heterogeneous pedunculated mass (4.1 × 2.2 cm) in left atrium (LA). She was

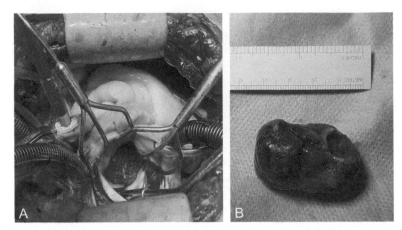

**FIG. 30.1**

(A) Expose the left atrium via ministernotomy and LA tumor. (B) Gross feature of Myxoma.

operated by ministernotomy and excision of LA mass near of mitral annulus and LA appendage was done. Left internal mammary artery harvested and then anastomosed on LAD. Pathology was LA myxoma (Fig. 30.1).

## Case 2

A 33-year-old female with chief complaints of palpitation and dyspnea with history of urinary bladder papillary cell carcinoma that was treated by resection through cystoscopy and BCG therapy and also has hyperthyroidism. Echocardiography shows EF: 55%, homogenous pedunculated semimobile mass ($2.1 \times 1.3$ cm) in left atrium (LA) attached to interatrial septum. She was operated by minimally invasive approach (minithoracotomy and femoral vessels cannulation) and excision of LA mass with safe margin and repair of septum. Pathology was LA myxoma (Fig. 30.2).

## Case 3

A 79-year-old male with chief complaint of dyspnea for 6 months without important medical history. Echocardiography reported EF: 35%–40%, large pericardial effusion and round heterogeneous mass ($3.1 \times 2.1$ cm) with septation and calcification in left atrium (LA) that attached to interatrial septum. He was operated by ministernotomy, excision of LA mass, and repair of septum by pericardial patch and also

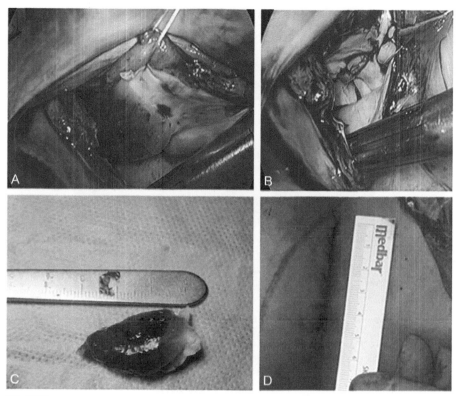

**FIG. 30.2**

(A) expose the left atrium and tumor via minimally invasive procedure by camera. (B) Left atrium after resection of tumor. (C) Small incision on the lower margin of right breast. (D) Gross feature of myxoma.

modified MAZE procedure. Pathology was LA myxoma with extensive hyalinization, calcification, and metaplastic bone formation (Fig. 30.3).

## Case 4

A 57-year-old female with chief complaint of dyspnea. Echocardiography shows EF: 55%, heterogeneous multilobulated, calcified, and semimobile mass (3.5 × 5.2 cm) in left atrium (LA) attached to interatrial septum. She was operated by minimally invasive approach (minithoracotomy and femoral vessels cannulation) and excision of LA mass with safe margin and repair of septum. Pathology was LA myxoma (Fig. 30.4).

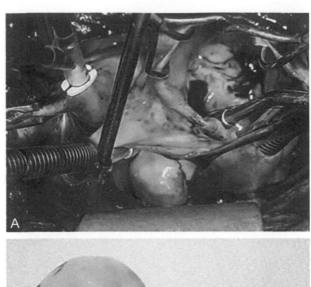

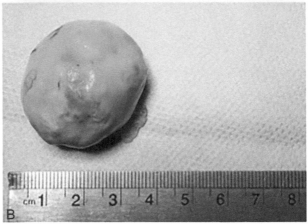

**FIG. 30.3**

(A) Expose the left atrium via ministernotomy and LA tumor. (B) Gross feature of calcified myxoma.

## Case 5

A 21-year-old female with chief complaint of chest discomfort without important medical history. Echocardiography reported EF: 40%, large and shaped homogeneous mass (5.7 × 3.1 cm) located in left ventricle apex with some attachment to LV myocardium and some compression effect on left ventricle. Based on MRI and echocardiography the primary diagnosis was hemangioma. He was operated

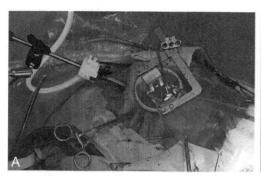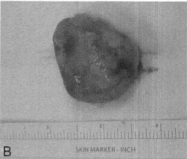

**FIG. 30.4**

(A) Expose the left atrium via minimally invasive procedure and position of instruments.
(B) Gross feature of myxoma.

by lower ministernotomy. Excision of left and right ventricle mass and repair of ventricles wall were done. Also we separated of LAD and other coronary arteries from mass without injury to them. Femoral vessels cannulated for CPB. Pathology Fibroma (Fig. 30.5).

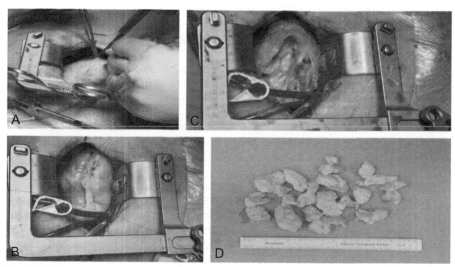

**FIG. 30.5**

(A) Expose the cardiac via ministernotomy and massive cardiac tumor. (B) Surface of left and right ventricles after resection of tumors and preserve of left anterior descending coronary artery. (C) Repair of left and right ventricles. (D) Feature of cardiac fibroma.

## References

[1] Dieberg G, Smart NA, King N. Minimally invasive cardiac surgery: a systematic review and meta-analysis. Int J Cardiol 2016;223:554–60. https://doi.org/10.1016/j.ijcard.2016.08.227. 27557486.

[2] Doenst T, Diab M, Sponholz C, Bauer M, Färber G. The opportunities and limitations of minimally invasive cardiac surgery. Dtsch Arztebl Int 2017;114(46):777–84. https://doi.org/10.3238/arztebl.207.0777. 29229038.

[3] Lamelas J, Aberle C, Macias AE, Alnajar A. Cannulation strategies for minimally invasive cardiac surgery. Innovations (Phila) 2020;15(3):261–9. https://doi.org/10.1177/1556984520911917. 32437215.

[4] Di Bacco L, Miceli A, Glauber M. Minimally invasive aortic valve surgery. J Thorac Dis 2021;13(3):1945–59. https://doi.org/10.21037/jtd-20-1968. 33841981.

[5] Devanabanda AR, Lee LS. Papillary fibroelastoma. In: StatPearls [Internet]. Treasure Island, FL: StatPearls Publishing; 2021. p. 2021. 31751019.

[6] Parnell A, Prince M. Anaesthesia for minimally invasive cardiac surgery. BJA Educ 2018;18(10):323–30. https://doi.org/10.1016/j.bjae.2018.06.004. 33456797.

[7] Morgant MC, Malapert G, Petrosyan A, Pujos C, Jazayeri S, Bouchot O. Comparison of automated fastener device Cor-Knot versus manually-tied knot in minimally-invasive isolated aortic valve replacement surgery. J Cardiovasc Surg (Torino) 2020;61(1):123–8. https://doi.org/10.23736/S0021-9509.19.10792-6. 31599141.

[8] Nguyen T, Vaidya Y. Atrial myxoma. In: StatPearls [Internet]. Treasure Island, FL: StatPearls Publishing; 2021. 32310500.

[9] Luo C, Zhu J, Bao C, Ding F, Mei J. Minimally invasive and conventional surgical treatment of primary benign cardiac tumors. J Cardiothorac Surg 2019;14(1):76. https://doi.org/10.1186/s13019-019-0890-2.

[10] Iribarne A, Easterwood R, Russo MJ, Yang J, Cheema FH, Smith CR, Argenziano M. Long-term outcomes with a minimally invasive approach for resection of cardiac masses. Ann Thorac Surg 2010;90(4):1251–5. https://doi.org/10.1016/j.athoracsur.2010.05.050. 20868822.

[11] Karagöz A, Keskin B, Karaduman A, Tanyeri S, Adademir T. Multidisciplinary approach to right ventricular myxoma. Braz J Cardiovasc Surg 2021;36(2):257–60. https://doi.org/10.21470/1678-9741-2020-0177. 33355796.

[12] Pineda AM, Santana O, Cortes-Bergoderi M, Lamelas J. Is a minimally invasive approach for resection of benign cardiac masses superior to standard full sternotomy? Interact Cardiovasc Thorac Surg 2013;16(6):875–9. https://doi.org/10.1093/icvts/ivt063.

[13] Kenawy A, Abdelbar A, Zacharias J. Minimally invasive resection of benign cardiac tumors. J Thorac Dis 2021;13(3):1993–9. https://doi.org/10.21037/jtd-20-1201.

[14] Taguchi S. Comprehensive review of the epidemiology and treatments for malignant adult cardiac tumors. Gen Thorac Cardiovasc Surg 2018;66(5):257–62. https://doi.org/10.1007/s11748-018-0912-3. 29594875.

[15] Endo Y, Nakamura Y, Kuroda M, et al. Treatment of malignant primary cardiac lymphoma with tumor resection using minimally invasive cardiac surgery. J Cardiothorac Surg 2018;13(97). https://doi.org/10.1186/s13019-018-0778-6.

# Fetal echocardiography in cardiac tumors

# 31

**Avisa Tabib**

*Heart Valve Disease Research Center, Rajaie Cardiovascular Medical and Research Center, Iran University of Medical Sciences, Tehran, Iran*

## Key points

- Fetal cardiac tumors are extremely rare and most are benign.
- They tend to appear between 20 and 30 weeks of pregnancy.
- The most common types of fetal cardiac tumors are rhabdomyomas, teratomas, and fibromas respectively.
- Fetal cardiac tumors may cause important complications, including arrhythmias, ventricular outflow or inflow obstruction, atrioventricular valve insufficiency, heart failure, and hydrops fetalis.
- Cardiac tumors are generally easy to diagnose prenatally by fetal echocardiography.
- Due to possible life-threatening complications, all cases should be referred to the perinatal center.
- Pregnancy should be continued as long as possible if there are no significant cardiovascular complications.
- The outcome of affected fetuses depends on the type of tumor and also on its location, size, number, cardiovascular complications, and associated extracardiac disorders.

## Introduction

Fetal cardiac tumors are relatively rare, representing 0.02% to 0.13% of cases in fetal cardiac series. They tend to appear between 20 and 30 weeks of pregnancy [1–5]. Most fetal cardiac tumors are benign, but they may cause important complications, including arrhythmias, ventricular outflow or inflow obstruction, atrioventricular valve insufficiency, heart failure, and hydrops fetalis [1,2,5,6]. Rarely, interference with the coronary arterial circulation may cause sudden fetal death [7].

Heart tumors are generally easy to diagnose prenatally by fetal echocardiography. Due to possible life-threatening complications, all cases should be referred to the perinatal center [7].

**Multimodal Imaging Atlas of Cardiac Masses.** https://doi.org/10.1016/B978-0-323-84906-7.00010-8

## Fetal primary cardiac tumors

Among the various histological types, the three most common types of fetal cardiac tumors are rhabdomyomas, teratomas, and fibromas, respectively [2,4,6,8]. Most fetal primary cardiac tumors (FPCTs) are benign and fetal malignant and metastatic cardiac tumors are very rare [2].

## Cardiac rhabdomyoma

Cardiac rhabdomyomas are the most common fetal cardiac tumors accounting for 70%–80% of cases in fetal cardiac series [1,7]. Cardiac rhabdomyomas are benign tumors of striated muscle cells. Echocardiography shows a homogeneous, well-circumscribed mass that is significantly more echogenic relative to the myocardium [1,3,6,7].

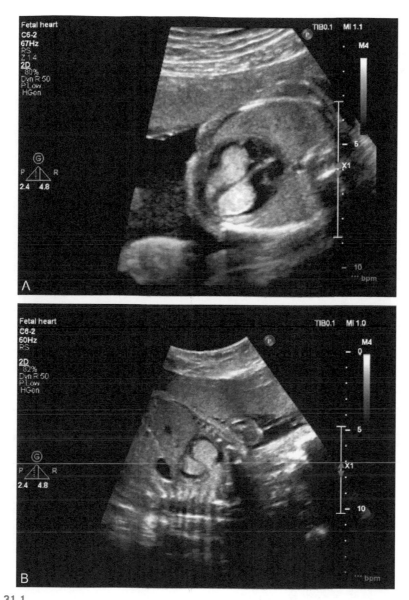

**FIG. 31.1**

Fetal echocardiography at 26 weeks of gestation in 4-chamber (A) and short-axis view of ventricles (B) showing intracavitary rhabdomyomas (Supplementary Video 31.1).

Cardiac rhabdomyoma may be intracavitary or intramural, found within the ventricular free wall or septum, the apex, the outflow tract, the conus papillary muscles, or rarely, within the atria. They are multiple tumors in 90% of cases, with variable sizes, usually sessile but can occasionally be mobile [1,2,6,7,9].

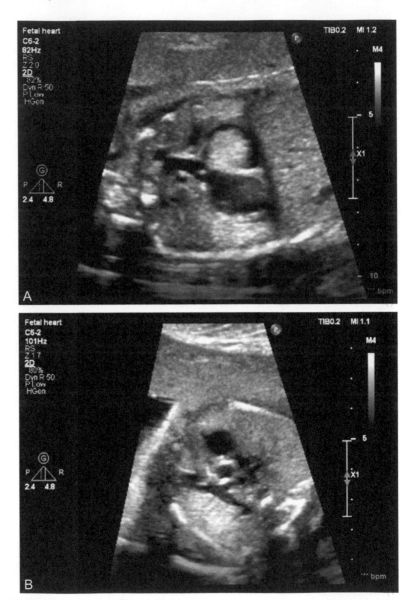

**FIG. 31.2**

Left ventricular outflow tract (A) and right ventricular outflow tract (B) views of the same fetus as shown in Fig. 31.1. Despite the presence of two large intracavitary tumors, there is no obstruction in the outflow tracts (Supplementary Video 31.2).

Cardiac rhabdomyoma may grow in size prior to 32 weeks and regress thereafter. Therefore serial assessment of an affected fetus is important particularly prior to 32 weeks [1,3]. Symptoms depend on the size, number, and location of the rhabdomyomas. An intervention is only necessary when serious complications occur [1–3].

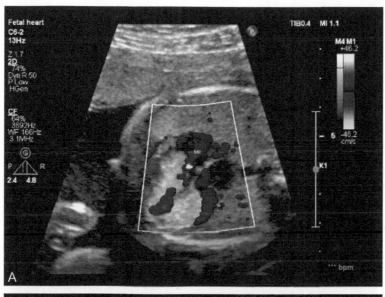

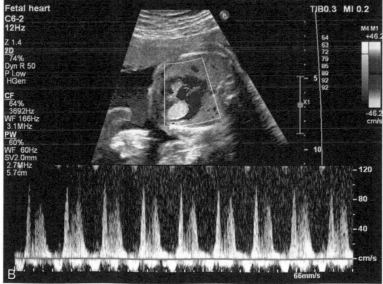

**FIG. 31.3**

Twenty-six weeks fetus with moderate tricuspid regurgitation due to large intracavitary rhabdomyoma in right ventricle. (A) Color Doppler and (B) pulsed Doppler flow of tricuspid regurgitation jet (Supplementary Video 31.3).

Despite the large size of tumors and flow obstruction or valve insufficiency, fetal hemodynamic compromise is rare in rhabdomyomas [7].

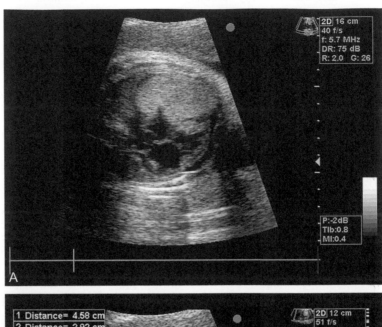

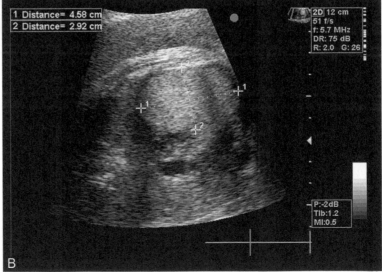

**FIG. 31.4**

Fetal echocardiography (four-chamber view) at 24 weeks, showing large rhabdomyoma of LV with mild pericardial effusion (A), the maximum diameter is approximately 46 mm (B). Several small tumors are also seen in RV free wall and right atrium (Supplementary Video 31.4).

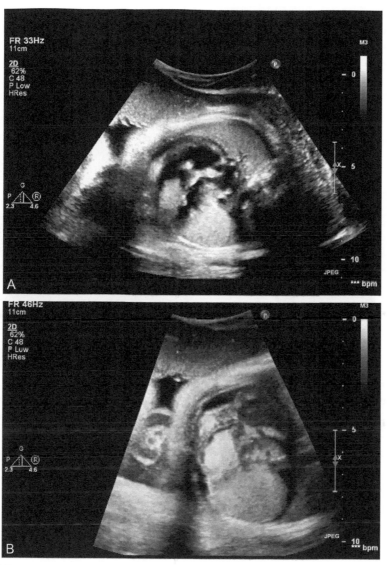

**FIG. 31.5**

Multiple rhabdomyomas in 36 weeks fetus with arrhythmias (A) 4-chamber view
(B) pericardial effusion (Supplementary Video 31.5).

Fetal outcome depends on the tumor size, impairment of flow, and rhythm disturbances. Early delivery at a viable age may be necessary for fetal hydrops with plans for neonatal intervention [1,7].

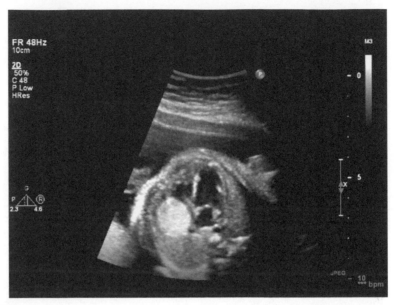

**FIG. 31.6**

Twenty-five weeks fetus with multiple rhabdomyomas. Four-chamber view shows a very large right atrial tumor without significant hemodynamic disturbance (Supplementary Video 31.6).

Rhabdomyomas are benign lesions and grow in utero due to the transmission of maternal estrogens to the fetus [3]. In general, they tend to shrink after birth and an operation is rarely necessary [7].

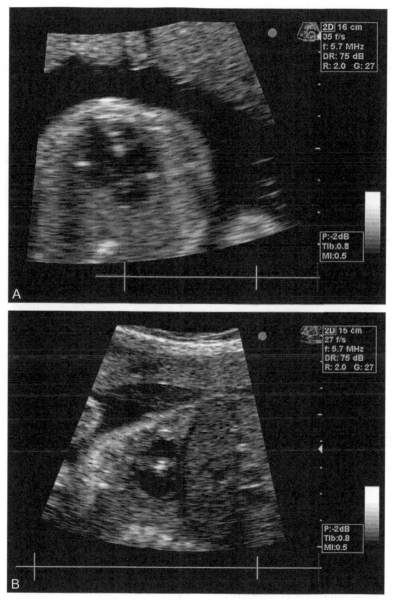

**FIG. 31.7**

Early detection of cardiac rhabdomyomas in 20 weeks fetus. Four-chamber view (A) and basal short-axis view (B) show multiple small rhabdomyoma in LV and RV free wall, interventricular septum, and right atrium (Supplementary Video 31.7).

It should be noted that small tumors, when located in the septum or ventricular cavity, often mimic an echogenic focus, thus leading to difficulty in recognizing them through early ultrasonographic screening [6] (Supplementary Videos 31.1–31.7 in the online version at https://doi.org/10.1016/B978-0-323-84906-7.00010-8).

## Fetal pericardial teratomas

Pericardial teratomas account for 10%–15% of cardiac tumors in fetal life and are usually benign. Teratomas are derived from two or three germinal cell layers and are typically extracardiac masses [1,2].

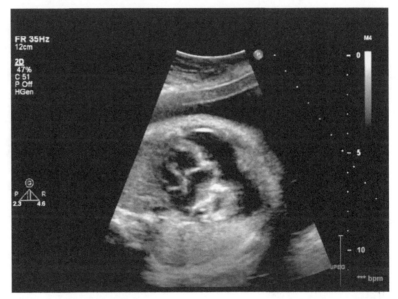

**FIG. 31.8**

Pericardial teratoma, 4-chamber image of 32 weeks fetus shows a large extracardiac mass with significant pericardial effusion (Supplementary Video 31.8).

Teratomas are typically extracardiac masses found within the pericardial reflection at the junction of the SVC, right atrium, and near the aorta and pulmonary artery. They are large encapsulated, irregularly shaped mass of heterogeneous echo texture, with calcified and cystic elements and usually single. Teratomas can also be found in other locations, including the mediastinum and rarely within the heart. Fetal teratomas can be multifocal [1–3,6,9,10].

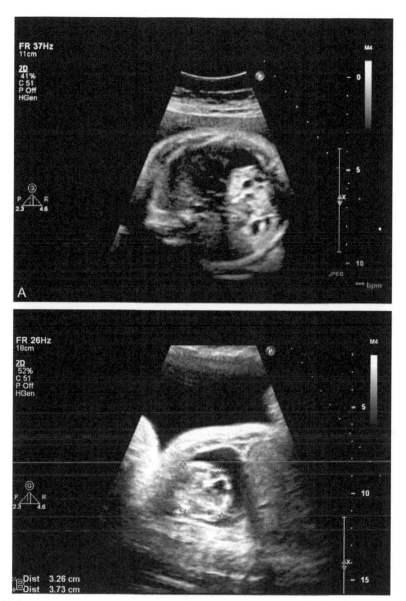

**FIG. 31.9**

Pericardial teratoma: axial (A) and sagittal (B) views of 32 weeks fetus with large intrapericardial teratoma and pericardial effusion.

Fetuses with pericardial teratomas are usually symptomatic, with pericardial effusions which are often significant and in 70%–80% of cases complicated by cardiac compression and hydrops fetalis [1,2,6]. In the presence of larger masses, fetal hydrops usually occurs in the second and third trimesters. Hydrops fetalis can be managed by pericardiocentesis, thoracoamniotic shunt, or elective delivery. Recently intrauterine surgical resection is possible with good results [1,2,10] (Supplementary Video 31.8 in the online version at https://doi.org/10.1016/B978-0-323-84906-7.00010-8).

## Fetal myocardial fibroma

Myocardial fibromas are rarely present during fetal life with an incidence of 5%–10% of fetal cardiac tumors [1,6]. They are benign connective tissue tumors derived from fibroblasts and myofibroblasts [1,2].

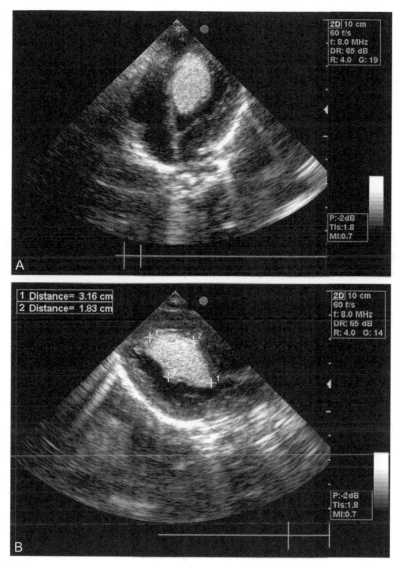

**FIG. 31.10**

Echocardiography in the first day of birth shows a single large echogenic tumor in ventricular septum protruding into left ventricle without outflow obstruction. (A) 4-chamber view, (B) LV long-axis view.

Myocardial fibromas are typically single intramural tumors that are often found within the ventricular septum, but they may also be found within the ventricular free walls [1–3,6].

Fetuses may present with hemodynamic disturbances, obstructions, and arrhythmias. By echocardiography, they are typically echogenic relative to the surrounding myocardium but often less than rhabdomyomas. Occasionally they are associated with calcification and cystic central degeneration, which results in the heterogeneous appearance [1,2,6,10].

Fibromas require clinical follow-up after birth. Unlike rhabdomyomas, fibromas do not regress and in some cases may lead to sudden cardiac death. They require surgical intervention to partially or completely remove the tumor [1–3,6]. Because they are large tumors, in some cases resection may be difficult and rarely heart transplantation is indicated [6].

## Fetal cardiac myxomas

Cardiac myxomas are composed of primitive connective tissue and are rarely identified in the fetus. After birth, they are usually single and associated with the atrial septum and atrial free walls, but in fetal myxomas, the left ventricle is the most common and the left atrium is the least common site [1,2,11].

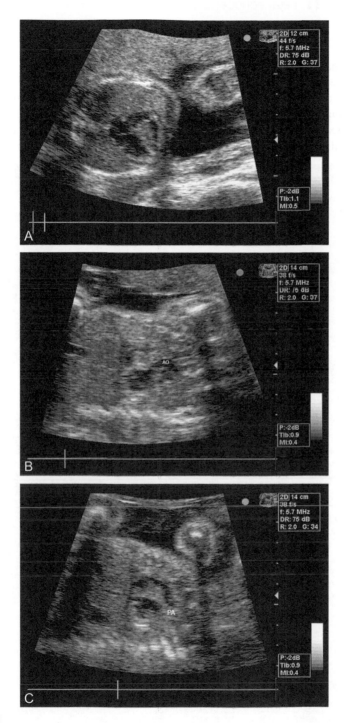

**FIG. 31.11**

Right ventricle myxoma in 25 weeks fetus without outflow obstruction. (A) 4-chamber view, (B) LV outflow tract, and (C) RV outflow tract (Supplementary Video 31.11).

Myxomas may be intracavitary or intramural, and they can rarely be epicardial. Tumor size and site could be predictors of adverse cardiac events. They are often, but not always, pedunculated. When pedunculated, movement in and out of the heart valves or outflow tracts can result in obstruction or atrioventricular valve regurgitation [1,11]. Myxomas may be echogenic relative to the myocardium and maybe well circumscribed or amorphous. They can rarely be associated with pericardial effusions [1].

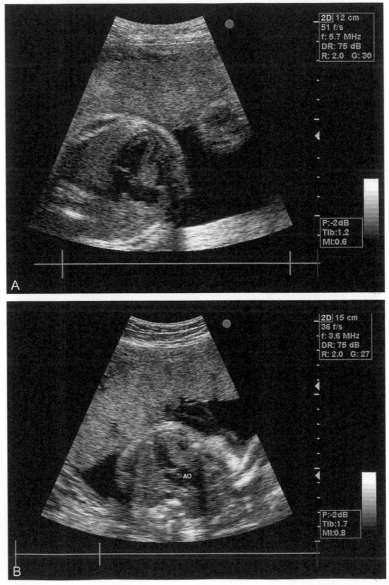

**FIG. 31.12**

Follow-up echo of the same fetus presented in Fig. 31.11 at 32 weeks shows a slight decrease in tumor size in proportion to the rest of the cardiac size. (A) 4-chamber view, (B) LV outflow tract (Supplementary Video 31.12).

Management strategies should be individualized based on the fetal condition. Their clinical courses are often benign. Small and nonmobile tumors may warrant close follow-up, and large tumors with obstruction signs or embolic potentials should be surgically treated during pregnancy [2,11] (Supplementary Videos 31.11 and 31.12 in the online version at https://doi.org/10.1016/B978-0-323-84906-7.00010-8).

## Fetal cardiac hemangiomas

Cardiac hemangiomas are rare in the fetus, with an incidence of 6%–7% [1,2].

Hemangiomas are vascular tumors and based on the size of the vessel lumen can be classified into three main types [1].

**Table 31.13** Classification of hemangiomas.

| Type | Texture |
| --- | --- |
| Cavernous hemangioma | Dilated thin-walled vessels |
| Capillary hemangioma | Lobules of smaller vessels |
| Mixed hemangioma | Composed of both types |

Fetal cases can be asymptomatic, but they can also be a cause of arrhythmia and hydrops fetalis. Spontaneous regression has been rarely reported in cardiac hemangiomas. Large cardiac hemangiomas may be associated with high cardiac output failure, arrhythmias, and consumption of blood products. Pericardial effusions and cardiac tamponade can be present with increasing age. Surgical resection is the most common treatment option for those with rapid tumor growth and heart failure, with good early and long-term outcomes and a small risk of recurrence. Steroid therapy should be reserved for unresectable tumors [1,2].

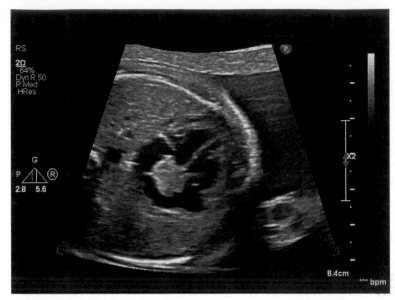

**FIG. 31.14**

Fetal echocardiography at 26 weeks gestation shows a single large homogeneous hyperechoic mass occupying biatrial cavities.

Cardiac hemangiomas are usually single tumors, which may be homogeneous or may have mixed cystic and solid components. The most common site of cardiac hemangiomas is the base of the heart adjacent to the right atrium, with an intracavitary component and pericardial effusion [1,2,9]. Occasionally in fetal echocardiography, the feeding vessel may be visible by color Doppler, and when highly vascular and large, power Doppler interrogation helps to make a correct diagnosis [1].

## Malignant fetal cardiac tumor

Primary malignant fetal cardiac tumor, such as fibrosarcomas and rhabdomyosarcomas, is extremely rare. There were only a few reports regarding malignant germ cell tumors in young children. Surgical biopsy or resection may be performed depending on the site and size of tumors. Surgical resection may offer symptomatic relief and life prolongation [1,2,4].

**Table 31.15** Echo characteristics of the most common fetal cardiac tumors.

| Tumor type | Most common location | Echo characteristic | Number |
|---|---|---|---|
| Rhabdomyoma | IVS, LV, RV free wall, papillary muscles, atria Intramural, epicardial, endocardial | Very echogenic, homogeneous, well circumscribed | Multiple in different size, single |
| Pericardial teratoma | SVC, AO pericardial reflection | Heterogeneous, echogenic, solid, and cystic elements, pericardial effusion | Single |
| Myocardial fibroma | IVS, LV, RV | Echogenic, homogeneous or heterogeneous, cystic degeneration, intramural | Single |
| Myxoma | LV, RV, atria | Echogenic, well circumscribed or amorphous, sessile or pedunculate | Single |
| Hemangioma | Right atrium | Lobulated and sessile, homogeneous or mixed echogenicity, may see vascularity with Doppler | Single |

## Benign structures mimicking cardiac masses
### Chiari network and crista terminalis

Advances in fetal imaging have resulted in more frequent reporting of primitive right atrial structures which can sometimes mimic cardiac tumors in prenatal echocardiography. Prominent crista terminalis and Chiari network are examples of these structures. They preferentially direct highly oxygenated blood coming from umbilical vein and inferior vena cava to the left atrium via foramen ovale. The similar echogenicity to the adjacent atrial tissue and the location are clues for differentiation of these normal structures from pathological entities [8].

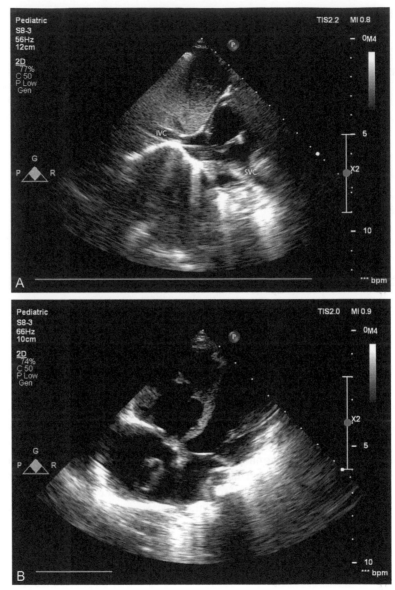

**FIG. 31.16**

Transthoracic image shows Chiari network. (A) Subcostal bicaval view, (B) apical 4-chamber view (Supplementary Video 31.14).

Chiari network results from the failure of resorption of the right valve of the sinus venosus during fetal life. A Chiari network is typically seen as a "whip-like" echogenic membrane with fenestrations in the right atrium. It can be identified by its attachment to the orifice of the inferior vena cava [8] (Supplementary Video 31.14 in the online version at https://doi.org/10.1016/B978-0-323-84906-7.00010-8).

## Echogenic intracardiac foci

Echogenic intracardiac foci are small discrete echogenic structures found within the ventricles in the region of the papillary muscles or chordae tendinae. They occur in 3% to 5% of the normal population and are correlated with areas of mineralization. They are not associated with structural heart disease and hemodynamic disturbance [12].

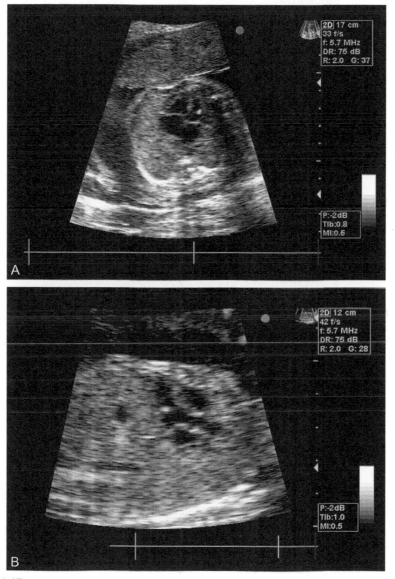

**FIG. 31.17**

Twenty-five weeks fetus images show single echogenic focus in LV. (A) Apical 4-chamber view. (B) LV long-axis view (Supplementary Video 31.15).

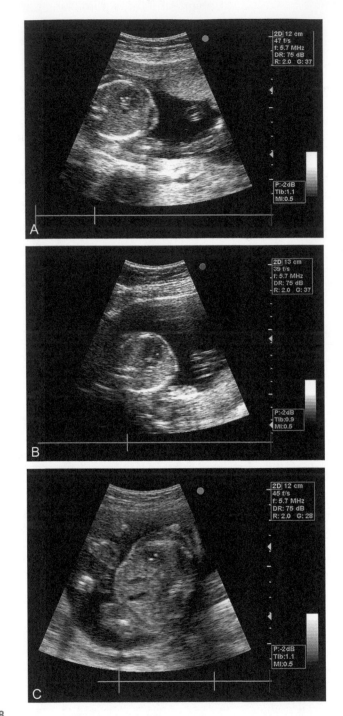

**FIG. 31.18**

Different location and number of echogenic foci in fetal cardiac images. (A). Apical 4-chamber view shows three echogenic foci in left ventricle. (B). Apical 4-chamber view shows a small echogenic focus in right ventricle. (C). Left ventricle short-axis view shows two echogenic foci on papillary muscles.

In 90% of cases, echogenic foci are seen in left ventricle but may also be identified in the right ventricle or bilaterally [12] (Supplementary Video 31.15 in the online version at https://doi.org/10.1016/B978-0-323-84906-7.00010-8).

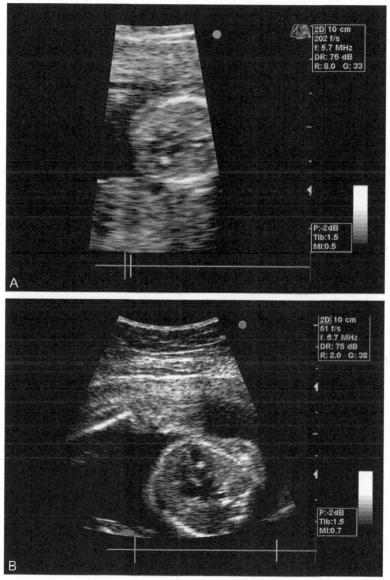

**FIG. 31.19**

Follow-up images of fetal cardiac mass (Supplementary Video 31.17). (A) Fifteen weeks fetus with large single echogenic mass in left ventricle. It was located at the site of papillary muscles, but it was obviously larger than the usual size of echogenic focus and had the appearance of a rhabdomyoma. (B) Follow-up echo at 22 weeks shows a significant change in tumor size in proportion to the LV size. In postnatal echocardiography, the echogenic focus is a papillary muscle with multiple chordae tendinae connecting to the area of echogenicity.

## Pitfalls

The pitfalls associated with prenatal echocardiographic diagnosis of cardiac tumors include the following:

— Cardiac tumor may be too small to be visualized in the early second trimester or even later in gestation.
— Echogenicity resulting from extracardiac structures or masses near the heart may falsely appear as tumors.
— Intracardiac echogenic foci may mimic rhabdomyomas [9].

The echogenic foci, particularly those in the papillary muscles, can be hypertrophic and may mimic rhabdomyomas. A follow-up scan is necessary for demonstrating the chordae tendinae attached to the papillary muscles, which move with the valves in the cardiac cycle [2] (Supplementary Video 31.17 in the online version at https://doi.org/10.1016/B978-0-323-84906-7.00010-8).

## Perinatal counseling and management for fetal cardiac tumors

**Counseling** for fetal tumors requires knowledge of the cardiac tumors, associated cardiac and extracardiac disorders, possibility of progression or regression, and risks of arrhythmias and other cardiovascular complications. It also requires understanding the indication of surgical intervention before or after birth. Due to the high risk of tuberous sclerosis complex in rhabdomyoma, in these cases consultation with a prenatal geneticist is recommended [1].

**Management** of fetuses with cardiac tumors requires serial echocardiograms, and the approach will vary according to the complications. Pregnancy should be continued as long as possible if there are no significant cardiovascular complications. Early delivery at a viable age may be necessary in case of hydrops fetalis with plans for neonatal intervention. In cases with critical obstruction of a ventricular inflow or outflow tract with reverse flow in the ascending aorta and pulmonary trunk, preterm delivery should be avoided except in cases with severe hemodynamic disorders. Initiation of a prostaglandin infusion after birth is necessary to stabilize theses neonate before surgical resection. In cases of fetal hydrops, with massive effusion, intrauterine pericardiocentesis or early delivery at a viable age may be necessary. In cases of malignant arrhythmias, drug treatment with antiarrhythmia agents should be started immediately [1,2,6].

**Prognosis** of affected fetuses depends on the type of tumor and also on its location, size, number, cardiovascular complications, and associated extracardiac disorders. They may cause arrhythmias including tachy or bradyarrhythmias, intracardiac flow obstruction, alteration of heart valves function, cardiac dysfunction, fetal hydrops, or even fetal death [1,2,9].

# References

[1] Hornberger LK, McBrien A. Fetal cardiac tumors. In: Yagel S, Silverman NH, Gembruch U, editors. Fetal cardiology: embryology, genetics, physiology, echocardiographic evaluation, diagnosis, and perinatal management of cardiac diseases. 3rd ed. CRC Press; 2019. p. 465–71.

[2] Yuan SM. Fetal primary cardiac tumors during perinatal period. Pediatr Neonatol 2017;58:205–10.

[3] Sarff B, Floyd R, Bildner A, Stormo J, Fisher K. Fetal echocardiographic detection of cardiac tumors: a case report of multiple fetal cardiac rhabdomyomas. J Diagn Med Sonogr 2019;35:426–30.

[4] Chen J, Wang J, Sun H, Gu X, Hao X, Fu Y, et al. Fetal cardiac tumor: echocardiography, clinical outcome and genetic analysis in 53 cases. Ultrasound Obstet Gynecol 2019;54:103–9.

[5] Saada J, Hadj RS, Fermont L, Le BJ, Bernardes LS, Martinovic J, et al. Prenatal diagnosis of cardiac rhabdomyomas: incidence of associated cerebral lesions of tuberous sclerosis complex. Ultrasound Obstet Gynecol 2009;34:155–9.

[6] Carrilho MC, Tonni G, Araujo JE. Fetal cardiac tumors: prenatal diagnosis and outcomes. Rev Bras Cir Cardiovasc 2015;30:VI–VII.

[7] Abuhamad A, Chaoui R. Fetal cardiomyopathies and fetal heart tumors. In: A practical guide to fetal echocardiography: normal and abnormal hearts. 3rd ed. Wolters Kluwer; 2016. p. 537–46.

[8] Bhatia S, Qasim A, Jiwani AK, Aly AM. Benign structures mimicking right atrial masses on prenatal ultrasound. Case Rep Pediatr 2021;2021:8889941.

[9] Zhou QC, Fan P, Peng QH, Zhang M, Fu Z, Wang CH. Prenatal echocardiographic differential diagnosis of fetal cardiac tumors. Ultrasound Obstet Gynecol 2004;23(2):165–71.

[10] Rychik J, Khalek N, Gaynor JW, Johnson MP, Adzick NS, Flake AW, et al. Fetal intrapericardial teratoma: natural history and management including successful in utero surgery. Am J Obstet Gynecol 2016;215(6):780.e1–7.

[11] Yuan SM. Fetal cardiac myxomas. Z Geburtshilfe Neonatol 2017;221(4):175–9.

[12] Bachman TM, Barrett HS. Congenital cardiac masses. In: Drose JA, editor. Fetal echocardiography. 2nd ed. Saunders: Elsevier; 2010. p. 268–80.

# Index

Note: Page numbers followed by *f* indicate figures, *t* indicate tables, and *b* indicate boxes.